Rasch Models in Health

Rasch Models in Health

Edited by
Karl Bang Christensen
Svend Kreiner
Mounir Mesbah

iSTE

WILEY

First published 2013 in Great Britain and the United States by ISTE Ltd and John Wiley & Sons, Inc.

ISTE Ltd
27-37 St George's Road
London SW19 4EU
UK

www.iste.co.uk

John Wiley & Sons, Inc.
111 River Street
Hoboken, NJ 07030
USA

www.wiley.com

Library of Congress Control Number: 2012950096

British Library Cataloguing-in-Publication Data
A CIP record for this book is available from the British Library
ISBN: 978-1-84821-222-0

MIX
Paper from responsible sources
FSC® C013604

Table of Contents

Preface

The family of statistical models known as Rasch models started with a simple model for responses to questions in educational tests presented together with a number of related models that the Danish mathematician Georg Rasch referred to as models for measurement. Since the beginning of the 1950s the use of Rasch models has grown and has spread from education to the measurement of health status. This book contains a comprehensive overview of the statistical theory of Rasch models.

Because of the seminal work of Georg Rasch [RAS 60] a large number of research papers discussing and using the model have been published. The views taken of the model are somewhat different. Some regard it as a measurement model and focus on the special features of measurement by items from Rasch models. Other publications see the Rasch model as a special case of the more general class of statistical models known as item response theory (IRT) models [VAN 97]. And, finally, some regard the Rasch model as a statistical model and focus on statistical inference using these models.

The statistical point of view is taken in this book, but it is important to stress that we see no real conflict between the different ways that the model is regarded. The Rasch model is one of the several measurement models defined by Rasch [RAS 60, RAS 61] and is, of course, also an IRT model. And even if measurement is the only concern, we need observed data and statistical estimates of person parameters to calculate the measures.

The statistical point of view is thus unavoidable. From this point of view, the sufficiency of the raw score is crucial and, following in the footsteps of Georg Rasch and his student Erling B. Andersen, we focus on methods depending on the conditional distribution of item responses given the raw score. The relationship between Rasch models and the family of multivariate models called graphical models [WHI 90, LAU 96] is also highlighted because this relationship enables analysis and modeling of properties like local dependence and non-differential item functioning in a very transparent way.

The book is structured as follows: Part I contains the probabilistic definition of Rasch models; Part II describes estimation of item and person parameters; Part III is about the assessment of the data-model fit of Rasch models; Part IV contains applications of Rasch models; Part V discusses how to develop health-related instruments for Rasch models; and Part VI describes how to perform Rasch analysis and document results.

The focus on the Rasch model as a statistical model with a latent variable means that little will be said about other IRT models, such as the two parameter logistic (2PL) model and the graded response model. This does not reflect a strong "religious" belief, that the Rasch model is the only interesting and useful IRT or measurement model, but only reflects our choice of a point of view for this book.

The book owes a lot to discussions at a series of workshops on Rasch models held in Stockholm (Sweden, 2001), Leeds (UK, 2002), Perth (Australia, 2003), Skagen (Denmark, 2005), Vannes (France, 2006), Bled (Slovenia, 2007), Perth (Australia, 2008 and 2012), Copenhagen (Denmark, 2010) and Dubrovnik (Croatia, 2011). Many of the authors have taken part and have helped create an atmosphere where topics relating to the Rasch model could be discussed in an open, friendly and productive manner.

The participants do not agree on everything and do not share all the points of views expressed. However, everyone agrees on the importance of Rasch's contributions to measurement and statistics, and it is fair to say that this book would not exist if it had not been for these workshops.

Karl Bang CHRISTENSEN, Svend KREINER and Mounir MESBAH
Copenhagen, November 2012

Bibliography

[LAU 96] LAURITZEN S. *Graphical Models*, Clarendon Press, 1996.

[RAS 60] RASCH G., *Probabilistic Models for Some Intelligence and Attainment Tests*, Danish National Institute for Educational Research, Copenhagen, 1960.

[RAS 61] RASCH G., "On general laws and the meaning of measurement in psychology", *Proceedings of the 4th Berkeley Symposium on Mathematical Statistics and Probability*, University of California Press, Berkeley, CA, pp. 321–334, 1961.

[VAN 97] VAN DER LINDEN W.J., HAMBLETON R.K., *Handbook of Modern Item Response Theory*, Springer-Verlag, New York, NY, 1997.

[WHI 90] WHITTAKER J., *Graphical Models in Applied Multivariate Statistics*, Wiley, Chichester, UK, 1990.

PART 1

Probabilistic Models

Introduction

This part introduces the models that are analyzed in the book. The Rasch model was originally formulated by Georg Rasch for dichotomous items [RAS 60]. This model is described in Chapter 1, where different parameterizations are also introduced. The sources of polytomous Rasch models are less clear. Georg Rasch formulated a quite general polytomous model where each item measures several latent variables [RAS 61]. However, this model has seen little use. Later, several authors [AND 77, AND 78, MAS 82] formulated models where items with more than two response categories measure a single underlying latent variable.

Bibliography

[AND 77] ANDERSEN E.B., "Sufficient statistics and latent trait models", *Psychometrika*, vol. 42, pp. 69–81, 1977.

[AND 78] ANDRICH D., "A rating formulation for ordered response categories", *Psychometrika*, vol. 43, pp. 561–573, 1978.

[MAS 82] MASTERS G.N., "A Rasch model for partial credit scoring", *Psychometrika*, vol. 47, pp. 149–174, 1982.

[RAS 60] RASCH G., *Probabilistic Models for Some Intelligence and Attainment Tests*, Danish National Institute for Educational Research, Copenhagen, 1960.

[RAS 61] RASCH G., "On general laws and the meaning of measurement in psychology", *Proceedings of the Fourth Berkeley Symposium on Mathematical Statistics and Probability, IV*, University of California Press, Berkeley, CA, pp. 321–334, 1961.

Chapter 1

The Rasch Model for Dichotomous Items

1.1. Introduction

The family of statistical models, which is known as Rasch models, was first introduced with a simple model for responses to dichotomous items (questions) in educational tests [RAS 60]. It was presented together with a number of related models that the Danish mathematician Georg Rasch called models for measurement. Since then, the family of Rasch models has grown to encompass a number of statistical models.

1.1.1. *Original formulation of the model*

All Rasch models share a number of fundamental properties, and we introduce this book with a brief recapitulation of the very first Rasch model: the Rasch model for dichotomous items. This model was developed during the 1950s when Georg Rasch got involved in educational research. The model describes responses to a number of items by a number of persons assuming that responses are stochastically independent, depending on unknown items and person parameters. In Rasch's original conception of the model (see Figure 1.1), the structure of the model was multiplicative. In this model, the probability of a positive response to an item depends on a *person parameter* ξ and an *item parameter* δ in such a way that the probability of a positive response to an item depends on the product of the person parameter and the item parameter.

Chapter written by Svend KREINER.

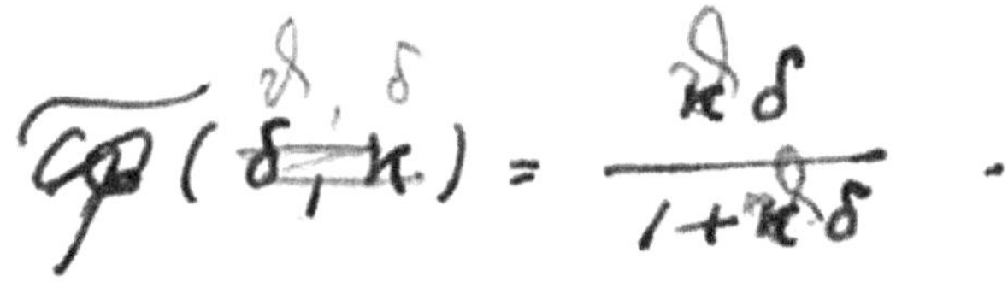

Figure 1.1. *The Rasch model 1952/1953*

If we refer to the response of person v to item i as X_{vi} and code a positive response as 1 and a negative response as 0, the Rasch model asserts that

$$Pr(X_{vi} = 1) = \frac{\xi_v \delta_i}{1 + \xi_v \delta_i} \quad [1.1]$$

where both parameters are non-negative real numbers. It follows from [1.1] that

$$Pr(X_{vi} = 0) = 1 - Pr(X_{vi} = 1) = \frac{1}{1 + \xi_v \delta_i} \quad [1.2]$$

The interpretation of the parameters in this model is straightforward: the probability of a positive response increases as the parameters increase toward infinity. In educational testing, the person parameter represents the ability of the student and the item parameter represents the easiness of the item: the better the ability and the easier the item, the larger the probability of a correct response to the item. In health sciences, the person parameter could represent the level of depression whereas the item parameters could represent the risk of experiencing certain symptoms relating to depression.

EXAMPLE 1.1.– Consider the following dichotomous items intended to measure depression:

1) Did you have sleep disturbance every day for a period of two weeks or more?

2) Did you have a loss or decrease in activities every day for a period of two weeks or more?

3) Did you have low self-esteem every day for a period of two weeks or more?

4) Did you have decreased appetite every day for a period of two weeks or more?

Items like these appear in several questionnaires. According to the Rasch model, responses to these items depend on the level of depression measured by the ξ parameter and on four item parameters δ_1–δ_4. In a recent study, the item parameters were found to be 2.57, 1.57, 0.52 and 0.48, respectively [FRE 09, MES 09]. The interpretation of these numbers is that sleep disturbance is the most common and loss of appetite is the least common of the four symptoms. To better understand the role of the item parameters, we have to look at the relationships between the probabilities of positive responses to two questions. This is shown in Table 1.1, where it can be seen that the *ratio* between the two item parameters is the odds ratio (OR) comparing the odds of encountering the symptoms described by the items *irrespective* of the level of depression ξ of the persons. This interpretation should be familiar to persons with a working knowledge of epidemiological methods. According to the Rasch model, the level of depression does not modify the *relative* risk of the symptoms. In the theory of Rasch models, this is sometimes called *no item-trait interaction*.

Item	parameter	$P(X=0)$	$P(X=1)$	Odds
1	δ_1	$\frac{1}{1+\xi_v\delta_1}$	$\frac{\xi_v\delta_1}{1+\xi_v\delta_1}$	$\xi_v\delta_1$
2	δ_2	$\frac{1}{1+\xi_v\delta_2}$	$\frac{\xi_v\delta_2}{1+\xi_v\delta_2}$	$\xi_v\delta_2$
				OR $= \frac{\delta_2}{\delta_1}$

Table 1.1. *Response probabilities for two items when the person parameter is* ξ_v

EXAMPLE 1.2.– Since the item parameters for the first two items are 2.57 and 1.57, we see that the odds ratio relating the risk of loss of or reduction of activities to the risk of sleep disturbances is equal to $1.57/2.57 = 0.613$. Because of the symmetry in formula [1.1] the same argument applies to comparisons of persons. Table 1.2 considers the risk of encountering a specific symptom for each of two persons with different levels of depression. As for the items, we interpret the ratio between the person parameters as the odds ratio comparing the risk for person two to the risk for person one.

Person	Parameter	$P(X=0)$	$P(X=1)$	Odds
1	ξ_1	$\frac{1}{1+\xi_1\delta_i}$	$\frac{\xi_1\delta_i}{1+\xi_1\delta_i}$	$\xi_1\delta_i$
2	ξ_2	$\frac{1}{1+\xi_2\delta_i}$	$\frac{\xi_2\delta_i}{1+\xi_2\delta_i}$	$\xi_2\delta_i$
				OR $= \frac{\xi_2}{\xi_1}$

Table 1.2. *Response probabilities for an item with an item parameter equal to* δ_i

To measure the level of depression, we have to estimate the parameter ξ based on observed item responses. However, this parameter is not identifiable in absolute terms because the probabilities [1.1] depend on the product of the person and item parameters. Multiplying all person parameters by a constant κ and dividing all item parameters by the same constant results in a reparameterized model

$$P(X_{vi}=1) = \frac{(\xi_v\kappa)(\delta_i/\kappa)}{1+(\xi_v\kappa)(\delta_i/\kappa)} \quad [1.3]$$

$$P(X_{vi} = 0) = \frac{1}{1 + (\xi_v \kappa)(\delta_i / \kappa)} \qquad [1.4]$$

with exactly the same formal structure and the same probabilities as the original model, and where the odds ratio comparing response probabilities for the two persons is the same as in Table 1.2. To identify the parameters, we consequently have to impose restrictions on the parameters. The standard way of doing this is to fix the parameters such that the product of the item parameters is equal to one. The parameters of the depression items above were fixed in this way. Another way that may be more natural for an epidemiologist would be to select a reference item where the item parameter is equal to one. The item parameters for other items are then interpretable as ORs comparing the item to the reference item (see Table 1.1). Because of the symmetry in formula [1.1], similar arguments apply to the person parameters, that is requiring that the product of the person parameters be equal to one or fixing the value for a single (reference) person. All these parameterizations are valid and characterized by invariant ratios of both the person parameters and item parameters.

Multiplication of quantitative measurements with a constant corresponds to a change of unit of the measurement scale on which the values are measured. Because ratios of person parameters are the same for all choices of a measurement unit, the measurement scale on which ξ is measured is a ratio scale. This argument was very important for Georg Rasch who repeatedly stressed the similarity with measurement in physics, stating [RAS 60]

> If for any two objects we find a certain ratio of their accelerations produced by one instrument, then the same ratio will be found for any other instruments.

Measurement using Rasch models is relative rather than absolute. We can use estimates of ξ to compare the level of depression for two persons, but we cannot use a single ξ measure to say that a person has a high or a low level of depression. Michell [MIC 97] claims that "scientific measurement is properly defined as the estimation of the ratio of some magnitude of a quantitative attribute to a unit of the same attribute" and also points out that measurement is relative rather than absolute depending on the choice of unit.

One further aspect of Rasch models is worth mentioning. Persons and items are completely symmetrical in the sense that there is no major difference between inference on item parameters and inference on person parameters using the simple model [1.1]. However, in the majority of applications, we will not exchange persons and items. The main purpose of constructing depression items like those discussed above is to measure a trait or the property of persons, whereas the risks associated with the four symptoms are of no special significance being only the means to the ends. Typically, covariates like age, gender and socioeconomic status are attached to people but not to items. Hence, conceptually there is a big difference between persons and items.

1.1.2. *Modern formulations of the model*

Over time, as the use of the model spread from educational testing to other research areas, the formal representation and the terminology associated with the model got changed. Today, the model is typically written as an additive logistic model, replacing ξ by $\theta = \log(\xi)$ and δ by $\beta = -\log(\delta)$. Furthermore, the unobservable (latent) nature of the person parameter is acknowledged by stating that Θ_v is a latent variable and θ_v is the unobserved realization of Θ_v and formulating the model in terms of the conditional probabilities

$$P(X_{vi} = 1|\Theta_v = \theta_v) = \frac{\exp(\theta_v - \beta_i)}{1 + \exp(\theta_v - \beta_i)} \qquad [1.5]$$

and thus

$$P(X_{vi} = 0|\Theta_v = \theta_v) = \frac{1}{1 + \exp(\theta_v - \beta_i)} \qquad [1.6]$$

In the above formulation, β_i is called an *item threshold parameter* or an *item location parameter*. The logit function $\text{logit}(p) = \log(p/(1-p))$ of the probability of a positive response is

$$\text{logit}\left(P(X_{vi} = 1|\Theta_v = \theta_v)\right) = \theta_v - \beta_i \qquad [1.7]$$

and therefore θ_v and β_i are often said to be on a logit scale. This terminology is not justifiable because the logit is a function of probabilities and we could argue that it is the *difference* between θ_v and β_i that is measured on a logit scale, similarly as probabilities are measured on a probability scale, but the name is popular and probably difficult to avoid. The two different representations of the model, [1.1] and [1.5], are mathematically equivalent. During statistical analysis of data by the Rasch model, it does not matter whether you use one or the other representation.

The scale on which θ is measured is often claimed to be an interval scale. This is not difficult to understand because changing the unit of the original ratio scale measure and then taking logarithms to get the value of θ after the change of the unit of ξ means changing the origin of the scale on which ξ is measured. When the unit on the multiplicative ξ scale is arbitrary, it follows that the origin on the θ scale is also arbitrary.

The symmetry of persons and items in the Rasch models and the fact that the probabilities in the Rasch models depend on the difference between person and item parameters show that items and persons are measured on the same scale. An item threshold can be interpreted as the person parameter value for which the probability of a positive response equals 0.5.

EXAMPLE 1.3.– The thresholds of the depression items are $\beta_1 = -\log(2.57) = -0.94$, $\beta_2 = -\log(1.57) = -0.45$, $\beta_3 = -\log(0.52) = 0.65$ and $\beta_4 = -\log(0.48) = 0.73$. Because the multiplicative parameters are restricted such that the product is equal to one, it follows that the sum of item thresholds is equal to zero (disregarding rounding error). Again, the risk of suffering from sleep disturbances is larger than the risk of loss of appetite, and the threshold of sleep disturbances is lower than the threshold of loss of appetite.

Finally, the assumption that the complete matrix consists of stochastically independent item responses has been replaced by the assumption that the set of item responses for a person is jointly *conditionally* independent given the variable Θ_v

$$P(\mathbf{X_v} = \mathbf{x}|\Theta_v = \theta_v) = \prod_{i=1}^{k} \frac{\exp(x_{vi}(\theta_v - \beta_i))}{1 + \exp(\theta_v - \beta_i)} \qquad [1.8]$$

where $\mathbf{X_v} = (X_{v1}, \ldots, X_{vk})$ and $\mathbf{x} = (x_1, \ldots, x_k)$. Of course, responses from different persons are also considered to be independent.

The assumption of joint conditional independence means that any subset of item responses is jointly independent given Θ_v and therefore items are pairwise conditionally independent; but the reverse is not true, meaning that pairwise conditional independence does not imply joint conditional independence. We will return to this topic in section 1.9.

1.1.3. *Psychometric properties*

Viewed as a statistical model, the latent variable Θ in the model [1.5] can be characterized as a random effect explaining the covariation among items. In statistical models with random effects, we are rarely interested in the actual value of the random effect variables, and in this sense, the Rasch model is a different kind of model. The main purpose of the model is to estimate either the θ_v values or functions of the θ_v values.

On the basis of this, it is more useful to describe the Rasch model as a member of the class of statistical models known as item response theory (IRT) models [VAN 97]. Before we proceed to the discussion of the statistical features of the Rasch model, we summarize a number of requirements of IRT models that also apply to items from the Rasch model.

1.1.3.1. *Requirements of IRT models*

Unidimensionality: The Rasch model [1.5] is a unidimensional latent trait model since Θ is a single scalar. Had Θ been a vector of variables, we would have said that the model is multidimensional.

Monotonicity: Because the probability [1.5] of a positive response to an item is a monotonously increasing function of θ, we say that the items satisfy the requirement of monotonicity.

Homogeneity: For any value of θ, the ordering of the item in terms of the probabilities is the same. Therefore, the set of items is called homogeneous. In the context of an educational test, this means that the easiest item is easiest for everybody.

Local independence: The assumption that item responses are conditionally independent given Θ is called by psychometricians the assumption of *local independence*.

Consistency: Psychometricians call a set of positively correlated items a consistent set of items. Because unidimensionality, monotonicity and local independence imply that all monotonously increasing functions of item responses – including the items in themselves – are positively correlated [HOL 86], it follows that items from Rasch models are consistent.

Absence of differential item functioning (DIF): Note, that the Rasch model only contains two types of variables: the latent variable and the items. When used, it is implicitly assumed that the model applies to all persons within a specific population (often called a specific frame of reference) and that partitioning into subpopulations does not change the model. If the frame of reference contains both men and women, it is assumed that the model [1.5] and the set of item parameters are the same for both men and women. This property is called the property of no DIF.

Criterion validity: The results concerning positive correlations among functions of items extend to relationships with other variables: if an exogenous variable is positively correlated with the latent variable; if items are unidimensional, monotonous and locally independent; and if there is no DIF, it follows that the exogenous variable must be positively correlated to all monotonous functions of the items, including the total score on all items. This result lies behind the psychometric notion of criterion validity.

Criterion-related construct validity: The ultimate requirement of measurement by items from IRT models is that the measurement is *construct* valid. Construct validity can be defined in several ways, for example by reference to an external *nomological* network of variables that theory insists are related to Θ [CRO 55], or by requirements of the way in which item responses depend on Θ. Rosenbaum collects all these points of views in a definition of criterion-related construct validity [ROS 89]. According to Rosenbaum, indirect measurement by a set of item responses is criterion-related construct valid if the requirements unidimensionality, monotonocity, local independence and absence of DIF are met by the items. Therefore, we claim that measurement by Rasch model items is construct valid.

1.2. Item characteristic curves

The functions $\theta \mapsto P(X_{vi} = 1|\Theta_v = \theta)$ are called *item characteristic curves* (ICCs). Figure 1.2 shows the item characteristic curves of the four depression items under the Rasch models. In addition to being monotonous, those curves never cross. IRT models with this property are called *double monotonous* IRT models. In fact, the curves are not only double monotonous but also parallel.

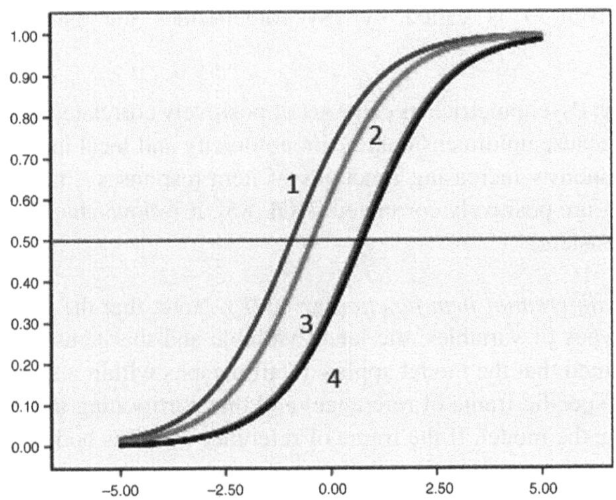

Figure 1.2. *Item characteristic curves for four depression items under the Rasch model. Thresholds are −0.94 (1), −0.45 (2), 0.65 (3) and 0.74 (4)*

Because the items are double monotonous, the rank of the items with respect to the probabilities of positive responses to items is the same for all values of θ. At all levels of θ, the probability of a positive response to item two is smaller than the probability of a positive response to item one, but larger than the probability of a positive response to item three. Items from Rasch models are therefore homogeneous.

1.3. Guttman errors

Homogeneity is closely related to the notion of Guttman errors. Let X_{va} and X_{vb} be two item responses and assume that $\beta_a < \beta_b$. We say that a Guttman error occurs when a person has a positive response to the item with the largest threshold and a negative response to the other item, $X_{va} = 0$ and $X_{vb} = 1$. Analyses of Guttman errors play an important role in IRT models with homogeneous double monotonous items.

In Rasch models, the risk of Guttman errors depends on both item and person parameters. The closer the thresholds of the two items a and b, the larger the risk of a Guttman error. The larger the numerical value of the person parameter, the smaller the risk of a Guttman error. The risk of Guttman errors for pairs of depression items across the level of depression is shown in Figure 1.3.

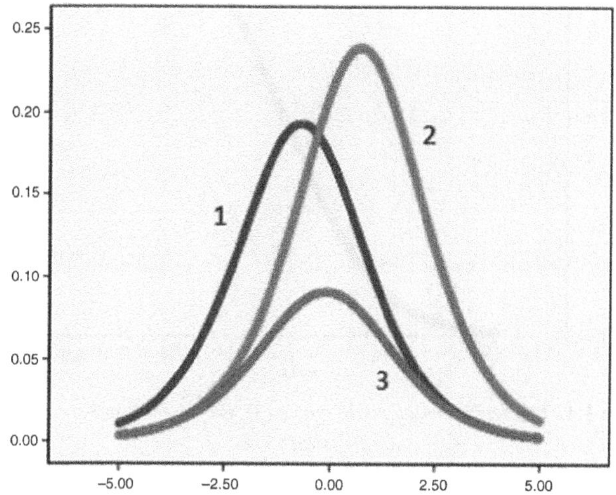

Figure 1.3. *The risk of Guttman errors among responses to items 1 and 2 (1), items 3 and 4 (2) and items 1 and 4 (3)*

1.4. Test characteristic curve

From the score probabilities, it is easy to calculate the expected (mean) score of R for different values of ξ. These are called true scores and the function describing the true score as a function of $\theta = \log(\xi)$ is called the test characteristic curve (TCC). The TCC for the four depression items is shown in Figure 1.4. Note that the TCC is not linear.

1.5. Implicit assumptions

In statistical terms, the requirement of no DIF can best be described as the requirement that item responses $(X_{v1}, \ldots, X_{vk})$ are conditionally independent of all exogenous variables $(Z_{v1}, \ldots, Z_{vk})$ given Θ. The absence of DIF is a fundamental validity assumption in psychometrics. The Rasch model shares this assumption, but only as an implicit assumption, because the exogenous variables do not enter this model at all. Similarly, the Rasch model also shares the property of criterion validity implicitly because criterion variables do not appear in the Rasch model.

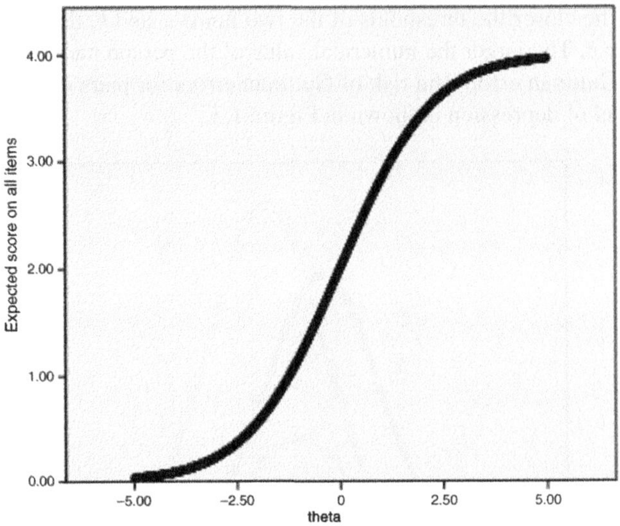

Figure 1.4. *The test characteristic curve (TCC) for the total score on four depression items*

1.6. Statistical properties

We return to the discussion of the Rasch model seen as a statistical model. When convenient, we will disregard the reference to stochastic variables writing x_{vi} rather than $X_{vi} = x_{vi}$ and θ_v rather than $\Theta_v = \theta_v$. The joint conditional distribution of item responses $\mathbf{x_v}$ for a single person in [1.8] is given by

$$P(\mathbf{x}_v|\theta_v) = \frac{\exp(r_v\theta_v - \sum_{i=1}^{k} x_{vi}\beta_i)}{\prod_{i=1}^{k}(1+\exp(\theta_v - \beta_i))} \quad [1.9]$$

where $r_v = \sum_{i=1}^{k} x_{vi}$. This formula is among the most important in the theory of Rasch models. It states that the total score $R_v = \sum_{i=1}^{k} X_{vi}$ is statistically sufficient for θ_v in the conditional distribution of item responses given θ_v since the joint probability is a product of one factor that depends on θ_v and R_v, one factor that depends on item responses and item parameters, and a normalizing factor that does not depend on data.

The fact that R_v is sufficient, means that all information about θ_v is collected in the total score and that the *conditional* distribution of the item responses given R_v does not depend on θ_v. If item parameters are known, the maximum likelihood estimate of θ_v is a function of r_v. If the only purpose is to measure θ_v, the pattern of item responses can therefore be ignored after the calculation of the total score. The formal symmetry of items of persons means that the same applies for items. Let $(X_{1i}, \ldots, X_{vi})$ be the vector of responses to item i and $M_i = \sum_{v=1}^{N} X_{vi}$ denote the item margin (the total number of positive responses). The joint distribution of this vector decomposes in exactly the same way as in formula [1.9], and from this it follows that M_i is statistically sufficient for β_i and that all information about the item parameter is contained in the item margin.

1.6.1. *The distribution of the total score*

The total score is important and it is of interest to derive its distribution. Doing so is less cumbersome using the multiplicative parameterization with $\xi_v = \exp(\theta_v)$ and $\delta_i = \exp(-\beta_i)$. We will look at the distribution of the score for a single person and will ignore the subscript referring to persons. Let $\mathbf{X} = (X_1, \ldots, X_k)$ and $\mathbf{x} = (x_1, \ldots, x_k)$ denote the vector of item responses and let $R = \sum_{i=1}^{k} X_i$. The probability of a given score r can be computed as the sum of over the set

$$X^{(r)} = \{(x_1, \ldots, x_k)|x_1 + \cdots + x_k = r\} \qquad [1.10]$$

of all response vectors with total score r

$$P(R = r|\xi) = \sum_{\mathbf{x} \in X^{(r)}} \prod_{i=1}^{k} \frac{(\xi\delta_i)^{x_i}}{1 + \xi\delta_i} = \sum_{\mathbf{x} \in X^{(r)}} \frac{\xi^r \prod_{i=1}^{k} \delta_i^{x_i}}{\prod_{i=1}^{k}(1 + \xi\delta_i)} \qquad [1.11]$$

If we define the so-called *score parameters*

$$\gamma_r = \sum_{\mathbf{x} \in X^{(r)}} \prod_{i=1}^{k} \delta_i^{x_i} \qquad [1.12]$$

and denote $\Gamma = \prod_{i=1}^{k} (1 + \xi\delta_i)$, we can rewrite [1.11] as

$$P(R = r|\xi) = \frac{\xi^r \gamma_r}{\Gamma} \qquad [1.13]$$

We note that the score parameters are functions of the item parameters and should be written as $\gamma_r = \gamma_r(\delta_1, \ldots, \delta_k)$. The distribution given by formula [1.13] is a power series distribution [NOA 50, JOH 69].

1.6.2. *Symmetrical polynomials*

The score parameters defined in [1.13] are functions of the item parameters

$$\gamma_r = \gamma_r(\delta_1, \ldots, \delta_k)$$

and are sometimes called symmetrical polynomials because they are defined as sums of products of the parameters,

$$\gamma_0 = 1$$

$$\gamma_1 = \delta_1 + \delta_2 + \cdots + \delta_k$$

$$\gamma_2 = \delta_1\delta_2 + \delta_1\delta_3 + \cdots + \delta_{k-1}\delta_k$$

$$\gamma_3 = \delta_1\delta_2\delta_3 + \delta_1\delta_2\delta_4 + \cdots + \delta_{k-2}\delta_{k-1}\delta_k$$

$$\vdots$$

$$\gamma_k = \Pi_{i=1}^k \delta_i$$

Note that $\gamma_k = 1$, if the parameters of the model are restricted in the standard way. The recursion formula

$$\gamma_r(\delta) = \gamma_r(\delta^{(i)}) + \delta_i\gamma_{r-1}(\delta^{(i)}) \qquad [1.14]$$

where $\delta = (\delta_1, \ldots, \delta_k)$ and $\delta^{(i)} = (\delta_1, \ldots, \delta_{i-1}, \delta_{i+1}, \ldots, \delta_k)$, is often useful. The intuition behind it is a division of the set $X^{(r)}$ of all response vectors with sum r into those with $X_i = 1$ and those with $X_i = 0$.

EXAMPLE 1.4.– Using these formulas and the item parameters of the depression items, it is easy to derive the distribution of the total score on the four depression items. The probabilities are

$$P(R = 0|\xi) = 1/\Gamma$$

$$P(R = 1|\xi) = 5.07 \cdot \xi/\Gamma$$

$$P(R = 2|\xi) = 8.42 \cdot \xi^2/\Gamma$$

$$P(R = 3|\xi) = 5.14 \cdot \xi^3/\Gamma$$

$$P(R = 4|\xi) = \xi^4/\Gamma$$

The normalizing constant $\Gamma = 1 + 5.07 \cdot \xi + 8.42 \cdot \xi^2 + 5.14 \cdot \xi^3 + \xi^4$ ensures that the probabilities add to one.

1.6.3. *Partial credit model parameterization of the score distribution*

In this section, we reparameterize the power series distribution [1.13] to illustrate the relation with another important distribution in the theory of Rasch models. Logarithmic transformation of parameters $\theta = \log(\xi)$ and $\lambda_r = \log(\gamma_r)$ yields

$$P(R = r|\xi) = \frac{\exp(r\theta + \lambda_r)}{\Gamma}$$

and defining $\beta_i = \lambda_{i-1} - \lambda_i$ for $i = 1, \ldots, k$, we can write $\lambda_r = -\sum_{i=1}^{r} \beta_i$, yielding

$$P(R = r|\theta) = \frac{\exp(r\theta - \sum_{i=1}^{r} \beta_i)}{\Gamma} = \frac{\exp(\sum_{i=1}^{r} (\theta - \beta_i))}{\Gamma} \quad [1.15]$$

This distribution appears in the theory of Rasch models in connection with the models for polytomous items called partial credit models, which is discussed in the next chapter. Therefore, we refer to distributions defined by formula [1.15] as partial credit *distributions*, but note that this is just another name for the power series distributions given by formula [1.13].

The parameters of this distribution are sometimes called threshold parameters and interpreted in these terms in the context of polytomous Rasch models. We therefore point out that the derivation of the partial credit distribution only sees these parameters as a transformation of the score parameters of power series distributions, and that interpretation beyond this is not warranted.

EXAMPLE 1.5.– The thresholds of the score on the depression items are $\beta_1 = -1.62$, $\beta_2 = -0.51$, $\beta_3 = 0.49$ and $\beta_4 = 1.64$. Note that the thresholds are increasing. This is always the case for scores from Rasch models for dichotomous items. This property is a property of the mathematical structure of the Rasch model and should not be interpreted as intrinsic properties of the scores that can be achieved on the set of items.

1.6.4. *Rasch models for subscores*

If a set of items fits a Rasch model, then the same is true for any subset of the items. This is due to the fact that formula [1.5] applies to any subset and that formula [1.8] also applies to any subset because joint independence of a set of variables implies joint independence of any subset of variables. The practical consequence of this is that when a set of questionnaire items fits the Rasch model, we do not need to check the fit of the items of a short form to the Rasch model. The short form must necessarily also concur with the Rasch model. Despite this, if you attempt to check the fit of the short form to the Rasch model and find that the fit is inadequate, then the analysis of the complete set of items that confirm the fit to the Rasch model must be erroneous in some way.

1.7. Inference frames

The sufficiency of the total score for the person parameter and of the item margins for the item parameters is a powerful feature of the Rasch model with very strong implications for the way data can be analyzed. This was pointed out by Rasch [RAS 61] himself who argued that (1) inference about item parameters should be based on the *conditional* distribution of item responses given person scores, because person parameters have been eliminated from these probabilities, (2) inference about person parameters should be based on the *conditional* distribution of item responses given the item margins because these probabilities do not depend on unknown item parameters and (3) the fit of the set of items to the Rasch models should be assessed in the *conditional* distribution of item responses given both person scores and item margins since this distribution does not depend on any unknown parameters [RAS 61].

We will return to the inference frames in the second part of this book (Chapters 3–9), but for now it will be useful to take a closer look at the conditional probabilities that can be derived from the Rasch model. Using the multiplicative parameterization, the joint distribution of the set of item responses for a person v is

$$P(X_{v1} = x_{v1}, \ldots, X_{vk} = x_{vk} | \xi_v) = \frac{\xi_v^{r_v} \prod_{i=1}^{k} \delta_i^{x_i}}{\Gamma}$$

Dividing this probability with the probability of the total score, formula [1.13], gives us the conditional distribution of the items given the total score

$$P(\mathbf{X_v} = \mathbf{x_v} | R_v = r) = \frac{\prod_{i=1}^{k} \delta_i^{x_{vi}}}{\gamma_r} \qquad [1.16]$$

The conditional probability of the response to item i given the total score can be calculated by summing [1.16] over all items except i. This yields

$$P(X_{vi} = 1 | R_v = r) = \frac{\delta_i \gamma_{r-1}(\delta_1, \ldots, \delta_{i-1}, \delta_{i+1}, \ldots, \delta_k)}{\gamma_r(\delta_1, \ldots, \delta_k)} \qquad [1.17]$$

and

$$P(X_{vi} = 0 | R_v = r) = \frac{\gamma_r(\delta_1, \ldots, \delta_{i-1}, \delta_{i+1}, \ldots, \delta_k)}{\gamma_r(\delta_1, \ldots, \delta_k)}$$

A plot of the function

$$r \mapsto P(X_{vi} = 1 | R_v = r)$$

is called the *conditional item characteristic curve* (CICC). To see the connection to the ICC function, we use the recursion formula [1.14] to rewrite the denominator in [1.17] and obtain

$$P(X_{vi} = 1 | R_v = r) = \frac{\delta_i \left[\frac{\gamma_{r-1}(\delta_1, \ldots, \delta_{i-1}, \delta_{i+1}, \ldots, \delta_k)}{\gamma_r(\delta_1, \ldots, \delta_{i-1}, \delta_{i+1}, \ldots, \delta_k)} \right]}{1 + \delta_i \left[\frac{\gamma_{r-1}(\delta_1, \ldots, \delta_{i-1}, \delta_{i+1}, \ldots, \delta_k)}{\gamma_r(\delta_1, \ldots, \delta_{i-1}, \delta_{i+1}, \ldots, \delta_k)} \right]}$$

Letting $\beta_i = -\log(\delta_i)$ and

$$\varphi_{ir} = \log\left[\frac{\gamma_{r-1}(\delta_1,\ldots,\delta_{i-1},\delta_{i+1},\ldots,\delta_k)}{\gamma_r(\delta_1,\ldots,\delta_{i-1},\delta_{i+1},\ldots,\delta_k)}\right]$$

yields

$$P(X_{vi} = 1|R_v = r) = \frac{\exp(\phi_{ir} - \beta_i)}{1 + \exp(\phi_{ir} - \beta_i)} \qquad [1.18]$$

Formula [1.18] is similar to formula [1.5] defining the ICC, but there are subtle differences that may lead to problems if they are not recognized. The most important of these is that the ICC is a function of θ_v whereas the CICC is a function of ϕ_{ir}, which itself is a function of a subset of item parameters. We will return to this problem in Chapter 5.

EXAMPLE 1.6.– The ICC and the CICC for the first depression item are

– $\theta_v = -1.229$, true score = 1, ICC = 0.102, CICC = 0.077;

– $\theta_v = -0.004$, true score = 2, ICC = 0.270, CICC = 0.216;

– $\theta_v = 1.227$, true score = 3, ICC = 0.571, CICC = 0.500;

where ICC values have been calculated for the three values of θ with true scores (expected scores) equal to 1, 2 and 3, respectively. The CICC values are the probabilities of a positive response to the item, given that the observed score is equal to the true score.

The conditional probabilities of item responses given the total item margins are similar to the probabilities of item responses given the person scores. Calculation of γ functions of person parameters is more challenging than the calculation of γ functions of item parameters because typically the number of persons is larger than the number of items. But apart from this, nothing more needs to be said at this point.

The joint probability of the complete matrix of item responses

$$X = (X_{v,i})_{i=1,\ldots,k;v=1,\ldots,n}$$

is given by

$$P(X = x|\theta) = \frac{\prod_{v=1}^{n}\exp(r_v\theta_v)\prod_{i=1}^{k}\exp(-m_i\beta_i)}{\prod_{v=1}^{n}\prod_{i=1}^{k}(1 + \exp(\theta_v - \beta_i))} \qquad [1.19]$$

where $\theta = (\theta_1,\ldots,\theta_n)$. Because of the sufficiency of the person scores and item margins, the probability depends only on the observed responses through these summary statistics. It follows that all data matrices with the same margins have the same probability so that the conditional distribution of the matrix of item responses given the person scores and item margins is uniform. Let $\mathbf{r} = (r_v)_{v=1,\dots,n}$ and $\mathbf{m} = (m_i)_{i=1,\dots,k}$ denote the margins and let $K(\mathbf{s}, \mathbf{m})$ denote the number of matrices with these margins. Because all matrices fitting the margins have the same conditional probability, it follows that

$$P(X = x|\mathbf{r}, \mathbf{m}) = \frac{1}{K(\mathbf{r}, \mathbf{m})} \qquad [1.20]$$

1.8. Specific objectivity

The Rasch model is one among several psychometric models that may be used to provide valid measurement of the outcomes of a latent variable. Most of the features of the Rasch models are shared by all conventional IRT models. From a statistical point of view, the Rasch model stands apart because it can be shown that the Rasch model is the only unidimensional IRT model with locally independent items and a sufficient total person score [AND 73]. From a methodological point of view, the Rasch model is the only unidimensional model with locally independent items that provide what Rasch called specific objectivity.

Let us define the notion of specific objectivity. To do this we have to provide answers to two questions: what exactly did Rasch mean by objectivity and why did he talk of *specific* objectivity and not just objectivity in general?

Rasch's concept of objectivity requires that comparison of persons is unbiased by the choice of items and that comparison of items is not biased by the sampling of persons for the statistical study.

Because conditional inference frames separate item parameters from person parameters, it follows that inference about item parameters does not depend on the sampling of persons and inference about person parameters does not depend on the choice of items. It is needless to say that sample sizes and the number of items will have an effect on standard errors of measurement and on the power of test statistics, but apart from that it does not matter which items are used and which persons are sampled. The sample of persons need not be representative as long as the inference is performed within a conditional frame of inference. Because Rasch models are the only IRT models with conditional inference frames, Rasch argued that the Rasch model is the only model providing objective measurement and that objectivity is only obtained if inference is conditional.

The term "specific" reflects the concern that statistical models only apply within specific frames of reference, for example in specific subpopulations or at specific time points. A measurement instrument shown to provide valid and objective measurement of the degree of paranoia among the mentally ill cannot automatically be assumed to provide objective measurement in a normal population. Referring to objectivity as *specific* objectivity is nothing more and nothing less than a cautious warning that you must never automatically assume that your results of a statistical analysis apply in all settings.

1.9. Rasch models as graphical models

In section 1.1.3, it was remarked that conditional independence of item pairs does not imply that all items are jointly conditionally independent and therefore also locally independent. It can be shown, however, that if all pairs of items are conditionally independent given Θ together with the responses to all the other items, then and only then will items be jointly locally independent. This result comes from the theory of graphical models [LAU 96, WHI 90]. Graphical models are defined by assumptions that certain pairs of variables are conditionally independent given all the other variables of the model. Graphical models are characterized by independence or Markov graphs, where variables are represented by nodes, conditional dependencies by edges or arrows, and conditional independence by missing edges/arrows between variables. The Rasch model is a graphical model. The independence graph of the Rasch model for the depression items is shown in Figure 1.5.

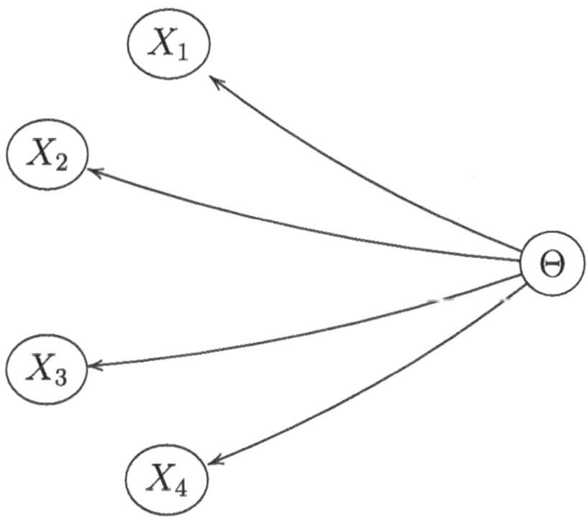

Figure 1.5. *Markov IRT graph of the four depression items*

This graph has a number of interesting properties that may be useful during the statistical analysis. For now, we focus on the visual display that, for us, is a very transparent way to illustrate the notion that items depend only on the latent variable. In the discussion of DIF, it was mentioned that the absence of DIF is an implicit assumption of Rasch models. To make this assumption more explicit, we add exogenous variables to the model to obtain *graphical Rasch models* [KRE 02]. These consist of items $X_1, \ldots, X_k$, the latent variable θ and exogenous variables $Z_1, \ldots, Z_p$, where items and exogenous variables are assumed to be conditionally independent given Θ. The graph for such a model is illustrated in Figure 1.6 where exogenous variables Z_1 and Z_2 AGE have been added to the Rasch model for the depression items.

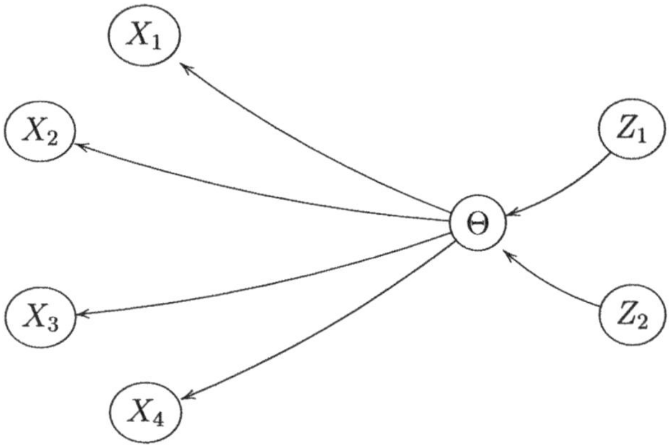

Figure 1.6. *The IRT graph of the graphical Rasch model containing depression items and two exogenous variables*

The graphs in Figures 1.5 and 1.6 encapsulate the assumptions of unidimensionality, local independence and absence of DIF. Because these assumptions apply to all IRT models we refer to the graphs in these figures as *IRT graphs*.

To illustrate the sufficiency of the total score R, we note that the sufficiency of R implies that items are conditionally independent of Θ and the exogenous variables given R. Adding R to the model results in a new Markov graph called a *Rasch graph*, where items are separated from all other variables by R. This is illustrated in Figure 1.7. Note that the edges have been added between items because they are not conditionally independent given the total score.

1.10. Summary

The Rasch model for dichotomous items is a statistical model for responses to a set of items that depend on a latent variable representing a trait or a property of the person responding. In the conditional distribution of items given the latent variable, the value of the latent variable appears as a person parameter and an estimate of this parameter is regarded as an indirect measure of the trait or property represented by the latent variable. The properties of the model can be discussed from both a statistical and a psychometric point of view.

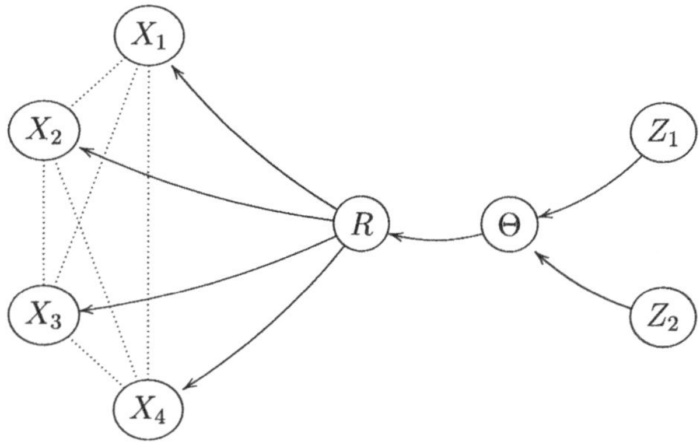

Figure 1.7. *The Rasch graph of the graphical Rasch model for the depression items*

From the psychometric point of view, we note that measurement is a criterion-related construct valid because the requirements of unidimensionality, monotonicity, local independence, consistency, homogeneity and absence of DIF are met. Furthermore, psychometricians would also note that indirect measurement by items from Rasch models is characterized by specific objectivity. Because, the Rasch models satisfy all known psychometric requirements of validity in addition to providing objective measurements, we can claim that measurement by Rasch model items can be regarded as ideal psychometric measurement.

From the statistical point of view, the Rasch model can be parameterized in several different but equivalent ways. In this book, we consider both the original multiplicative parameterization and the more commonly used logistic parameterization because each of them has its own advantages.

The total person scores and item margins are statistically sufficient for, respectively, the person and item parameters of the model. From this, it follows that we can define three different conditional frames of inference for the analysis of data where nuisance parameters have been eliminated. The specific objective in Rasch models is a consequence of this result. Measurement is only objective if estimates are calculated in the conditional frame of inference.

In addition to the conditional frames of inference, the Rasch model also permits analysis in two other inference frames. In the joint unconditional frame of inference, all parameters are regarded as fixed parameters that have to be jointly estimated. In the marginal frame of inference, person parameters are regarded as random effects with a specific type of statistical distribution – typically a normal distribution – whose parameters are estimated together with the item parameters. The statistical analyses in the different frames of inference will be described and compared in Chapters 4 and 5.

The distribution of the total score on a set of Rasch items is, in particular, simple. Under the different parameterizations of the model, we would describe the distribution as either a power series distribution or a partial credit distribution with ordered thresholds.

We finally noted that the Rasch model is a graphical model and briefly outlined the notion of graphical Rasch models where exogenous person covariates are added to the Rasch model. Graphical models have a number of properties that are very useful during the statistical analysis. In Chapter 5 on item fit statistics and Chapter 8 on tests of local independence on statistical analyses by Rasch models, it will be shown how these properties can be made useful.

1.11. Bibliography

[AND 73] ANDERSEN E.B., "Conditional inference for multiple-choice questionnaires", *British Journal of Mathematical and Statistical Psychology*, vol. 26, pp. 31–44, 1973.

[CRO 55] CRONBACH L.J., MEEHL L.J., "Construct validity in psychological tests", *Psychological Bulletin*, vol. 52, pp. 281–302, 1955.

[FRE 09] FREDOUILLE J., LAPORTE E., MESBAH M., "Housing and mental health", in ORMANDY D. (ed.), *Housing and Health in Europe. The Who Lares Project*, Taylor and Francis, Boston, 2009.

[HOL 86] HOLLAND P.W., ROSENBAUM P.R., "Conditional association and unidimensionality in monotone latent variable models", *The Annals of Statistics*, vol. 14, pp. 1523–1543, 1986.

[JOH 69] JOHNSON N.L., KOTZ S., *Discrete Distributions*, John Wiley & Sons, New York, 1969.

[KRE 02] KREINER S., CHRISTENSEN K.B., "Graphical rasch models", in MESBAH M., LEE M.-T., COLE B.F. (eds), *Statistical Methods for Quality of Life Studies: Design, Measurements and Analysis*, Kluwer Academic Publishers, pp. 187–203, 2002.

[LAU 96] LAURITZEN S., *Graphical Models*, Clarendon Press, 1996.

[MES 09] MESBAH M., "Building quality of life related housing scores using LARES study – a methodical approach to avoid pitfalls and bias", in ORMANDY D. (ed.), *Housing and Health in Europe. The Who Lares Project*, Taylor and Francis, Boston, 2009.

[MIC 97] MICHELL J., "Quantitative science and the definition of measurement in psychology", *British Journal of Psychology*, vol. 88, pp. 355–383, 1997.

[NOA 50] NOACK A., "A class of random variables with discrete distributions", *Annals of Mathematical Statistics*, vol. 21, pp. 127–132, 1950.

[RAS 60] RASCH G., *Probabilistic Models for Some Intelligence and Attainment Tests*, Danish National Institute for Educational Research, Copenhagen, 1960.

[RAS 61] RASCH G., "On general laws and the meaning of measurement in psychology", in *Proceedings of the Fourth Berkeley Symposium on Mathematical Statistics and Probability, IV*, University of California Press, Berkeley, CA, pp. 321–334, 1961.

[ROS 89] ROSENBAUM P., "Criterion-related construct validity", *Psychometrika*, vol. 54, pp. 625–633, 1989.

[VAN 97] VAN DER LINDEN W.J., HAMBLETON R.K., *Handbook of Modern Item Response Theory*, Springer-Verlag, New York, NY, 1997.

[WHI 90] WHITTAKER J., *Graphical Models in Applied Multivariate Statistics*, Wiley, Chichester, 1990.

Chapter 2

Rasch Models for Ordered Polytomous Items

2.1. Introduction

Chapter 1 presented the models for dichotomous items, where the response X_{vi} of person v to item i is within a set of two possibilities, "yes" or "no" and "agree" or "disagree". The random variable X_{vi} is a Bernoulli variable, with a natural coding: $X_{vi} = 0$ or $X_{vi} = 1$, but the probability $Pr(X_{vi} = 1)$ is not constant across values of v and i.

In health sciences, for patient-reported outcomes and/or other purposes, we often use "polytomous" items with more than two ordered responses by categories. So, if we denote the response by X_{vi}, the possible responses are usually coded as $X_{vi} = 0, 1, 2, \ldots, m_i$, where the number of response categories of item i is $m_i + 1$. Note that in applications like these, there is a natural prespecified ordering and that dichotomous items can be considered as a special case where $m_i = 1$.

2.1.1. *Example*

The Diabetes Health Profile (DHP) questionnaire [MEA 96] includes items that diabetic patients must answer in order to assess their level of disinhibited eating (DE). The DE dimension reflects the effects of emotional arousal on eating behavior (e.g. eating extra when feeling bored or fed up), as well as responses to external food cues (e.g. finding it difficult to saying no to food). The items are shown in Table 2.1. Data from a French translation of the questionaire [CHW 07, BOI 10] are used for illustration.

Chapter written by Mounir MESBAH and Svend KREINER.

Item	Wording	Response options
Dhp32	Do you wish there were not so many nice things to eat?	a) "Not at all" b) "A little" c) "A lot" d) "Very much"
Dhp34	How likely are you to eat something extra when you feel bored or fed up?	a) "Not at all likely" b) "Not very likely" c) "Quite likely" d) "Very likely"
Dhp36	When you start eating how easy do you find it to stop?	a) "Very easy" b) "Quite easy" c) "Not very easy" d) "Not at all easy"
Dhp38	Do you have problems keeping to your diet because you eat to cheer yourself up?	a) "Never" b) "Sometimes" c) "Usually" d) "Always"
Dhp39	Do you have problems keeping to your diet because you find it hard saying no to food you like?	a) "Never" b) "Sometimes" c) "Usually" d) "Always"

Table 2.1. *The items of the disinhibited eating (DE) subscale in the Diabetes Health Profile (DHP) questionnaire*

2.1.2. *Ordered categories*

For each item, all response categories are ordered. Consider, for instance, item Dhp32 "Do you wish there were not so many nice things to eat?" We expect that a person answering "not at all" (a) is *more* inhibited with eating than a person answering "a lot" (c). The ordering of the categories should be coherent with the level of a person on the latent continuum defined by the construct "inhibition with eating" we want to measure. A lower category will correspond to a lower level, and a higher category will correspond to a higher level. This is a *monotonicity* property.

Modeling such responses is not straightforward. In the statistical literature, there are many published papers, presenting various models, but only a few can be considered as polytomous Rasch models (PRMs), even if some of those models can be considered as generalization of the dichotomous Rasch model.

Usually, we use a simple coding as, for instance, $X_{vi} = 0$ if the response choice is (a), $X_{vi} = 1$ if the response choice is (b), $X_{vi} = 2$ if the response choice is (c) and $X_{vi} = 3$ if the response choice is (d). Of course, such a choice does not mean that the distance between modality "c" and modality "a" is twice the distance between modality "d" and modality "a". The only assumption made is about the ordering of categories.

In the dichotomous case, we considered probabilities $P(X = 1|\theta)$ that are increasing as θ increases. However, we could also consider probabilities $P(X = 0|\theta)$. This is shown in Figure 2.1, where β_i is the item parameter in the dichotomous Rasch model, which is also called the threshold parameter. Its value corresponds in the latent continuum to the value of θ, where these two curves cross, that is where the probability equals 0.5.

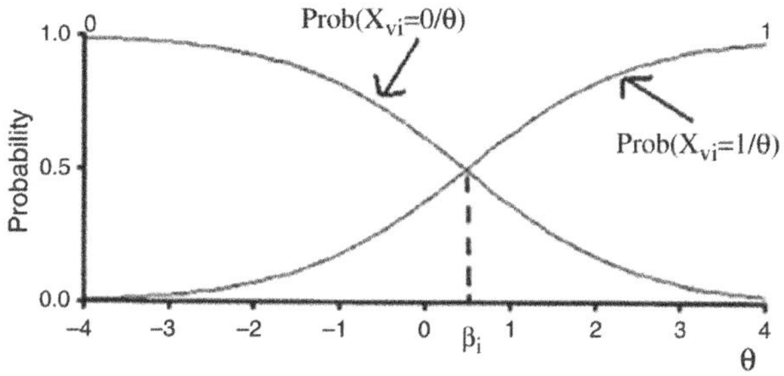

Figure 2.1. *Probability function for dichotomous item i with item parameter β_i*

Of course, in this situation, there is a simple relation

$$P(X = 0) = 1 - P(X = 1)$$

between the probabilities.

If, for instance, the number of categories is three, we will have three probability functions, each corresponding to conditional probabilities of a category given the latent variable. These are usually called the *category characteristic curves* (CCCs). An example is shown in Figure 2.2.

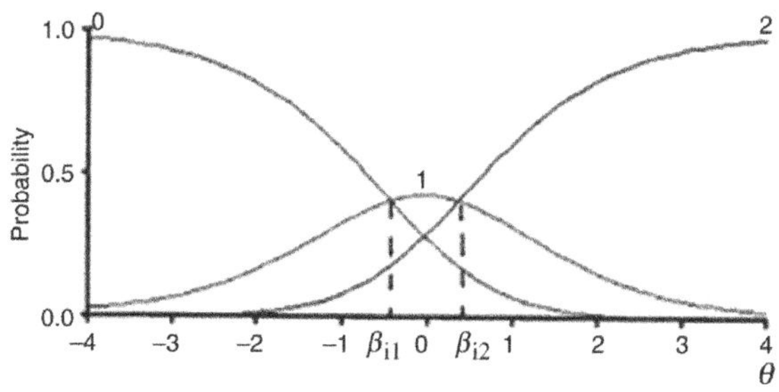

Figure 2.2. *Category characteristic curves (CCCs): probability function of each category for an item with three categories (0, 1, 2)*

It is intuitively clear that as θ increases, the probability of the low category (0) will decrease and similarly that, for the high category (2), the probability function increases. The probability function of the middle category (1) can be obtained by subtraction, so it is easy to show that it looks like the one in Figure 2.2. Based on Figure 2.2, we define two parameters: β_{i1}, which corresponds to the θ value where the first (category 0) and the second (category 1) probability functions intersect, and β_{i2}, which corresponds to the intersection between the second (category 1) and the last (category 2) probability function. It turns out that these parameters can be used to define the PRM.

Andersen [AND 77] defines the following model:

$$P(X_{vi} = x|\Theta = \theta_v) = \frac{\exp(\theta_v x + \psi_{ix})}{\sum_{h=0}^{m_i} \exp(\theta_v h + \psi_{ih})} \qquad [2.1]$$

This is the PRM. It is for some purposes convenient to rewrite [2.1] as

$$P(X_{vi} = x|\Theta = \theta) = \frac{\exp(\theta_v x + \sum_{z=0}^{m_i} \psi_{iz} 1_{(X_{vi}=z)})}{\sum_{h=0}^{m_i} \exp(\theta_v h + \psi_{ih})} \qquad [2.2]$$

using indicators $1_{(X_{vi}=z)}$ taking the value one if the response to item i by person v is z and zero otherwise. Indicators are shown in Table 2.2, where the number of categories for an item is four.

Response to item i		X_{vi}	$1_{(X_{vi}=1)}$	$1_{(X_{vi}=2)}$	$1_{(X_{vi}=3)}$
Lowest category	a)	0	0	0	0
	b)	1	1	0	0
	c)	2	0	1	0
Highest category	d)	3	0	0	1

Table 2.2. *Indicators: nominal, ordinal or multinomial coding*

The first column gives the label of the category response as it usually appears in the questionnaire form, in its natural ordering: from the lowest (a) to the highest (d). The second column gives a simple ordinal coding from 0 to 3. The three last columns give the indicator variable coding, indicating clearly that the item responses in the polytomous context are multivariate with three dependent Bernoulli variable responses. This kind of coding of categorical variables is common in statistical software. Multinomial variables belong to the exponential family distribution, so it is usual to analyze such data with generalized linear models [MCC 83, AGR 84]. Under this framework, we have to specify the probability distribution, the link function and the linear predictor. Similar to the dichotomous case, for each person v, multiple correlated responses correspond to each item response. For instance, in the DE subscale data, we observe for each person five responses corresponding to the five given questions. These five responses cannot be considered as independent; so, we need to specify precisely the joint probability distribution for the vector of the five responses. Latent variable models to which the Rasch model belongs specify such joint distributions through conditional probabilities of observed item responses given the latent variable and an assumption of conditional independence of the items given the latent variable.

Formula [2.2] makes it easy to understand the sufficiency properties of the model; however, the relation to the category probability functions is less clear. Defining

$$\beta_{iz} = \psi_{i(z-1)} - \psi_{iz} \tag{2.3}$$

we can rewrite [2.2] as

$$P(X_{vi} = x) = \frac{\exp(\theta_v x - \sum_{z=1}^{x} \beta_{iz})}{\sum_{h=0}^{m_i} \exp(\theta_v h - \sum_{z=1}^{h} \beta_{iz})} \tag{2.4}$$

This is the *partial credit model* (PCM) proposed by Masters [MAS 82] and it is easy to see that the βs defined by [2.3] correspond to the intersection between adjacent category probability curves in Figure 2.2. Often β_{iz} are called *threshold parameters*, and sometimes *centralized thresholds*

$$\beta_{iz}^{*} = \beta_{iz} - \sum_{h=1}^{m_i} \beta_{ih} \tag{2.5}$$

are also considered.

An important feature of this model is that the probability of each category of response depends on all thresholds locations. This feature illustrates that the described process is not sequential, that is it goes from category 0 to the chosen category. It is rather a simultaneous process, which takes into consideration the difficulty of all thresholds and fixes on the most suitable category.

2.1.3. *Properties of the polytomous Rasch model*

The model [2.1] has several nice properties.

Monotonicity: it is easy to see from [2.1] that for any x the probabilities

$$P(X_{vi} \geq x | \Theta_v = \theta) = \sum_{z=x}^{m_i} P(X_{vi} = z | \Theta_v = \theta)$$

and the expected scores $E(X_{vi}|\theta)$ are increasing as a function of θ.

Sufficiency: from

$$\log P(X_{vi} = x|\Theta_v = \theta; \psi_{ih}) = \theta_v x_i + \sum_{z=0}^{m_i} \psi_{iz} 1_{(X_{vi}=z)} - K_i(\theta)$$

with $K_i(\theta)$ given by

$$K_i(\theta) = \sum_{h=0}^{m_i} \exp(\theta_v h + \psi_{ih})$$

we recognize an exponential family and for this reason the Rasch model has several sufficiency properties, most importantly that the total score R is sufficient for θ. This property of the Rasch model is not shared by any other IRT model.

Invariance of parameters: consider the probabilities of two adjacent categories of an item for two persons with θ values θ_1 and θ_2, respectively. The probabilities in Table 2.3 yield an odds ratio that has a simple structure:

$$\frac{\exp(\theta_1(x-1) + \psi_{i(x-1)}) \times \exp(\theta_2 x + \psi_{ix})}{\exp(\theta_1 x + \psi_{ix}) \times \exp(\theta_2(x-1) + \psi_{i(x-1)})} = \exp(\theta_2 - \theta_1)$$

This is similar to the dichotomous Rasch model.

Category	$P(\cdot\|\theta_1)$	$P(\cdot\|\theta_2)$
x − 1	$\frac{\exp(\theta_1(x-1) + \psi_{i(x-1)})}{K_i(\theta_1)}$	$\frac{\exp(\theta_2(x-1) + \psi_{i(x-1)})}{K_i(\theta_2)}$
x	$\frac{\exp(\theta_1 x + \psi_{ix})}{K_i(\theta_1)}$	$\frac{\exp(\theta_2 x + \psi_{ix})}{K_i(\theta_2)}$

Table 2.3. *Odds ratios in the polytomous Rasch model*

The logarithm of the odds ratio, when it moves from an item level $x - 1$ to the adjacent level x and from an ability θ_1 to another ability θ_2, equals the difference between the latent values $\theta_1 - \theta_2$ and the odds ratio is invariant across items. Furthermore, this local comparison is also invariant over values of x. Similar results apply when we compare two persons relative to response options that are not adjacent.

We see that this local comparison is also invariant over the values of x. A similar result applies when comparing two items since if we move from x_1 to x_2, we get

$$\frac{\exp(\theta_1 x_1 + \psi_{ix_1}) \times \exp(\theta_2 x_2 + \psi_{ix_2})}{\exp(\theta_1 x_2 + \psi_{ix_2}) \times \exp(\theta_2 x_1 + \psi_{ix_1})} = \exp((\theta_2 - \theta_1)(x_2 - x_1))$$

The logarithm of the odds ratio, when it moves from $x-1$ to x and from person location θ_1 to θ_2, is equal to the difference between latent values $\theta_1-\theta_2$, whereas the logarithm of the odds ratio, when it moves from level x_1 to level x_2 and from θ_1 to θ_2, equals the difference $\theta_1-\theta_2$ between latent values weighted by the level difference x_1-x_2.

2.1.4. *Assumptions*

Several assumptions are made in the PRM:

1) The latent trait θ is a scalar; so that the latent trait is unidimensional.

2) The individuals are mutually independent.

3) The items are locally independent, that is they are conditionally independent given the latent trait.

In Figure 2.2, we have seen two new parameters β_{i1} and β_{i2}. These are called thresholds and indicate points where the probability of adjacent response categories is equal. For dichotomous items, the only threshold is the unique item parameter, also called item difficulty in educational context, which is the point where the probability of either zero or one is the same. In the case of three categories, there are two threshold parameters.

2.2. Derivation from the dichotomous model

The PRM [2.1] was first proposed by Andersen, who was a student of Rasch. Andrich proposed another version of this model [AND 78], while Masters derived the same model with a different parameterization [MAS 82]. The idea is to rewrite the probabilities of the dichotomous Rasch model in such a way that the generalization to a score greater than one appears clearly as a function of the differences between the latent parameter and the successive threshold parameters, that is as a function of quantities like $\theta_v-\beta_{ix}$ (with $x=0,1,\ldots,m_i$) similar to the dichotomous Rasch model. First, we rewrite the dichotomous model

$$P(X_{vi}=0)=\frac{e^{0(\theta_v-\beta_i)}}{e^{0(\theta_v-\beta_i)}+e^{1(\theta_v-\beta_i)}}$$

$$P(X_{vi}=1)=\frac{e^{1(\theta_v-\beta_i)}}{e^{0(\theta_v-\beta_i)}+e^{1(\theta_v-\beta_i)}}$$

Generalizing this model to a model with possible scores equal to zero, one and two suggests that when the response is $x_{vi}=2$, we will expect that:

$$P(X_{vi}=2)=\frac{e^{2(\theta_v-\beta_i)}}{e^{0(\theta_v-\beta_i)}+e^{1(\theta_v-\beta_i)}+e^{2(\theta_v-\beta_i)}} \qquad [2.6]$$

A similar but more general model that includes, as a special case, the dichotomous Rasch model is

$$P(X_{vi}=0)=\frac{e^{0(\theta_v-\beta_i)}}{e^{0(\theta_v-\beta_i)}+e^{-\beta_{i1}+1(\theta_v-\beta_i)}+e^{-\beta_{i1}-\beta_{i2}+2(\theta_v-\beta_i)}}$$

$$P(X_{vi}=1)=\frac{e^{-\beta_{i1}+1(\theta_v-\beta_i)}}{e^{0(\theta_v-\beta_i)}+e^{-\beta_{i1}+1(\theta_v-\beta_i)}+e^{-\beta_{i1}-\beta_{i2}+2(\theta_v-\beta_i)}}$$

$$P(X_{vi}=2)=\frac{e^{-\beta_{i1}-\beta_{i2}+2(\theta_v-\beta_i)}}{e^{0(\theta_v-\beta_i)}+e^{-\beta_{i1}+1(\theta_v-\beta_i)}+e^{-\beta_{i1}-\beta_{i2}+2(\theta_v-\beta_i)}}$$

A direct consequence of these equations is the clear interpretation of the threshold parameters as latent values corresponding to the intersection of adjacent category probability curves.

$$P(X_{vi}=0)=P(X_{vi}=1) \qquad \Rightarrow \beta_{i1}=\theta_v-\beta_i$$

$$P(X_{vi}=1)=P(X_{vi}=2) \qquad \Rightarrow \beta_{i2}=\theta_v-\beta_i$$

Figure 2.3 is a copy of Figure 2.2, where the category probabilities are shown as functions of $\theta_v-\beta_i$ instead of θ_v. The horizontal axis is divided into three intervals: $I_0=]-\infty,\beta_{i1}]$; $I_1=[\beta_{i1},\beta_{i2}[$ and $I_2=[\beta_{i2},\infty[$.

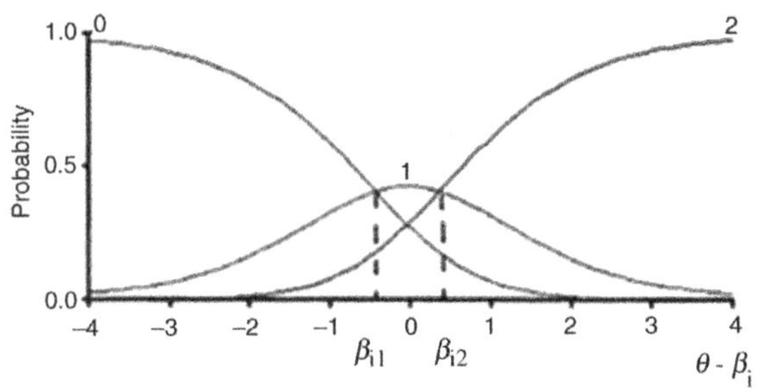

Figure 2.3. *Centralized probability function of each category for an item with three categories (0, 1, 2)*

This relates to the centralized thresholds [2.5]. Note that $P(X_{vi}=0)$ is greater than $P(X_{vi}=1)$ and $P(X_{vi}=2)$ in I_0, while $P(X_{vi}=1)$ is the greater probability function in I_1 and $P(X_{vi}=2)$ is the greater probability function in I_2.

More generally, when the number of categories is m_i, the probability function of category x can be written as:

$$P(X_{vi}=x)=\frac{e^{x(\theta_v-\beta_i)-\sum_{z=1}^{x}\beta_{iz}}}{\sum_{h=0}^{m_i}e^{h(\theta_v-\beta_i)-\sum_{z=1}^{h}\beta_{ih}}} \qquad [2.7]$$

This is the PRM [AND 77, AND 78]. The most popular form of [2.7] is the partial credit model [MAS 82] derived using the fact the probability of category x conditional of being in x or in $x-1$ is

$$\frac{P(X_{vi}=x)}{P(X_{vi}=x)+P(X_{vi}=x-1)}=\frac{e^{-\beta_{ix}+(\theta_v-\beta_i)}}{1+e^{(\theta_v-\beta_i-\beta_{ix})}} \qquad [2.8]$$

which is a dichotomous Rasch model with item parameter $\beta_i+\beta_{ix}$.

The latent conditional probability of succeeding at threshold x, which is a dichotomous response given that the response is in $x-1$ or x, is a dichotomous Rasch model and the location at which the success or failure is obtained is the threshold qualified by the overall location of the item. In the above equations, the thresholds sum to zero around the overall difficulty of the item. To reference the threshold to scale as a whole, the location of the item has to be added to the thresholds in the above equations. The response at each threshold that we inferred algebraically above never happens. We only have a single response in one of the categories. This is the kind of response, we can imagine, that happens behind the process. It is called the *latent response*. There is one latent response at each threshold. For $m_i=3$

$$\begin{aligned}
P(X_{vi}=0)&=P(L_{1vi}=0,L_{2vi}=0,L_{3vi}=0)\\
P(X_{vi}=1)&=P(L_{1vi}=1,L_{2vi}=0,L_{3vi}=0)\\
P(X_{vi}=2)&=P(L_{1vi}=1,L_{2vi}=1,L_{3vi}=0)\\
P(X_{vi}=3)&=P(L_{1vi}=1,L_{2vi}=1,L_{3vi}=1)
\end{aligned}$$

written

$$\begin{aligned}
P(X_{vi}=0)&=e^{0(\theta_v-(\beta_i+\beta_{i1}))}e^{0(\theta_v-(\beta_i+\beta_{i2}))}e^{0(\theta_v-(\beta_i+\beta_{i3}))}/d_{vi}\\
P(X_{vi}=1)&=e^{1(\theta_v-(\beta_i+\beta_{i1}))}e^{0(\theta_v-(\beta_i+\beta_{i2}))}e^{0(\theta_v-(\beta_i+\beta_{i3}))}/d_{vi}\\
P(X_{vi}=2)&=e^{1(\theta_v-(\beta_i+\beta_{i1}))}e^{1(\theta_v-(\beta_i+\beta_{i2}))}e^{0(\theta_v-(\beta_i+\beta_{i3}))}/d_{vi}\\
P(X_{vi}=3)&=e^{1(\theta_v-(\beta_i+\beta_{i1}))}e^{1(\theta_v-(\beta_i+\beta_{i2}))}e^{1(\theta_v-(\beta_i+\beta_{i3}))}/d_{vi}
\end{aligned}$$

where d_{vi} is a normalizing factor (the sum of the numerators). This means that the score $X_{vi}=x$ arises from the following pattern of latent responses at the thresholds.

Thus, the score of $X_{vi}=x$ arises from exactly x successes at the first x thresholds and m_i-x failures at the remaining thresholds. This is called the *Guttman pattern*: an ordered polytomous response defined by a multinomial response in a constrained space, where values like $\{0,1,0\}$, $\{0,0,1\}$ or $\{0,1,1\}$ are impossible. A success at level two implies that a preliminary success at level one was obtained. Figure 2.4 shows of the interpretation of the model parameters.

Response to item i by person v		X_{vi}	L_{1vi}	L_{2vi}	L_{3vi}
Lowest category:	a)	0	0	0	0
	b)	1	1	0	0
	c)	2	1	1	0
Highest category:	d)	3	1	1	1

Table 2.4. *Latent responses*

The parameter β_{iz} of formula [2.7] can be thought of as an item step difficulty associated with the location on the underlying trait where categories $z - 1$ and z intersect. This parameter expresses the attractiveness of the respective response category z of item i. This attractiveness is assumed to be the same for all subjects. If the thresholds are ordered, these parameters provide a partition of the latent continuum into $m_i + 1$ sections where one response category has the highest probability. Thus, the probability of a respondent v endorsing category z for item i is a function of the difference between their level on the underlying trait and the step difficulty.

Table 2.5 summarizes the different ways that the Rasch model for polytomous items can be parameterized. We have added the power series formalization described in Chapter 1. This formulation is convenient because formulas based on this parameterization are less cumbersome than formulas based on the PRM formalization and much less cumbersome than formulas based on the PCM parameterization. The power series formalization also avoids the problems with non-observed item categories because $\gamma_{iz} = 0$ is permitted. The PRM and PCM parameterizations require that $\gamma_{iz} > 0$.

The PCM formalization is the most popular because it looks like a simple generalization of the logistic IRT models for dichotomous variables. Also, thresholds and locations are measured on the same (interval) scale as person parameters. Finally, many think that threshold parameters are easier to interpret than score parameters, but it is an open question whether or not these interpretations are correct. Masters' interpretation is wrong.

Rasch models can be defined by imposing restrictions on the thresholds

$$\beta_{iz} = \sum_{h=0}^{d} \delta_{ih} z^h$$

Such a model with $d = 2$ was defined by Leunbach who referred to it as a normal distribution for discrete variables [LEU 76]. A discussion of these restricted models has been presented by von Davier and Rost [VON 95, p. 375]. The computer program RUMM [AND 10] uses models of this kind.

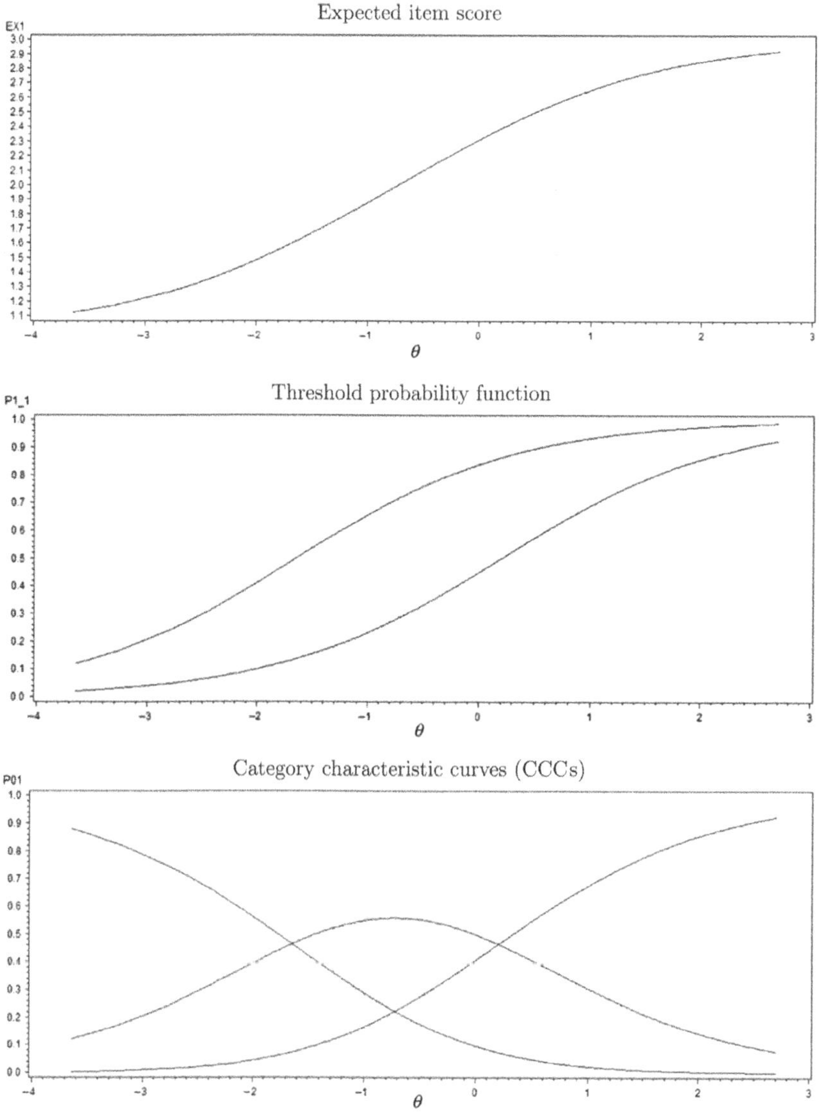

Figure 2.4. *Expected item score, threshold probability function and category characteristic curves (CCCs) for an item with three response options. Threshold parameters are* $\beta_{i1} = -1.65$ *and* $\beta_{i2} = 0.20$

2.3. Distributions derived from Rasch models

To simplify the notation in this section, we disregard the subscript referring to persons in this section and refer to *θ* as the outcome of the latent variable Θ_v.

	PCM	PCM location	PRM	Multiplicative power series
Person parameter	θ	θ	θ	$\xi = \exp(\theta)$
$P(X_{vi} = x \mid \Theta_v = \theta)$	$\frac{\exp(x\theta - \sum_{z=1}^{x} \beta_{iz})}{\sum_{x=0}^{m_i} \exp(x\theta - \sum_{z=1}^{x} \beta_{iz})}$	$\frac{\exp(x(\theta - \bar{\beta}_i) - \sum_{z=1}^{x} \bar{\beta}_{iz})}{\sum_{x=0}^{m_i} \exp(x(\theta - \bar{\beta}_i) - \sum_{z=1}^{x} \bar{\beta}_{iz})}$	$\frac{\exp(x\theta + \psi_{ix})}{\sum_{x=0}^{m_i} \exp(x\theta - \psi_{ix})}$	$\frac{\xi^x \gamma_{ix}}{\sum_{x=0}^{m_i} \xi^x \gamma_{ix}}$
Constraint	$\beta_{i0} = 0$ and $\sum_{i=1}^{k} \sum_{h=1}^{m_i} \beta_{ih} = 0$	$\sum_{i=1}^{k} (\bar{\beta}_i + \bar{\beta}_{im}) = 0$ or $\sum_{i=1}^{k} \bar{\beta}_i = 0$	$\psi_{i0} = 0$ and $\sum_{i=1}^{k} \psi_{im_i} = 0$	$\gamma_{i0} = 1$ and $\prod_{i=1}^{k} \gamma_{im_i} = 1$

Notes:

$\bar{\beta}_i$ is sometimes called the location of item i.

PCM is sometimes written as $P(X_{vi} = x \mid \Theta_v = \theta) = \frac{\exp(\sum_{z=1}^{x}(\theta - \beta_{iz}))}{\sum_{x=0}^{m_i} \exp(\sum_{z=1}^{x}(\theta - \beta_{iz}))}$.

PCM = partial credit model, PRM = polytomous Rasch model.

Table 2.5. *Different parameterizations of the Rasch model for polytomous items*

Let $X = (X_1, \ldots, X_k)$ be a set of locally independent Rasch items depending on θ with maximum item scores equal to $(m_1, \ldots, m_k)$. The total person score is $R = \sum_{i=1}^{k} X_i$. Subscores over subsets of items $V \subseteq \{1, \ldots, K\}$ are equal to $R_V = \sum_{i \in V} X_i$ and rest scores for the same subset of items are referred to as $R^{(V)} = R - R_V$. The item margins counting the number of responses in separate response categories defined by $C_{ix} = \sum_{v=1}^{n} 1_{(X_{vi}=x)}$ are sufficient statistics for the item parameters.

2.3.1. *The score distribution*

The distributions of scores, subscores and rest scores and the conditional distributions of items given these scores are central to the theory of Rasch models. To derive these, we rewrite the PRM as a multiplicative power series model

$$P(X_i = x|\theta) = \frac{\xi^x \gamma_{ix}}{\sum_{h=0}^{m_i} \xi^h \gamma_{ih}} \qquad [2.9]$$

where $\xi = \exp(\xi)$ and $\gamma_{ix} = 0$ for $x < 0$ and $x > m_i$. Denote the total score on two items by $R_{(i,i')} = X_i + X_{i'}$. The distribution of this sum can be calculated as

$$P(R_{(i,i')} = r|\xi) = P(X_i + X_{i'} = r|\xi) = \sum_{x=0}^{m_i} P(X_i = x|\xi)P(X_{i'} = r - x|\xi) \qquad [2.10]$$

Inserting [2.9] yields

$$P(R_{(i,i')} = r|\xi) = \frac{\xi^r \sum_{x=0}^{m_i} \gamma_{ix}\gamma_{i',r-x}}{D} \qquad [2.11]$$

where $D = \left(\sum_{h=0}^{m_i} \xi^h \gamma_{ih}\right)\left(\sum_{h'=0}^{m_{i'}} \xi^{h'} \gamma_{i'h'}\right)$. Define

$$\omega_r = \sum_{x=0}^{m_i} \gamma_{ix}\gamma_{i',r-x} \qquad [2.12]$$

and rewrite [2.11] as

$$P(X_i + X_{i'} = r|\xi) = \frac{\xi^r \omega_r}{D} \qquad [2.13]$$

with

$$D = \sum_{r=0}^{m_i+m_{i'}} \xi^r \omega_r \qquad [2.14]$$

Thus, the distribution of the sum of two items of PRM is again the distribution of a polytomous Rasch item. Using this result recursively shows that the same can be said for scores over any subset of items from a Rasch model, including the total score $\sum_{i=1}^{k} X_i$

$$P(R = r|\theta) = \frac{\exp(r\theta + \varphi_r)}{\sum_{h=0}^{m.} \exp(h\theta + \varphi_h)} \qquad [2.15]$$

where $m_. = \sum_{i=1}^{k} m_i$. Adding items together therefore does not introduce the need for a new type of statistical distribution. The distribution of the single items of the PRM therefore covers everything and, where convenient, we can regard scores, subscores and restscores as polytomous Rasch items.

The score parameters of the model can, if necessary, be written as explicit functions of the parameters of the original items. Recall that $\gamma_{i0} = 1$ for all items. From this and the recursion formula [2.12], it follows that the score parameters for the sum of two polytomous items are, for instance, given by $\omega_0 = 1, \omega_1 = \gamma_{i1} + \gamma_{i'1}, \delta_2 = \gamma_{i2} + \gamma_{i1}\gamma_{i'1} + \gamma_{i'2}$. For dichotomous items, these are called γ polynomials, or symmetrical polynomials.

The recursive procedure is easily programmable requiring only a few lines of code. Historically, these calculations created problems due to the lack of precision of the computers of the 1960s and 1970s. Today, these procedures never create problems with the typical number of items in health-related scales.

2.3.2. *Conditional distribution of item responses given the total score*

The result about the conditional distribution of X_i given $X_i + X_{i'}$ extends to the joint conditional distribution of all items and to the conditional distribution of a single item given the total score on all items. This can be rewritten in terms of exponential score parameters

$$P(\mathbf{X} = \mathbf{x}|R = r) = \frac{\exp(\sum_{i=1}^{k} \psi_{ix_i})}{\exp(\varphi_r)}$$

and

$$P(X_i = x|R = r) = \frac{\exp(\psi_{ix} + \varphi_{r-x}(R^{(i)}))}{\exp(\varphi_r)}$$

where φ_s are the exponential score parameters of the distribution of the score on all items and $\varphi_r(R^{(i)})$ are the exponential score parameters of the rest score without X_i. Note that similar results apply to any item subset V by replacing R with R_V. Conditional score distributions play a central role during conditional inference and this is discussed in Chapter 3. The role of the score distribution in the estimation of person parameters is discussed in Chapter 4.

2.4. Bibliography

[AGR 84] AGRESTI A., *Analysis of Ordinal Categorical Variables*, Wiley, New York, NY, 1984.

[AND 77] ANDERSEN E.B., "Sufficient statistics and latent trait models", *Psychometrika*, vol. 42, pp. 69–81, 1977.

[AND 78] ANDRICH D., "A rating formulation for ordered response categories", *Psychometrika*, vol. 43, pp. 561–573, 1978.

[AND 10] ANDRICH D., SHERIDAN B., LUO G., RUMM2030 Computer software and manual, RUMM Laboratory, Perth, Australia, 2010.

[BOI 10] BOINI S., ERPELDING M.L., FAGOT-CAMPAGNA A., MESBAH M., CHWALOW J., PENFORNIS A., COLICHE V., MOLLET E., MEADOWS K., BRIANÇON S., "Factors associated with psychological and behavioral functioning in people with type 2 diabetes living in France". *Health and Quality of Life Outcomes (HQLO)*, vol. 8, p. 124, 2010, available at http://www.hqlo.com/content/8/1/124.

[CHW 07] CHWALOW J., MEADOWS K., MESBAH M., COLICHE V., MOLLET E., "Empirical validation of a quality of life instrument: empirical internal validation and analysis of a quality of life instrument in French diabetic patients during an educational intervention", in HUBER C., LIMNIOS N., MESBAH M., NIKULIN N. (eds), *Mathematical Methods in Survival Analysis, Reliability and Quality of Life*, Hermes, London, 2007.

[LEU 76] LEUNBACH G., *A Probabilistic Measurement Model for Assessing Whether Instruments Measure the Same Personal Factor*, Danish Institute for Educational Research, Copenhagen, 1976.

[MAS 82] MASTERS G.N., "A Rasch model for partial credit scoring", *Psychometrika*, vol. 47, pp. 149–174, 1982.

[MCC 83] MCCULLAGH P., NELDER J., *Generalized Linear Models*, Chapman and Hall, London, 1983.

[MEA 96] MEADOWS K., STEEN N., MCCOLL E., ECCLES M., SHIELS C., HEWISON J., HUTCHINSON A., "The Diabetes Health Profile (DHP): a new instrument for assessing the psychosocial profile of insulin requiring patients – development and psychometric evaluation", *Quality of Life Research*, vol. 5, pp. 242–254, 1996.

[RAS 60] RASCH G., *Probabilistic Models for Some Intelligence and Attainment Tests*, Danish National Institute for Educational Research, Copenhagen, 1960.

[VON 95] VON DAVIER M., ROST J., "Polytomous mixed Rasch models", in FISCHER G.H., MOLENAAR I.W. (eds), *Rasch Models, Foundations, Recent Developments, and Applications*, Springer, New York, pp. 371–382, 1995.

PART 2

Inference in the Rasch Model

Introduction

There are many ways to analyze data from the Rasch models and it is easy to become confused while trying to compare and evaluate the different methods. The best way to explain why methods are so different is to say that the different methods analyze the data from and within very different frames of inference. Therefore, and because the sufficiency of the Rasch model makes it unique among IRT models by permitting a range of inference frames that do not exist for the other models, we introduce Part 2 with a short discussion of the available frames of inference for item analysis by Rasch models.

Persons and items are completely symmetrical in the Rasch model, so there is no major difference between inference on item parameters and inference on person parameters using the simple model [1.1]. In applications, they are not exchangeable. Typically, item parameter estimation is done first, followed by model checks based on these estimates. In the final step, the person parameters, which are the main reason for collecting the data, are estimated and regarded as "measurements" of properties of the person.

Other reasons to distinguish between item and person parameter estimation are that the estimation procedures and the quality of the estimates are very different. In the proper inference frames, item parameter estimates are consistent in the sense that bias and unsystematic error disappear as the number of persons increases. In order for person parameter estimates to be consistent, we would require that the number of items approaches infinity. Because the number of items in health-related scales usually is quite low, it follows that person parameter estimates are likely to be imprecise with uncomfortably large standard errors and – depending to some extent on the choice of technique – non-ignorable bias.

Several estimates of the parameters have been suggested. The best of them are based on maximum likelihood paradigms, but they differ because they assess the likelihood within different frames of inference. As such frames are important when we want to understand the different approaches of Rasch analyses found in the literature, the following section gives a brief introduction on this notion.

Inference frames

Assume that we have a statistical model that depends on a set of unknown parameters. We refer to a statistical model that has been derived from the original model by a set of mathematical arguments as a frame of inference. A frame of inference is supposed to depend on a subset of parameters of the original model so that inference on the subset of parameters can be performed within the derived model. It was one of the fundamental insights used by Georg Rasch [RAS 60] that it is possible to derive three different conditional frames of inference by conditioning with the sufficient person and item scores of the model. Let $X = (X_{vi})$, $R = (R_v)$ and $C = (C_{ih})$ denote the item responses, person scores and item category counts, respectively. The three frames of inference are defined by the conditional distribution of X, given one or two sets of sufficient margins.

Rasch suggested that $P(X|R)$ is the frame of inference in which item parameters should be estimated, $P(X|C)$ is the frame of inference in which person parameters should be estimated and $P(X|R, C)$ is the frame of inference in which the model should be fitted. These suggestions have only been followed to a certain degree due to technical problems related to the conditional distributions. The problems with analysis in the $P(X|R)$ inference frame were resolved in the early 1970s and it is now regarded as one of the standard frames of inference in Rasch models, being used for estimation of item parameters as described in Chapter 3 and for the analysis of model fit. The estimation of person parameters in the $P(X|C)$ inference frame has never been seriously attempted even though the technical problems are no hindrance with today's computers. Instead, person parameters are usually estimated under the assumption that item parameters are estimated with very small standard errors so that they can be used as essentially known item parameters during the estimation of person parameters.

The attractive property of the $P(X|R, C)$ inference frame is that the probabilities in this inference frame do not depend on any unknown parameters. The inference frame defined by $P(X|R, C)$ is a uniform distribution of all tables of item responses fitting the observed person and item margins. The number of item response tables fitting given margins is astronomical and undeterminable, making analysis in this inference frame impractical. Markov chain Monte Carlo techniques have been developed for the dichotomous Rasch model [BES 89, PON 01, CHE 05, CHR 10] but are rarely used.

In addition to the conditional frames of interference, two other inference frames are also commonly used. The joint inference frame $P(X)$ is simply the original

Rasch model itself where outcomes on the latent variables are treated as unknown parameters. The marginal inference frame $P_M(X) = \int P(X|\theta)dQ(\theta)$ makes the assumption that the latent variable follows a specific type of statistical distribution – typically a normal distribution – depending on a small set of population parameters. If we have confidence in the assumption concerning the distribution of the latent variable and if the data originated in a representative survey of subjects, then marginal inference is preferable to conditional inference. If this is not the case, then we prefer conditional to the marginal frames of inference. The joint framework is not recommended and model fitting within this framework is, therefore, not discussed in this book. Many of the notions of fit testing derived within the joint framework are, however, sound; it will be described how they can be altered to make them appropriate for conditional inference frames.

Bibliography

[BES 89] BESAG J., CLIFFORD P., "Generalized Monte Carlo significance tests", *Biometrika*, vol. 76, pp. 633–642, 1989.

[CHE 05] CHEN Y., SMALL D., "Exact tests for the Rasch model via sequential importance sampling", *Psychometrika*, vol. 70, pp. 11–30, 2005.

[CHR 10] CHRISTENSEN K.B., KREINER S., "Monte Carlo tests of the Rasch model based on scalability coefficients", *British Journal of Mathematical and Statistical Psychology*, vol. 63, pp. 101–111, 2010.

[PON 01] PONOCNY I., "Nonparametric goodness-of-fit tests for the Rasch model", *Psychometrika*, vol. 66, pp. 437–459, 2001.

[RAS 60] RASCH G., "On general laws and the meaning of measurement in psychology", *Berkeley Symposium on Mathematical Statistics and Theory of Probability*, vol. IV, 20/6–30/7, University of California Press, Berkeley, CA, pp. 321–333, 1960.

Chapter 3

Estimation of Item Parameters

3.1. Introduction

This chapter describes item parameter estimation in dichotomous and polytomous Rasch models. Three different ways of estimating item parameters are discussed: (1) conditional maximum likelihood (CML) estimation, (2) pairwise CML estimation and (3) marginal maximum likelihood (MML) estimation. Throughout this chapter, we will use the short notation $P(\cdot|\theta) = P(\cdot|\Theta_v = \theta)$, where convenient.

Recall that for dichotomous items the probability that an item response vector $\mathbf{X_v} = (X_{v1}, \ldots, X_{vk})$ is equal to $\mathbf{x_v} = (x_{v1}, \ldots, x_{vk})$ is given by

$$P(\mathbf{X_v} = \mathbf{x_v}|\theta) = \prod_{i=1}^{k} \frac{\exp\left(x_{vi}\left(\theta - \beta_i\right)\right)}{1 + \exp\left(\theta - \beta_i\right)} \qquad [3.1]$$

$$= \frac{\exp(r_v\theta - \sum_{i=1}^{k} x_{v,i}\beta_i)}{K(\theta, \beta)} \qquad [3.2]$$

where $\beta = (\beta_1, \ldots, \beta_k)$ is the vector of item parameters and

$$K(\theta, \beta) = \prod_{i=1}^{k} \left(1 + \exp\left(\theta - \beta_i\right)\right) \qquad [3.3]$$

is a normalizing constant. It can be seen from the above equation that for any integer a, using $\theta^* = \theta + a$ and $\beta_i^* = \beta_i + a$, for $i = 1, \ldots, k$, will yield the same probabilities, that is the model is overparameterized. Restrictions are needed to ensure that the model

---

Chapter written by Karl Bang CHRISTENSEN.

is identified and this can be done by placing a linear restriction either on the item parameters or on the person parameters.

The total sum score $R_v = \sum_{i=1}^{k} X_{vi}$ with realization $r_v = \sum_{i=1}^{k} x_{vi}$ is statistically sufficient for θ_v. The probabilities determining the distribution of the total sum score can be calculated by summation over all response vectors $\mathbf{x} = (x_1, \ldots, x_k)$ with $\sum_{i=1}^{k} x_{vi} = r$, yielding

$$P(R_v = r|\theta) = \sum_{\mathbf{x} \in X^{(r)}} P(\mathbf{X} = \mathbf{x}|\theta) = \frac{\exp(r\theta)\gamma_r}{K(\theta, \beta)} \tag{3.4}$$

where

$$\gamma_r = \gamma_r(\beta) = \sum_{\mathbf{x} \in X^{(r)}} \exp\left(\sum_{i=1}^{k} x_i \beta_i\right) \tag{3.5}$$

are symmetrical polynomials (also called γ polynomials) defined as sums of products of the parameters (see Chapter 1).

The polytomous Rasch model is a generalization where items $X_{v1}, \ldots, X_{vk}$ take values $x_{vi} = 0, 1, \ldots, m_i$. Note that this includes the dichotomous Rasch model as the special case m_i=1, for all i. The conditional probability given the value of the person parameter is

$$P(X_{vi} = x|\theta) = \exp(x\theta + \psi_{ix})/K_i(\psi_i, \theta) \tag{3.6}$$

for $x = 0, 1, \ldots, m_i$. Here, $\psi_{i0} = 0$, $\psi_i = (\psi_{i1}, \ldots, \psi_{im_i})$ is the vector of item parameters and

$$K_i(\psi_i, \theta) = \sum_{h=0}^{m_i} \exp(h\theta + \psi_{ih}) \tag{3.7}$$

is a normalizing constant. Where convenient, we will use the short notation $K_i = K_i(\psi_i, \theta)$. Note that this yields a monotonous relation between θ and the mean item score and that the model requires that the item parameters are the same for every person in the sample. The item parameters $\psi_i = (\psi_{i1}, \ldots, \psi_{im_i})$ can be interpreted through the locations of the thresholds between adjacent response categories

$$\beta_{ix} = -(\psi_{ix} - \psi_{ix-1}) \tag{3.8}$$

for $x = 1, \ldots, m_i$ (see Chapter 2). Without loss of generality, we will, where convenient in the remainder of this chapter, assume that $m_i = m$ for all i. The assumption

$$P(X_{v1} = x_1, \cdots, X_{vk} = x_k|\theta_v) = \prod_{i=1}^{k} P(X_{vi} = x_i|\theta_v) \tag{3.9}$$

of local independence yields the likelihood function

$$L(\psi_1, \ldots, \psi_k | \theta_v) = \frac{\exp(R_v \theta_v + \sum_{i=1}^{k} \psi_{ix_i})}{\prod_{i=1}^{k} K_i(\psi_i, \theta_v)} \qquad [3.10]$$

It is convenient to rewrite this as a function of indicator variables

$$(I_{vih})_{v=1,\ldots,n; i=1,\ldots,k; h=1,\ldots,m},$$

given by

$$I_{vih} = 1_{(X_{vi}=h)} \begin{cases} 1, & \text{if} \quad X_{vi} = h \\ 0, & \text{otherwise} \end{cases}$$

such that

$$L(\psi_1, \ldots, \psi_k | \theta_v) = \frac{\exp(r_v \theta_v + \sum_{i=1}^{k} \sum_{h=1}^{m} I_{vih} \psi_{ih})}{\prod_{i=1}^{k} K_i(\psi_i), \theta_v)} \qquad [3.11]$$

Again, restrictions are needed to ensure that the model is identified and this can be done by placing a linear restriction either on the item parameters or on the person parameters. Estimation of item parameters using the joint likelihood function

$$L_J(\psi_1, \ldots, \psi_k, \theta_1, \ldots, \theta_n) = \prod_{v=1}^{n} L(\psi_1, \ldots, \psi_k | \theta_v) \qquad [3.12]$$

leads to inconsistent item parameter estimates because the number of parameters increases with the number of persons [NEY 48]. Therefore, either a conditional or a marginal approach must be used when estimating item parameters.

3.2. Estimation of item parameters

The fundamental property of sufficiency can be used to overcome the problem of item parameter estimation. This can be done by conditioning on the sum R_v of the entire response vector $\mathbf{X_v} = (X_{v1}, \ldots, X_{vk})$ yielding CML inference or by conditioning on the sum of item pairs $\{(X_{vi}, X_{vi'}) | i \neq i'\}$ yielding pairwise conditional inference. Another way of estimating item parameters is to assume that the latent variables are sampled from a population and to introduce an assumption about the distribution of the latent variable. This approach yields MML inference.

3.2.1. *Estimation using the conditional likelihood function*

For a vector $\mathbf{X_v} = (X_{v1}, \ldots, X_{vk})$ from the Rasch model, the distribution of the score $R_v = \sum_{i=1}^{k} X_{vi}$ is given by the probabilities

$$P(R_v = r|\theta) = \sum_{\mathbf{x} \in X^{(r)}} P(\mathbf{X} = \mathbf{x}|\theta) \quad [3.13]$$

$$= \sum_{\mathbf{x} \in X^{(r)}} \frac{\exp(r\theta + \sum_{i=1}^{k} \psi_{ix_i})}{\prod_{i=1}^{k} K_i(\psi_i, \theta)} \quad [3.14]$$

where, as before, the summation is over the set $X^{(r)}$ of all response vectors $\mathbf{x} = (x_1, \ldots, x_k)$ with $\sum_{i=1}^{k} x_i = r$. The probability can be written as

$$P(R_v = r|\theta) = \frac{\exp(r\theta)}{\prod_{i=1}^{k} K_i(\psi_i, \theta)} \sum_{\mathbf{x} \in X^{(r)}} \exp(\sum_{i=1}^{k} \psi_{ix_i}) \quad [3.15]$$

Let the last sum be denoted by

$$\gamma_r = \gamma_r(\psi_1, \ldots, \psi_k) = \sum_{\mathbf{x} \in X^{(r)}} \exp\left(\sum_{i=1}^{k} \psi_{ix_i}\right) \quad [3.16]$$

The symmetrical function [3.16] generalizes the simple symmetrical (or γ) polynomials associated with the dichotomous Rasch model and has the following properties

$$\gamma_0 = 1$$

$$\gamma_1 = \exp(\psi_{11}) + \cdots + \exp(\psi_{k1})$$

$$\vdots$$

$$\gamma_{km.} = \exp(\psi_{1m_1} + \cdots + \psi_{km_k})$$

and because $x_{vi} = h$ implies that the sum of the other items is $r - h$, they are easily calculated using the recursive formula

$$\gamma_r(\psi_1, \ldots, \psi_k) = \sum_{x=1}^{m_i} \exp(\psi_{ix})\gamma_{r-x}^{(i)} + \gamma_r^{(i)} \quad [3.17]$$

where $\gamma_r^{(i)}$ denotes the function γ evaluated with item i omitted. Because the score is a sufficient statistic for θ, the item parameters can be estimated using the conditional distribution of the responses given the scores. The conditional distribution of the vector $\mathbf{X}_v = (X_{v1}, \ldots, X_{vk})$ of item responses given the score is given by the probabilities

$$P(\mathbf{X}_v = \mathbf{x}_v | R_v = r, \Theta_v = \theta_v) = \frac{\exp\left(\sum_{i=1}^{k} \psi_{ix_{vi}}\right)}{\gamma_r(\psi_1, \ldots, \psi_k)} \quad [3.18]$$

These do not depend on the value of θ_v and the *conditional likelihood function* is the product

$$L_C(\psi_1, \ldots, \psi_k) = \prod_{v=1}^{n} \frac{\exp(\sum_{i=1}^{k} \psi_{ix_{vi}})}{\gamma_{r_v}(\psi_1, \ldots, \psi_k)} \quad [3.19]$$

Again a linear restriction on the parameters is needed to ensure that the model is identified. Maximizing this likelihood yields item parameter estimates that are conditionally consistent. If, for each possible response vector $\mathbf{x} = (x_1, \ldots, x_k)$, we let $n(\mathbf{x})$ denote the number of persons with this response vector and for each possible score r and $n(r)$ denote the observed number of persons with this value of the score, this likelihood function can be written as

$$L_C(\psi_1, \ldots, \psi_k) = \frac{\prod_{\mathbf{x}} \exp(n(\mathbf{x}) \sum_{i=1}^{k} \psi_{ix_i})}{\prod_r \gamma_r(\psi_1, \ldots, \psi_k)^{n(r)}} \quad [3.20]$$

and, using the indicator functions $(I_{vih})_{v=1,\ldots,n;i=1,\ldots,k;h=1,\ldots,m}$ discussed earlier, this likelihood function can be rewritten as

$$L_C(\psi_1, \ldots, \psi_k) = \frac{\prod_{v=1}^{n} \exp(\sum_{i=1}^{k} \sum_{h=1}^{m} I_{vih}\psi_{ih})}{\prod_r \gamma_r(\psi_1, \ldots, \psi_k)^{n(r)}} \quad [3.21]$$

yielding the conditional log-likelihood function

$$l_C(\psi_1, \ldots, \psi_k) = \sum_{i=1}^{k} \sum_{h=1}^{m} I_{.ih}\psi_{ih} - \sum_{r=0}^{km} n(r) \log(\gamma_r(\psi_1, \ldots, \psi_k)) \quad [3.22]$$

where $I_{.ih} = \sum_{v=1}^{n} I_{vih}$ are the sufficient statistics for the item parameters. These sufficient statistics, called item margins, are the number of persons giving the response h to item i. The item parameters in this model can be estimated by solving the likelihood equations that equate the sufficient statistics $(I_{.ih})_{i=1,\ldots,k;h=1,\ldots,m}$ to their expected values conditional on the observed value $\mathbf{r} = (r_1, \ldots, r_n)$ of the vector $\mathbf{R} = (R_1, \ldots, R_n)$ of scores. These expected values have the form

$$E(I_{.ih}|\mathbf{R} = \mathbf{r}) = \sum_{v=1}^{n} P(X_{vi} = h|R_v = r_v) \quad [3.23]$$

and for an item i, these can be written in terms of the probabilities of having a score of $r - h$ on the remaining items yielding

$$E(I_{.ih}|\mathbf{R} = \mathbf{r}) = \exp(\psi_{ih}) \sum_{r=0}^{km} n(r) \frac{\gamma_{r-h}^{(i)}(\psi_1, \ldots, \psi_k)}{\gamma_r(\psi_1, \ldots, \psi_k)} \quad [3.24]$$

CML estimation was originally discussed by Andersen [AND 70]. Because these likelihood equations have the same form as those in a generalized linear model [KEL 84, TJU 82, AGR 93], the item parameters can be estimated using standard software like SPSS [TEN 93] or SAS [CHR 03, CHR 06]. Furthermore, these likelihood equations can be extended to models that impose a structure on the item parameters $(\psi_{ih})_{i=1,\ldots,k;h=1,\ldots,m}$ and therefore they can be used for estimation in a variety of models.

3.2.2. *Pairwise conditional estimation*

For a pair of dichotomous items (X_{v1}, X_{v2}), say, the distribution of the sum is given by

$$P(X_{v1} + X_{v2} = x|\Theta_v = \theta) = \frac{e^{x\theta}\gamma_x}{K_1 K_2}$$

and the conditional probabilities

$$\pi_{12} = P(X_{v1} = x_1, X_{v2} = x_2|X_{v1} + X_{v2} = x_1 + x_2, \theta) \qquad [3.25]$$

do not depend on θ. In fact

$$\pi_{12} = \frac{e^{-x_1\beta_1 - x_2\beta_2}}{\gamma_{x_1+x_2}}$$

and noting that for $X_{v1} + X_{v2} = 0$ the item pair (X_{v1}, X_{v2}) takes the value (0,0) with probability 1 and that for $X_{v1} + X_{v2} = 2$, the value is (1,1) with probability 1, we only have to consider the situation $X_{v1} + X_{v2} = 1$. Here, the conditional probabilities have the form

$$\pi_{12} = \begin{cases} \dfrac{e^{-\beta_1}}{e^{-\beta_1} + e^{-\beta_2}} & \text{for} \quad (x_1, x_2) = (1, 0) \\ \dfrac{e^{-\beta_2}}{e^{-\beta_1} + e^{-\beta_2}} & \text{for} \quad (x_1, x_2) = (0, 1) \end{cases}$$

So, for this item pair, the contribution to the conditional likelihood is

$$L(\beta_1, \beta_2) = \prod_{v=1}^{n} \frac{e^{-\beta_1 x_{v1} - \beta_2 x_{v2}}}{e^{-\beta_1} + e^{-\beta_2}} \qquad [3.26]$$

yielding the log-likelihood

$$l(\beta_1, \beta_2) = -\beta_1 x_{.1} - \beta_2 x_{.2} - \log(e^{-\beta_1} + e^{-\beta_2}) \qquad [3.27]$$

where $x_{.i} = \sum_{v=1}^{n} x_{vi}$ is a sufficient statistic for β_i, $i = 1, 2$. Combining the information from all item pairs

$$(X_{v1}, X_{v2}), \ldots, (X_{v,k-1}, X_{vk})$$

yields the *pairwise conditional log-likelihood function*

$$l(\beta_1, \ldots, \beta_k) = \sum_{i=1}^{k} \sum_{i'=i+1}^{k} \left(-\beta_i x_{.i} - \beta_{i'} x_{vi'} - n \log(e^{-\beta_i} + e^{-\beta_{i'}})\right) \quad [3.28]$$

Because the terms in this sum are not independent, this is a not a log-likelihood function, but a pseudo-log-likelihood function. Estimating the item parameters $(\beta_1, \ldots, \beta_k)$ by maximizing the pseudo-log-likelihood function yields consistent estimates [ZWI 95]. For the polytomous case $X_{vi} \in \{0, 1, \ldots, m_i\}$, the conditional probability is

$$\pi_{12} = \frac{e^{\psi_{1x_1} + \psi_{2x_2}}}{\gamma_{x_1+x_2}^{(1,2)}}$$

where

$$\gamma_r^{(1,2)} = \sum_{x=1}^{m_1} e^{\psi_{1x} + \psi_{2,r-x}} \quad [3.29]$$

This yields the log-likelihood

$$l(\psi_1, \psi_2) = \sum_{h_1=1}^{m_1} \psi_{1h_1} I_{.1h_1} + \sum_{h_2=1}^{m_2} \psi_{2h_2} I_{.2h_2} - \sum_{v=1}^{n} \log \gamma_{x_{v1}+x_{v2}}^{(1,2)} \quad [3.30]$$

where $(I_{.ih})_{i=1,2;h=1,\ldots,m_i}$ are sufficient statistics for $(\psi_{ih})_{i=1,2;h=1,\ldots,m_i}$, given by $I_{.ih} = \sum_{v=1}^{n} I_{vih}$ for $i = 1, 2$. Combining the information from all item pairs yields a pairwise conditional log-likelihood function with the form

$$l(\psi_1, \ldots, \psi_k) = \sum_{i=1}^{k} \sum_{i'=i+1}^{k} \left(A_i + A_{i'} - \log \Gamma_{x_1+x_2}^{(i,i')}\right)$$

where $A_i = \sum_{h=1}^{m_i} I_{.ih} \psi_{ih}$, for $i = 1, \ldots, k$, and

$$\Gamma_r^{(i,i')} = \sum_{x=1}^{m_i} \exp(\psi_{ix} + \psi_{i',r-x})$$

for $h + h' = 1, \ldots, m_i + m_{i'} - 1$. Computation of these coefficients is simpler than computing the full symmetric functions $\gamma_r(\psi_1, \ldots, \psi_k)$ and therefore maximizing the pairwise conditional likelihood function is simpler than maximizing the full conditional likelihood function.

Pseudo-likelihood was originally proposed by Besag [BES 74] for approximate inference in spatial processes, where the principal idea was to replace the joint density by a product of conditional densities that do not necessarily multiply to the joint distribution.

General results on the consistency and asymptotic normality of estimators obtained by maximizing pseudo-log-likelihood functions can be derived along the lines of classical proofs for maximum likelihood estimators [ARN 91] and their asymptotic covariance matrix can be approximated by a "sandwich estimator" $J^{-1}KJ^{-1}$, where

$$J = -\sum \frac{\partial^2 l(\psi)}{\partial\psi\partial\psi} \quad [3.31]$$

and

$$K = \sum_{\frac{\partial l(\psi)}{\partial\psi}} \frac{\partial l(\psi)}{\partial\psi} \quad [3.32]$$

Alternatively, an estimator of $E\left[-\frac{\partial^2 l(\partial\psi)}{\partial\psi\partial\psi}\right]$ that does not require the evaluation of second-order derivatives can be used. These estimators are likely to be less efficient than the maximum likelihood estimators because they rely on a restricted amount of information. It should be noted that items with the same margins may have different item parameter estimates.

Because the likelihood equations have the same form as those of the conditional log-likelihood function, the item parameters can be estimated using standard software like SAS, but this will not yield the correct standard errors of the item parameter estimates.

3.2.3. *Marginal likelihood function*

Let $\mathbf{X}_v = (X_{v1}, \ldots, X_{vk})$ denote the vectors of item responses for each person. Assuming the latent variable θ is normally distributed with mean μ and variance σ^2, the marginal probability $\pi(\mathbf{x}) = P(\mathbf{X}_v = \mathbf{x})$ of observing the response vector $\mathbf{x} = (x_1, \ldots, x_k)$ is

$$\pi(\mathbf{x}) = \int P(\mathbf{X}_v = x|\theta)\varphi\left(\frac{\theta-\eta}{\sigma}\right)d\theta \quad [3.33]$$

$$= \int \frac{\exp\left(r\theta + \sum_{i=1}^k \psi_{ix_i}\right)}{\prod_{i=1}^k K_i(\psi_i, \theta)}\varphi\left(\frac{\theta-\eta}{\sigma}\right)d\theta \quad [3.34]$$

where $r = \sum_{i=1}^k x_i$ and φ is the density of the standard normal distribution. This yields the *marginal likelihood function*

$$L_M(\psi_1, \ldots, \psi_k, \mu, \sigma) = \prod_{v=1}^n \int \frac{\exp\left(r_v\theta + \sum_{i=1}^k \psi_{ix_i}\right)}{\prod_{i=1}^k K_i(\psi_i, \theta)}\varphi\left(\frac{\theta-\mu}{\sigma}\right)d\theta \quad [3.35]$$

Restrictions are needed to ensure that the model is identified. If item parameters are restricted, the mean and variance can be estimated, and if the mean is set to zero, the variance and all item parameters can be estimated.

If, for each possible response vector $\mathbf{x} = (x_1, \ldots, x_k)$, we let $n(\mathbf{x})$ denote the number of persons with this response vector, the likelihood function can be written as

$$L_M(\psi_1, \ldots, \psi_k, \mu, \sigma) = \prod_{\mathbf{x}} \pi(\mathbf{x})^{n(\mathbf{x})} \qquad [3.36]$$

and the maximum likelihood estimation can be done using the parametric multinomial distribution, where the parametric representation of cell probabilities meets certain requirements [CRA 46, RAO 73].

Maximizing this log-likelihood by, for example, the Newton–Raphson method will thus yield maximum likelihood estimates that are asymptotically normally distributed and computation of the Fisher information will yield asymptotic standard errors.

Implementation in standard software for nonlinear random effects regression modeling is available by using PROC NLMIXED in SAS [CHR 06]. If the latent distribution is correctly specified, the maximum likelihood estimates of item parameters are consistent [ZWI 90] and likely to be superior to the CML estimates discussed below. If the distribution is not normal, the MML estimates are not consistent.

This likelihood can be calculated using numerical integration. Other assumptions about the distribution of the latent variable can be made, and any choice can, in principle, be implemented when choosing quadrature points and weights in the numerical integration. Much research interest has focused on the possibility of doing marginal inference without having to make distributional assumptions about the latent variable. This is discussed in the following section.

3.2.4. *Extended likelihood function*

Let Q denote the distribution of the latent variable in the population. The probabilities of the marginal score distribution are given by

$$\kappa_r = P(R_v = r) = \int P(R_v = r | \theta_v = \theta) dQ(\theta) \qquad [3.37]$$

and using Bayes' rule, the marginal probabilities in the distribution of the vector $\mathbf{X}_v = (X_{v1}, \ldots, X_{vk})$ of item responses can be written as

$$P(\mathbf{X}_v = \mathbf{x}) = P(\mathbf{X}_v = \mathbf{x}_v | R_v = r)\kappa_r \qquad [3.38]$$

or using indicators I_{vih}:

$$P(\mathbf{X}_v = \mathbf{x}_v) = \exp\left(\sum_{i=1}^{k} \psi_{ix_{vi}}\right)\frac{\kappa_r}{\gamma_r} = \exp\left(\sum_{i=1}^{k}\sum_{h=1}^{m} I_{vih}\psi_{ih}\right)\frac{\kappa_r}{\gamma_r} \quad [3.39]$$

The *extended likelihood function* is given by

$$L_E(\psi_1, \ldots, \psi_k, \kappa) = \prod_{v=1}^{n} P(\mathbf{X}_v = \mathbf{x}_v) \quad [3.40]$$

$$= \exp\left(\sum_{i=1}^{k}\sum_{h=1}^{m_i} I_{.ih}\psi_{ih}\right)\prod_{r}\left(\frac{\kappa_r}{\gamma_r}\right)^{n(r)} \quad [3.41]$$

where the last product is over the set of possible scores and $n(r)$ are the observed number of persons with each value of the score. This likelihood includes random person effects by using the probabilities as unrestricted parameters [TJU 82, AGR 93] and is identified if the item parameters are restricted and

$$\sum \kappa_r = 1$$

The maximum likelihood estimates in this model are the relative frequencies $\hat{\kappa}_r = n_r/n$ and the CML-estimates of the item parameters. If a score value is not observed, the estimate is 0, and even though this value might be considered reasonable it is not located in the interior of the parameter space, and standard asymptotic theory may not apply.

3.2.5. *Reduced rank parameterization*

The methods discussed in the previous section also apply in situations where further restrictions are put on the item parameters. This may be parameterized explicitly in terms of only the first two moments, for example

$$\tilde{\psi}_{ix} = -x\delta_i + x(m_i - x)\lambda_i \quad [3.42]$$

where the first parameter $\delta_i = \sum_{h=0}^{m_i} \psi_{ih}/m_i$ is the mean of the thresholds and the second parameter is the average half distance between successive thresholds of item i. This reparameterization imposes the constraint that the distance between successive thresholds is equal. When $m_i > 3$, this parameterization is effectively of reduced rank relative to the maximum rank m_i. Reduced rank parameterization using the first three moments or reduced rank parameterization using the first four moments is also feasible. These approaches are implemented in RUMM [AND 10] and are described in more detail by Andrich and Luo [AND 03].

3.2.6. *Parameter estimation in more general Rasch models*

Rasch models have been extended in two ways: (1) to include relations between items and covariates [KEL 84] yielding log-linear Rasch models and (2) to include relations between the latent variable and covariates [AND 77b, ZWI 91, ADA 97] yielding latent regression models. A log-linear Rasch model is an extension of the Rasch model, which includes uniform differential item functioning and uniform local dependence between items. The term "uniform" indicates that for all values of θ, the same relation between item parameters or between item parameters and covariates is included. In principle, the procedures for CML can be used to estimate the item parameters in these models, but because these are models for high-dimensional contingency tables with structural zeros, the estimation can be complicated [KEL 92]. The computer program DIGRAM [KRE 03] implements a simple iterative proportional fitting algorithm that estimates the parameters of log-linear Rasch models.

3.3. Example

We illustrate the methods using data from a study validating a French translation of the Diabetes Health Profile [CHW 07]. Again the five polytomous items of the disinhibited eating subscale are considered. Estimates of the 15 parameters $(\beta_{ih})_{i=1,\dots,5,h=1,2,3}$ are shown in Table 3.1 for each of the three estimation methods discussed.

	Item	β_1	β_2	β_3
CML	dhp32	−0.59	0.79	0.86
	dhp34	0.11	−0.56	−0.69
	dhp36	−0.21	−0.84	0.79
	dhp38	−0.50	1.86	−0.10
	dhp39	−1.89	1.29	−0.33
Pair-wise	dhp32	−0.65	0.85	0.90
	dhp34	−0.15	−0.84	−0.64
	dhp36	−0.23	−0.88	0.93
	dhp38	−0.58	2.05	0.18
	dhp39	−2.02	1.31	−0.24
MML	dhp32	−0.18	1.45	1.62
	dhp34	0.45	−0.32	−0.08
	dhp36	0.18	−0.38	1.53
	dhp38	−0.07	2.55	0.65
	dhp39	−1.54	1.90	0.36

Table 3.1. *Item parameter estimates for five items in the disinhibited eating (DE) subscale of the Diabetes Health Profile (DHP)*

We note that the CML estimates and the estimates from pairwise CML estimation are quite similar. At first glance, the MML estimates appear to be quite different from the CML and pairwise estimates. However, this arises largely from the fact that for the CML and the pairwise conditional we have required that

$$\sum_{i=1}^{5}\sum_{h=1}^{3}\beta_{ih}=0$$

in order to ensure that the model is identified. For the MML, we have required $\theta \sim N(0,\sigma^2)$ to ensure that the model is identified. It is easily seen that for the MML estimates $\sum_{i=1}^{5}\sum_{h=1}^{3}\beta_{ih})=0.54$, and that subtracting 0.54 from all of the βs yields estimates that are much closer to the other estimates. Note that this corresponds to $\theta \sim N(\mu,\sigma^2)$, where $\hat{\mu}=0.54$.

3.4. Bibliography

[ADA 97] ADAMS R.J., WILSON M.R., WANG W.C., "The multidimensional random coefficients multinomial logit model", *Applied Psychological Measurement*, vol. 21, pp. 1–24, 1997.

[AGR 93] AGRESTI A., "Computing conditional maximum likelihood estimates for generalized Rasch models using simple loglinear models with diagonals parameters", *Scandinavian Journal of Statistics*, vol. 20, pp. 63–71, 1993.

[AND 70] ANDERSEN E.B., "Asymptotic properties of conditional maximum likelihood estimators", *Journal of the Royal Statistical Society B*, vol. 32, pp. 283–301, 1970.

[AND 77a] ANDERSEN E.B., "Sufficient statistics and latent trait models", *Psychometrika*, vol. 42, pp. 69–81, 1977.

[AND 77b] ANDERSEN E.B., MADSEN M., "Estimating the parameters of the latent population distribution", *Psychometrika*, vol. 42, pp. 357–374, 1977.

[AND 03] ANDRICH D., LUO G., "Conditional pairwise estimation in the Rasch model for ordered response categories using principal components", *Journal of Applied Measurement*, vol. 4, pp. 205–221, 2003.

[AND 10] ANDRICH D., SHERIDAN B., LUO G., RUMM2030, Computer software and manual, RUMM Laboratory, Perth, Australia, 2010.

[ARN 91] ARNOLD B.C., STRAUSS D., "Pseudolikelihood estimation: some examples", *Sankhya B*, vol. 53, pp. 233–243, 1991.

[BES 74] BESAG J., "Spatial interaction and the statistical analysis of lattice systems", *Journal of the Royal Statistical Society. Series B*, vol. 36, pp. 192–236, 1974.

[CHR 03] CHRISTENSEN K.B., BJORNER J.B., SAS macros for Rasch based latent variable modelling, Research Report 13, Department of Biostatistics, University of Copenhagen, 2003.

[CHR 06] CHRISTENSEN K.B., "Fitting Polytomous Rasch Models in SAS", *Journal of Applied Measurement*, vol. 7, pp. 407–417, 2006.

[CHW 07] CHWALOW J., MEADOWS K., MESBAH M., COLICHE V., MOLLET E., "Empirical validation of a quality of life instrument: empirical internal validation and analysis of a quality of life instrument in French diabetic patients during an educational intervention", in HUBER C., LIMNIOS N., MESBAH M., NIKULIN N. (eds), *Mathematical Methods in Survival Analysis, Reliability and Quality of Life*, Hermes, London, 2007.

[CRA 46] CRAMÉR H., *Mathematical Methods of Statistics*, Princeton University Press, 1946.

[KEL 84] KELDERMAN H., "Loglinear Rasch model tests", *Psychometrika*, vol. 49, pp. 223–245, 1984.

[KEL 92] KELDERMAN H., "Computing maximum likelihood estimates of loglinear models from marginal sums with special attention to loglinear item response theory", *Psychometrika*, vol. 57, pp. 437–450, 1992.

[KRE 03] KREINER S., Introduction to DIGRAM, Research report 03/10, Copenhagen: Department of Biostatistics, University of Copenhagen, 2003.

[NEY 48] NEYMAN J., SCOTT E.L., "Consistent estimates based on partially consistent observations", *Econometrika*, vol. 16, pp. 1–32, 1948.

[RAO 73] RAO C.R., *Linear Statistical Inference and its Applications*, 2nd ed., John Wiley & Sons, New York, NY, 1973.

[TEN 93] TENVERGERT E., GILLESPIE M., KINGMA J., "Testing the assumptions and interpreting the results of the Rasch model using log-linear procedures in SPSS", *Behaviour Research Methods, Instruments, and Computers*, vol. 25, pp. 350–359, 1993.

[TJU 82] TJUR T., "A Connection between Rasch's item analysis model and a multiplicative Poisson model", *Scandinavian Journal of Statistics*, vol. 9, pp. 23–30, 1982.

[ZWI 90] ZWINDERMAN A.H., VAN DEN WOLLENBERG A.L., "Robustness of marginal maximum likelihood estimation in the Rasch model", *Applied Psychological Measurement*, vol. 14, pp. 73–81, 1990.

[ZWI 91] ZWINDERMAN A.H., "A generalized Rasch model for manifest predictors", *Psychometrika*, vol. 56, pp. 589–600, 1991.

[ZWI 95] ZWINDERMAN A.H., "Pairwise parameter estimation in Rasch models", *Applied Psychological Measurement*, vol. 19, pp. 369–375, 1995.

Chapter 4

Person Parameter Estimation and Measurement in Rasch Models

4.1. Introduction and notation

During analysis by Rasch models, estimates of person parameters are regarded as *measures* of unobservable latent traits and the bias and standard errors of the estimates are regarded as measurement bias and standard error of measurement (SEM). This chapter describes person parameter estimation in dichotomous and polytomous Rasch models, illustrates the methods using data from the disinhibited eating (DE) subscale of the Diabetes Health Profile (DHP) questionnaire [MEA 96] and finally discusses how to assess the quality of measurement provided by Rasch model items from a population point of view.

Parameter estimation in statistics is well described [LEH 83], especially in situations with independent and identically distributed data. Person parameter estimation in the Rasch model and other IRT models is a very different thing for several reasons: (1) there is one parameter θ_v for each person v, and this means that usual asymptotic theory does not apply, (2) the number of items is fixed and, in many applications, not very large and (3) for a given person, the observed item responses are independent only by the local independence assumption and are not identically distributed. This chapter uses the short notation $Pr(\cdot|\theta)$, omitting the subscript v.

Chapter written by Svend KREINER and Karl Bang CHRISTENSEN.

For dichotomous items, the probability that the vector $\mathbf{X} = (X_1, \ldots, X_k)$ of item responses takes the value $\mathbf{x} = (x_1, \ldots, x_k)$ is

$$P(\mathbf{X} = \mathbf{x}) = \exp(r\theta) \exp\left(-\sum_{i=1}^{k} x_i \beta_i\right) K(\theta, \beta)^{-1} \qquad [4.1]$$

where $r = \sum_{i=1}^{k} x_i$ is the score, $\beta = (\beta_1, \ldots, \beta_k)$ is the vector of item parameters and

$$K(\theta, \beta) = \prod_{i=1}^{k} (1 + \exp(\theta - \beta_i)) \qquad [4.2]$$

The score $R = \sum_{i=1}^{k} X_i$ with realization $r = \sum_{i=1}^{k} x_i$ is sufficient for θ and the probabilities determining its distribution can be computed by summation over all vectors $\mathbf{x} = (x_1, \ldots, x_k)$ with $\sum_{i=1}^{k} x_i = r$, yielding

$$P(R = r|\theta) = \exp(r\theta)\gamma_r(\beta) K(\theta, \beta)^{-1} \qquad [4.3]$$

where $\gamma_r(\beta)$ are the symmetrical polynomials defined as sums of products of the parameters (see Chapter 1).

The polytomous Rasch model, where $x = 0, 1, \ldots, m_i$, can be written as

$$P(X_i = x|\theta) = \exp(x\theta + \psi_{ix}) K_i(\theta, \psi_{\mathbf{i}})^{-1} \qquad [4.4]$$

where $\psi_{i0} = 0$, $\psi_{\mathbf{i}} = (\psi_{i1}, \ldots, \psi_{im_i})$ is the vector of item parameters for item i and $K_i(\psi_{\mathbf{i}}, \theta) = \sum_{h=0}^{m_i} \exp(h\theta + \psi_{ih})$ (see Chapter 2). The assumption

$$P(\mathbf{X} = \mathbf{x}|\theta) = \prod_{i=1}^{k} P(X_i = x_i|\theta) \qquad [4.5]$$

of local independence yields

$$P(\mathbf{X} = \mathbf{x}|\theta) = \exp\left(r\theta + \sum_{i=1}^{k} \psi_{ix_i}\right) \prod_{i=1}^{k} K_i(\theta, \psi_{\mathbf{i}})^{-1}$$

and the distribution of the score R, defined for $r = 0, 1, \ldots, m_.$, with $m_. = \sum_{i=1}^{k} m_i$, is given by

$$P(R = r|\theta) = \exp(r\theta)\gamma_r(\psi_{\mathbf{1}}, \ldots, \psi_{\mathbf{k}}) K(\theta)^{-1} \qquad [4.6]$$

where

$$K(\theta) = \prod_{i=1}^{k} K_i(\theta, \psi_{\mathbf{i}}) = \sum_{r=0}^{m_.} \exp(r\theta)\gamma_r(\psi_{\mathbf{1}}, \ldots, \psi_{\mathbf{k}}) \qquad [4.7]$$

is seen to have the same form as [4.3]. Because [4.3] and [4.6] are power series distributions [NOA 50, JOH 69], we can use standard results about exponential families for person parameter estimation.

4.2. Maximum likelihood estimation of person parameters

If the item parameters are known (or if consistently estimated values of the item parameters are inserted), standard theory tells us that the maximum likelihood estimate (MLE) of θ is the solution to the likelihood equation

$$s(\theta) = D_\theta \log P(R = r|\theta) = 0 \tag{4.8}$$

where R is the sufficient score. This equation has the form

$$r = E(R|\theta) \tag{4.9}$$

and the MLE is known to exist and to be unique. The Fisher information is

$$\begin{aligned} I(\theta) &= -E(D_\theta^2 \log P(R = r|\theta)) \\ &= V(D_\theta \log P(R = r|\theta)) \end{aligned} \tag{4.10}$$

and from standard asymptotic theory, the MLE of the person parameter is asymptotically normal with standard error (s.e.)

$$\text{s.e. } (\theta) = \frac{1}{\sqrt{I(\theta)}}. \tag{4.11}$$

This asymptotic result, however, requires that the number of items increases toward infinity in such a way that the probability of extreme scores goes toward zero. These assumptions are meaningless in situations with few items and MLE's are known to be biased unless the number of items is large. Furthermore, the MLE is not finite in situations where $r = 0$ or $r = m_.$. The values $-\infty$ and ∞ make sense intuitively, but are not always useful.

The distribution of the MLE of θ does not, however, require asymptotic results. To see this, let $\hat{\theta}_r$ be the person parameter estimate corresponding to a total score r on all items. It follows from the one-to-one relationship between r and $\hat{\theta}_r$ that the conditional probability of the person parameter estimate given $\hat{\theta}$ is equal to the conditional probability of r, $P(\hat{\theta}_r|\theta) = P(r|\theta)$, which is given by formula [4.6].

Given this result, it would be possible to calculate the exact values of bias and standard error of measurement (SEM) except for the fact that the MLE is not finite in situations where $r = 0$ or $r = m_. = \sum_{i=1}^{k} m_i$. These values make sense intuitively, but are not always useful because the means and the differences of the estimates are not defined. To overcome the problem of infinite estimates for extreme scores, we have to assign finite values of $\hat{\theta}_0$ and $\hat{\theta}_{m_.}$.

A simple way to do this is by setting $\hat{\theta}_0$ equal to a value corresponding to an expected score a little above zero and $\hat{\theta}_{m.}$ equal to a value with an expected score a little below $m_.$

$$\epsilon = E(R|\Theta = \hat{\theta}_0) \quad [4.12]$$

$$m_. - \epsilon = E(R|\Theta = \hat{\theta}_{m.}) \quad [4.13]$$

Defined in this way, the MLE can be regarded as a Bayes modal estimator corresponding to a uniform prior across the interval $[\hat{\theta}_0, \hat{\theta}_{m.}]$ and given such estimates exact values of bias, SEM and root mean square error (RMSE) for different values of θ can easily be calculated

$$\text{Bias}(\theta) = E(\hat{\theta}|\theta) - \theta = \sum_{r=0}^{m.} \hat{\theta}_r P(r|\theta) - \theta \quad [4.14]$$

$$\text{SEM}(\theta) = \sqrt{\sum_{r=0}^{m.} (\hat{\theta}_r - E(\hat{\theta}|\theta))^2 P(r|\theta)} \quad [4.15]$$

$$\text{RMSE}(\theta) = \sqrt{\sum_{r=0}^{m.} (\hat{\theta}_r - \theta)^2 P(r|\theta)}. \quad [4.16]$$

4.3. Item and test information functions

The Fisher information is a measure of how precisely θ is estimated because it is the variance of the score function

$$s(\theta) = D_\theta \log P(R = r|\theta)$$

used in the likelihood equation. Since the seminal work of Alan Birnbaum [BIR 68], who introduced Fisher information in IRT, the notion of item and test information has been central. The general definition of the item information function for a dichotomous item i given by Birnbaum is

$$I_i(\theta) = -E{D_\theta}^2 \log P(X_i = x_i|\theta)$$
$$= \frac{D_\theta P(X_i = 1|\theta)}{P(X_i = 1|\theta)P(X_i = 0|\theta)}$$

and the test information function is

$$I(\theta) = \sum_{i=1}^{k} I_i(\theta) \quad [4.17]$$

In the dichotomous Rasch model, the item information function reduces to

$$I_i(\theta) = P(X_i = 1|\theta)P(X_i = 0|\theta) = V(X_i|\theta) \quad [4.18]$$

The polytomous Rasch model is a power series distribution with score function

$$s(\theta) = x_i - E(X_i|\theta)$$

and the Fisher information is the variance of the score function, so the item information function becomes

$$I_i(\theta) = V(X_i|\theta)$$
$$= \sum_{x=0}^{m_i} x^2 \frac{\exp(x\theta + \psi ix)}{K_i(\psi_{\mathbf{i}}, \theta)} - \left(\sum_{x=0}^{m_i} x \frac{\exp(x\theta + \psi_{ix})}{K_i(\psi_{\mathbf{i}}, \theta)} \right)^2$$

Using the assumption of local independence, the test information function reduces to

$$I(\theta) = \sum_{i=1}^{k} I_i(\theta) = \sum_{i=1}^{k} V(X_i|\theta) = V(R|\theta) \quad [4.19]$$

which is valid for both the dichotomous and the polytomous Rasch models.

4.4. Weighted likelihood estimation of person parameters

The bias in the person parameter estimates can be avoided using *weighted maximum likehood estimation*, by maximizing

$$L(\theta) = P(R = r|\theta)\sqrt{I(\theta)} \quad [4.20]$$

The solution is called the weighted likelihood estimate, and using this estimate we can reduce the bias to a considerable degree [WAR 89]. Furthermore, this has the additional advantage that it provides finite estimates for extreme scores. This estimator can be viewed as a Bayes modal estimator, but it should be noted that no assumptions about the distribution of parameters are made because the prior $\sqrt{I(\theta)}$ only depends on the estimated item parameters. For more details, see [HOI 95] for information about person parameter estimation in the dichotomous Rasch model and see [WAN 01] and [PEN 05] for information about person parameter estimation in polytomous IRT models.

4.5. Example

We illustrate the MLE and the weighted maximum likelihood estimate (WMLE) using the data set from the DE subscale of the DIIP inventory. The data set and the items of the DE subscale are described in Chapter 2. The DE subscale is the sum of the item scores from five polytomous items with four response categories where zero represents no dysfunction. The estimation of item parameters has been discussed in Chapter 3. As described above, these estimates are considered as known parameters during the estimation of person parameters.

Table 4.1 provides information about the distribution of the score along with the score parameters of the score distribution [4.6], and the MLE and WMLE. To remind the reader that the score distribution [4.6] can be reparameterized as a partial credit distribution, we have included the partial credit thresholds next to the score parameters. Note that all thresholds are ordered even though some of the thresholds of the separate items were disordered.

r	$P(R=r)$	γ_r	τ_r	MLE	WMLE
0	0.058	1.00	−4.061		−3.512
1	0.069	15.70	−2.752	−2.493	−2.064
2	0.053	83.96	−1.672	−1.672	−1.437
3	0.116	276.58	−1.189	−1.203	−1.066
4	0.116	690.84	−0.912	−0.865	−0.787
5	0.095	1344.82	−0.663	−0.585	−0.545
6	0.090	2088.62	−0.437	−0.329	−0.316
7	0.138	2635.91	−0.229	−0.082	−0.084
8	0.116	2582.94	0.024	0.167	0.156
9	0.032	1921.42	0.299	0.420	0.404
10	0.048	1130.50	0.531	0.683	0.655
11	0.011	510.38	0.797	0.963	0.911
12	0.026	177.95	1.051	1.279	1.185
13	0.000	46.78	1.335	1.675	1.503
14	0.021	8.56	1.696	2.304	1.933
15	0.011	1.00	2.122		2.803

Table 4.1. *Marginal score distribution, score parameters (γ_r), partial credit thresholds (τ_r), and estimates of person locations for the disinhibited eating (DE) subscale of the Diabetes Health Profile (DHP)*

Note that although the MLE is not finite for $R = 0$ and $R = 15$, MLE estimates for extreme scores can be calculated by extrapolation, for example by choosing them in such a way that the expected scores are equal to 0.25 and 14.75. This or any other choice is, however, arbitrary.

The table shows that there are considerable differences between MLEs and WMLEs. Theoretically, WMLE should be less biased than MLE. In Figure 4.1, the exact bias of the two estimates is plotted against θ.

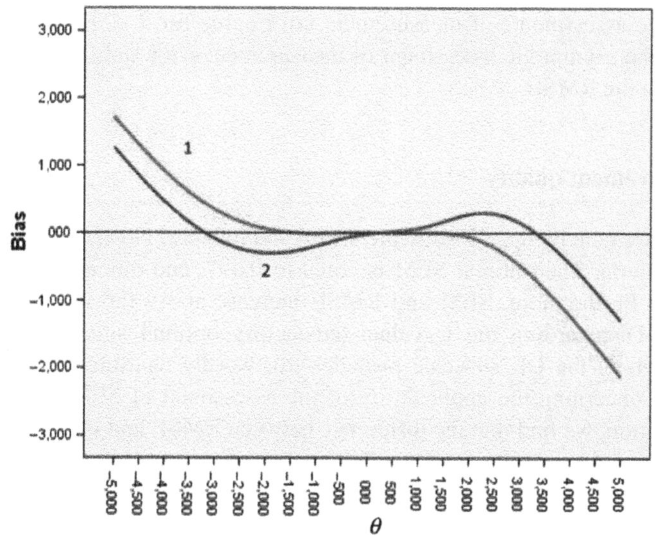

Figure 4.1. *Exact bias of WMLE (1) and MLE (2)*

The WMLE is virtually unbiased for $\theta \in [-2, 2]$ and less biased than MLE for $\theta \in [-2.5, 2.7]$. Beyond this range, the MLE is, however, less biased than WML. Figure 4.2 compares the asymptotic s.e. defined by the test information function to the exact s.e. and the RMSE defined by the exact distribution of the WMLE.

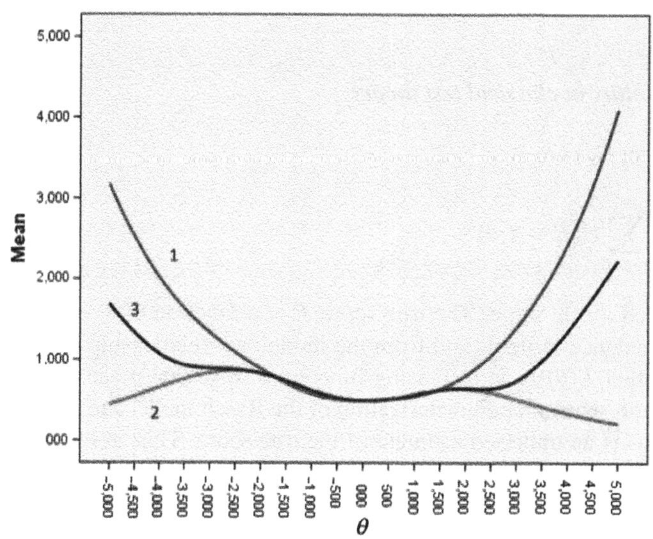

Figure 4.2. *Asymptotic s.e. (1), exact s.e. (2) and RMSE (3) of the WMLE*

The three assessments of measurement error agree for $\theta \in [-2.0, 1.6]$. Beyond this range, the asymptotic assessment of measurement error and (later) the exact s.e. departs from the RMSE.

4.6. Measurement quality

Is measurement by the DE subscale useful and reliable? Now, the answer depends on some criteria. The optimal SEM is equal to 0.497, and this is rarely considered satisfactory. Furthermore, SEM and RMSE increase above 0.6 for $\theta < -1.0$ and $\theta > 1.5$. Disregarding the less-than-satisfactory optimal situation, we see that the range where the DE subscale provides trustworthy measurements is relatively restricted. Concerning the applicability of the assessment of SEM as a function of test information, we find that the difference between RMSE and the asymptotic SEM is less than 0.5 for $\theta \in [-2.0, 1.6]$. The quality of measurement and the degree to which we can rely on the asymptotic results for the calculation of the SEM therefore depends on θ. Having seen that, the next issue to address is whether we can expect θ to lie within the range where person estimates are unbiased and precise with well-known standard errors. With such questions, the focus of interest changes from individual persons to populations and to the question whether the DE subscale is appropriate for the population in which it has been administered. Psychometrics has several ways to address this issue. One way to do it is by generalizing the indicators of measurement precision for individuals to the expected bias, test information, SEM and RMSE for the population as a whole. Another way is by using a set of techniques that originated in classical test theory (CTT) long before anybody had thought of item response theory and Rasch models.

4.6.1. *Reliability in classical test theory*

The expected score

$$T = \sum_{r=0}^{m.} P(R = r|\theta) \qquad [4.21]$$

is often called a *true* score. The true score T is a function of θ. It follows from the local independence of items and from the monotonic relationship between θ and the item scores that $T(\theta)$ is an increasing function of θ so that it can be argued that the true score represents a reparameterization of the Rasch model and that the total score over all items is an unbiased estimate of the true score. This, at least, is the point of view of CTT, where the true score is regarded as the natural person parameter and the possibility of alternative parameterizations is rarely acknowledged. CTT assumes that (1) $R = T + e$ and (2) the measurement error e is independent of T. Under this assumption, CTT defines the reliability of measurement in two different ways:

the first defines reliability as the ratio between the population variance of T and the population variance of R, whereas the second defines reliability as the correlation between repeated measurements, $R_1 = T+e_1$ and $R_2 = T+e_2$, under the assumption that the measurement errors e_1 and e_2 are independent and identically distributed. Thus, reliability is calculated as

$$\rho_1 = \frac{V(T)}{V(R)} \qquad [4.22]$$

$$\rho_2 = \text{corr}(R_1, R_2) \qquad [4.23]$$

Under the linear CTT model, it follows that $V(R) = V(T) + V(e)$ and $\rho_1 = \rho_2$. It follows from these definitions that CTT reliability is never a general statement of the quality of the measurement instrument, rather it is a statement of how the measurement instrument functions in a population where the variance of the true score is equal to $V(T)$. Reliability is high when the measurement error is small compared to the variation of the true scores and low if that is not the case.

Rasch was less enthusiastic when talking about reliability because he insisted that a statement concerning the properties of items and test scores should be independent of the study population providing data for the measurement instrument. We do not, however, share Rasch's reservations. We think that it is relevant and useful to study the way an instrument works in specific populations and both CTT definitions of reliability are, in our point of view, intuitive, attractive and meaningful. Our only reservation is with statements referring to reliability as general statements concerning the applicability of the instrument.

Apart from the lack of understanding that reliability depends on the study population, the only problem with CTT reliability lies in the fact that there is no easy way to estimate the population variance of the true scores because these scores are unknown parameters, and there is no way to collect repeated measurements in such a way that we can be sure that measurement errors are independent and identically distributed. However, there is a solution to this problem. If items are locally independent, it can be shown that CTT reliability is larger than a function of the average item score correlations called Cronbach's coefficient α [CRO 51]. Therefore, this coefficient is often used as a measure of reliability.

4.6.2. *Reliability in Rasch models*

The two definitions of reliability, [4.22] and [4.23], also make sense for Rasch models, but the two measures of reliability are not exactly the same and the errors depend on the true scores under the Rasch model because Rasch models are nonlinear models. This may sound complicated, but it is, in fact, the opposite. Given the Rasch model framework, it is possible not only to estimate both ρ_1 and ρ_2 so that Cronbach's coefficient α can be discarded, but also to come up with alternative measures of reliability that are intuitively more attractive than ρ_1 and ρ_2. To see how to do this, first consider first the problem of estimating ρ_1 under the Rasch model. Recall that the true score T is the expected score, $E(R|\theta)$ is a function of θ and θ is a random variable with density $f(\theta)$. If estimates of $f(\theta)$ are available, it follows that the population variance of the true score can be approximated by

$$\widehat{V(T)} = \int E(T|\theta)^2 \widehat{f(\theta)} d\theta - \left[\int E(T|\theta) \widehat{f(\theta)} d\theta \right]^2 \qquad [4.24]$$

The variance $V(R)$ of the score can be derived from the marginal score distribution

$$P(R = r) = \int P(R = r|\theta) f(\theta) d\theta \qquad [4.25]$$

from which $\rho_1 = V(T)/V(R)$. The test–retest correlation ρ_2 under conditional independence can be derived from the joint distribution

$$P(R_1 = r_1, R_2 = r_2) = \int P(R_1 = r_1|\theta) P(R_2 = r_2|\theta) f(\theta) d\theta \qquad [4.26]$$

There are, in principle, no restriction on the choice of the distribution of θ. In practice, it is usually assumed that the latent distribution is normal requiring estimates of the population mean and variance of θ.

EXAMPLE 4.1.– The population characteristics of the DE subscale of the DHP are as follows: $E(R) = 5.55$, $SD = 3.35$, $E(\theta) = -0.516$, $SD(\theta) = 0.855$, Cronbach's $\alpha = 0.69$, $\rho_1 = 0.71$ and $\rho_2 = 0.72$.

The Rasch model framework provides several common ways to modify CTT reliability. Within this framework, the estimates of the person parameters are regarded as the measures of the latent trait. Therefore, it may appear to be more common to define reliabilities [4.22] and [4.23] in terms of the person parameter estimates

$$\rho_3 = \frac{V(\theta)}{V(\hat{\theta})} \qquad [4.27]$$

$$\rho_4 = \text{corr}(\hat{\theta}_1, \hat{\theta}_2) \qquad [4.28]$$

Specifically, [4.28] is referred to as the person separation index (PSI) [AND 82]. In practice, there is seldom any large difference between [4.22] and [4.27] and between [4.23] and [4.28] because of the near-linear relationship between the person parameter estimates and R so that we can argue the distinction between the two sets of reliability coefficients has no practical importance.

Wright and Masters [WRI 82] refer to the ratio $G = SD(\theta)/SD(\hat{\theta})$ as the separation ratio and develop another measure

$$H = (4G + 1)/3$$

which they claim is a measure of discernable strata. Because G and H are simple monotonic functions of ρ_3 and because the interpretation of what these measures stand for is based on the CTT assumptions that the measurement error is normally distributed and independent of θ – assumptions that are false for the Rasch model – there is no reason to use G and/or H instead of ρ_3.

If it is required to extend the notion of reliability in Rasch models in ways that go beyond the way it is done in CTT, there are several ways to do it. This subsection presents two ways, carrying CTT reliability one step further without discarding the fundamental point of view, whereas the next subsection extends the notion of measurement error at the individual level to measurement error in populations as a whole.

One simple way to generalize reliability is by replacing the test–retest correlations [4.23] and [4.28] with the correlation that exists between the latent trait variable and the person parameter estimate

$$\rho_5 = \text{corr}(\theta, \hat{\theta}) \qquad [4.29]$$

This correlation will be stronger than the test–retest correlation and will present a more fair assessment of the quality of measurement. In the DE example discussed above, $\rho_5 = 0.84$.

The notion of person separation is important for clinical purposes where we would require that the rank of persons according to the estimates of the person parameters is the same as the rank order according to the true person parameters. Another way to formalize the notion of correct person separation is to calculate the probability that the scores (and therefore the person parameter estimates) rank two random persons in the same way as the true person parameters

$$\rho_6 = P(R_1 < R_2 | \theta_1 < \theta_2) = \int_{\theta_1 < \theta_2} P(R_1|\theta_1)P(R_2|\theta_2)f(\theta_1)f(\theta_2)d\theta_1 d\theta_2 \qquad [4.30]$$

we refer to ρ_6 as the correct person separation probability. The probability that the DE scale correctly separates two random persons from a population where $E(\theta) = -0.52$ and $SD(\theta) = 0.86$ in the correct way is $\rho_6 = 0.77$.

4.6.3. *Expected measurement precision*

Measurement precision in terms of bias, test information, SEM and RMSE is usually assessed at the person level. Because these statistics depend on θ, it is useful to assess these properties relative to a specific population by calculation of expected values of these statistics in the population

$$E(\text{Bias}) = \int |\text{Bias}(\theta)| f(\theta) d\theta$$

$$E(I) = \int I(\theta)f(\theta)d\theta$$

$$E(\text{SEM}) = \int \text{SEM}(\theta)f(\theta)d\theta$$

$$E(\text{RMSE}) = \int \text{RMSE}(\theta)f(\theta)d\theta$$

In addition to providing population information about the same kind of indicators that are used to evaluate measurement precision for individuals, these indicators have the additional advantage that they can be used to compare the performance of different person parameter estimates.

In the DE example, the maximum test information is equal to 4.05, but the expected average information for the whole population is $E(\text{info}) = 3.23$. Table 4.2 shows the expected bias, SEM and MSE of ML and WML estimates for the DE subscale of the DHP.

	E(Bias)	E(RMSE)	E(SEM)
ML	0.112	0.699	0.687
WML	0.011	0.592	0.591

Table 4.2. *Assessment of measurement precision for ML and WML estimates of person locations for the disinhibited eating (DE) subscale of the Diabetes Health Profile (DHP)*

The WML is supposed to reduce the bias of the person parameter estimate compared to the ML estimate, but it is known that bias of the WML estimate is larger than the bias of the ML estimate for extreme values of θ. Therefore, it does not automatically follow that the expected bias of the WML is smaller than the expected bias of the ML estimate. From Table 4.2, it is evident that in the population where the DE scale was administered, the WML estimator, as expected, performed better than the ML estimator. The expected bias of the WML estimate is close to zero and the RMSE of the WML estimate is smaller than the RMSE of the ML estimate.

4.6.4. *Targeting*

The issues addressed above, are called the issues of targeting. Targeting in Rasch models is usually addressed in an informal way by the so-called person–item location maps as shown in Figure 4.3, comparing the distribution of the person parameter estimates together with the distribution of the item thresholds.

Person–item location maps are useful to identify items with thresholds that are extreme compared to the persons of the study population. Such items are of interest because they provide very little item information in the population. Observing and including responses to such items will therefore have little impact on the precision of the person parameter estimates. These items are out of target.

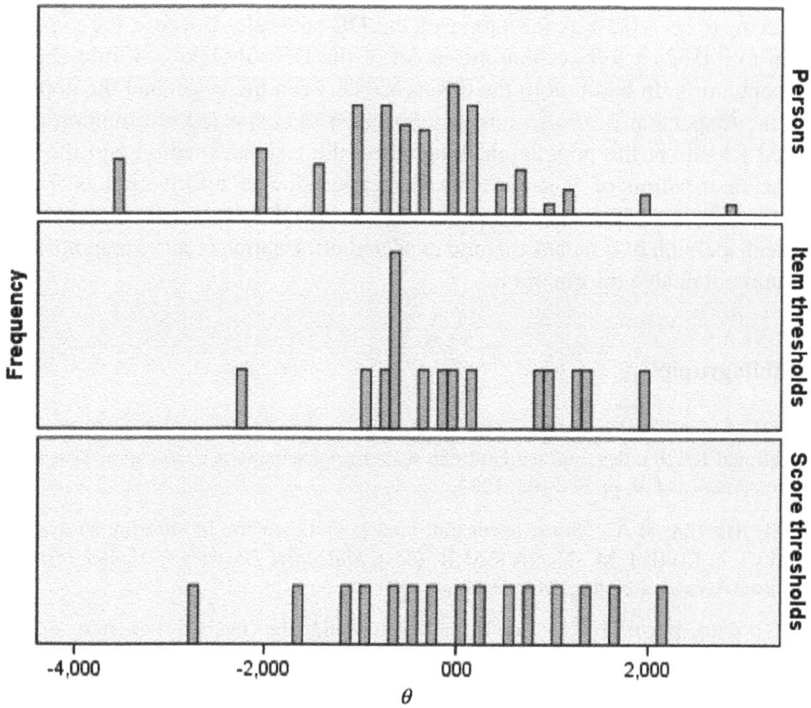

Figure 4.3. *Item map showing the distribution of person parameter estimates together with the distributions of the item thresholds and score thresholds over all items*

Figure 4.3 also shows the distribution of the thresholds of the partial credit distribution of the score R because it is the distribution of R that determines the properties of the person parameter estimates. In summary it is the presence of extreme score thresholds that signal the measurement instrument may be out of target.

In this example, the differences between the distributions of persons and items appear to be unimportant. The study population is well targeted by the DE subscale. In other studies, things are not so straightforward, making subjective assessment of item maps questionable. In such cases, it would be useful to have more formal numerical assessments of targeting. To develop such measures, we have to say precisely what we mean when we say that a population is targeted by a summated scale. We claim that a population is well targeted by a scale if the test information is high and the bias ignorable for the majority of the members of the population.

For the DE example, it is evident from Table 4.2 that the bias is ignorable if the person parameter estimate is a WML estimate. Examination of the test information function of the DE subscale shows that test information is maximized and RMSE is minimized at $\theta = -0.14$, where the test information is 4.04 and RMSE $= 0.50$. We refer to $\theta = -0.14$ as the target of the DE subscale. Because the expected θ is equal to -0.52, it follows that the target of the DE subscale is a little above the study population. In addition to the difference between the target and the population mean, the dispersion of θ also has an impact on the expected information and the expected RMSE in the population. Integrating the test information and the RMSE over the distribution of θ shows that the expected test information is 3.26 and $E(\text{RMSE}) = 0.59$. The distance between the target and the population mean together with the dispersion of θ means that the expected information is more than 80% of the maximum obtainable information.

4.7. Bibliography

[AND 82] ANDRICH D., "An index of person separation in latent trait theory, the traditional KR20 index, and the Guttman scale response pattern", *Education Research and Perspectives*, vol. 9, pp. 95–104, 1982.

[BIR 68] BIRNBAUM A., "Some latent trait models and their use in inferring an examinee's ability", in LORD F.M., NOVICK M.R. (eds), *Statistical Theories of Mental Test Scores*, Addison-Wesley, Reading, MA, 1968.

[CRO 51] CRONBACH L.J., "Coefficient alpha and the internal structure of tests", *Psychometrika*, vol. 16, pp. 297–334, 1951.

[HOI 95] HOIJTINK H., BOOMSMA A., "On person parameter estimation in the dichotomous rasch model", in FISCHER G.H., MOLENAAR I.W. (eds), *Rasch Models. Foundations, Recent Developments, and Applications*, Springer-Verlag, New York, NY, 1995.

[JOH 69] JOHNSON N.L., KOTZ S., *Discrete Distributions*, John Wiley & Sons, New York, NY, 1969.

[LEH 83] LEHMANN E.L., *Theory of Point Estimation*, John Wiley & Sons, New York, NY, 1983.

[MEA 96] MEADOWS K., STEEN N., MCCOLL E., ECCLES M., SHIELS C., HEWISON J., HUTCHINSON A., "The Diabetes Health Profile (DHP): a new instrument for assessing the psychosocial profile of insulin requiring patients – development and psychometric evaluation", *Quality of Life Research*, vol. 5, pp. 242–254, 1996.

[NOA 50] NOACK A., "A class of random variables with discrete distributions", *Annals of Mathematical Statistics*, vol. 21, pp. 127–132, 1950.

[PEN 05] PENFIELD R.D., BERGERON J.M., "Applying a weighted maximum likelihood latent trait estimator to the generalized partial credit model", *Applied Psychological Measurement*, vol. 29, pp. 218–233, 2005.

[WAN 01] WANG S., WANG T., "Precision of warm's weighted likelihood estimates for a polytomous model in computerized adaptive testing", *Applied Psychological Measurement*, vol. 25, pp. 317–331, 2001.

[WAR 89] WARM T., "Weighted likelihood estimation of ability in item response theory", *Psychometrika*, vol. 54, pp. 427–450, 1989.

[WRI 82] WRIGHT B.D., MASTERS G.N., *Rating Scale Analysis: Rasch Measurement*, MESA Press, Chicago, IL, 1982.

PART 3

Checking the Rasch Model

Introduction

This part of the book describes the methods that can be used to evaluate the fit of a data set to the Rasch model. A good fit is an important part of any statistical analysis, but in connection with the Rasch model it plays a special part. First, the Rasch model should be seen as a null hypothesis rather than as a statistical model. Second, the data–model relationship is very different from what is usually seen in a statistical analysis. Misfit often leads to the rejection of the data (because it does not live up to the requirements of the Rasch model), whereas in other applications it would lead to the rejection of the model.

Thus, any applications view the Rasch model as a prescriptive model in which we investigate *how the data fit the model* instead of the more classical statistical problem of *how the model fits the data* [BON 01].

The Rasch model applies in situations where the task is to find and discard flawed items, and can also be extended to models that incorporate deviations from the requirements of the original Rasch model.

Bibliography

[AND 04] ANDRICH D., "Controversy and the Rasch model: a characteristic of incompatible paradigms?", *Medical Care*, vol. 42, pp. 7–16, 2004.

[BON 01] BOND T.G., FOX C.M., *Applying the Rasch Model: Fundamental Measurement in the Human Sciences*, Lawrence Erlbaum Associates, Inc., Mahwah, NJ, 2001.

Chapter 5

Item Fit Statistics

5.1. Introduction

Items from Rasch models and items from other IRT models share a number of properties, and differ only with respect to the choice of functions describing how the probabilities of responses to items depend on the latent variable. The properties shared by all IRT models are unidimensionality, monotonicity, local independence and no differential item functioning. These properties are often motivated by subject matter theory about the latent variable that items are supposed to measure. The same can rarely be said about the choice of the specific probability function of the Rasch model and it is often argued that the parsimonious Rasch model is too simple to have a chance to fit real-life data. Therefore, it is important to provide strong empirical evidence supporting the claim that the Rasch model is adequate for data.

This chapter describes two types of item fit statistics that can be used for this purpose. The first type takes all the fundamental assumptions of the Rasch model as given and tries to assess the degree to which the separate items appear to have conditional response probabilities that do not depart from the Rasch model probabilities. The second type addresses the assumption of no differential item functioning, but does it one item at a time, assuming all the other items do not violate the Rasch model assumptions.

The methods described in this chapter always target separate items. It is therefore common that evidence against the data-model fit provided by these methods is often taken for evidence against specific items that do not fit the model, rather than against the fit of the model to data. The degree to which such a viewpoint

Chapter written by Karl Bang CHRISTENSEN and Svend KREINER.

is viable is controversial. We refer to Andrich [AND 04] for a discussion of these issues. What we want to stress here is that violations of the fundamental assumptions of unidimensionality, local independence and no DIF imply that the idea that the separate items should follow a Rasch model (or any other standard IRT model sharing these assumptions) looses its meaning. Before we dismiss an item because of its disagreement with the response probabilities of the model, we should always check the assumptions of unidimensionality, local response dependence and DIF among the other items. We will return to these issues at the end of the chapter.

Item response theory, in general, and Rasch models, in particular, contain a plethora of different item fit statistics. It is beyond the scope of this book to discuss these in detail, but we will discuss a number of item fit statistics that are useful and intuitive. The interested reader should refer to Glas and Verhelst [GLA 95a, GLA 95b] or Smith [SMI 04] for an overview.

There are a number of misunderstandings concerning how statistical methods work. For this reason, a number of concrete ideas for testing the fit of an item to the Rasch model have been implemented in ways that may produce erroneous results during the analysis. To make it easier to assess these issues, we discuss the Rasch model residuals, which compare observed responses with expected responses, and the way they should be used to test the fit of items to Rasch models.

5.2. Rasch model residuals

In statistics, residuals are defined as the difference between observed data and expected values under a specific model and/or hypothesis. The theory of Rasch models describes and uses two types of residuals: individual response residuals and group residuals. To clearly distinguish between the two types of residuals, we need first to introduce some notations.

5.2.1. *Notation*

Let X_{vi} denote the response of person v to item i and let $E_{vi} = E(X_{vi})$ denote its expectation. Under the Rasch model, E_{vi} is given by

$$E_{vi} = \sum_{x=0}^{m_i} x \frac{\exp(x\theta_v + \psi_{ix})}{K(\theta_v, \psi_{i0}, \ldots, \psi_{im_i})} \quad [5.1]$$

Because item and person parameters are unknown, it is common to use estimates of the parameters instead of the true parameter. This leads to *estimates* of expected item scores given by

$$\hat{E}_{vi} = \sum_{x=0}^{m_i} x \frac{\exp(x\hat{\theta}_v + \hat{\psi}_{ix})}{K(\hat{\theta}_v, \hat{\psi}_{i0}, \ldots, \hat{\psi}_{im_i})} \quad [5.2]$$

We use these when we want to make it clear that expected item scores are based on parameter estimates rather than known parameters.

Let $R_v = \sum_{i=1}^{k} X_{vi}$ denote the total score over all items. The maximum score over all items is $m_. = \sum_{i=1}^{k} m_i$. Let G_v denote a categorical variable with m_G categories. Finally, let S_v be an ordinal categorical variable defined by m_S score intervals.

Let n be the number of persons in the complete sample. To define group residuals, we refer to the number of persons in different groups. We do this in the following way: n_r denotes the number of persons with $R_v = r$, n_g denotes the number of persons with $G_v = g$, n_s denotes the number of persons with $S_v = s$, and n_{gr} denotes the number of persons with $G_v = g$ and $R_v = r$. Unless specifically stated, we always assume that persons with extreme scores (0 and $m_.$) are excluded from these counts because there is no information in the response profiles of these persons that are useful during the analysis of the fit of the items to the Rasch model.

At the group level, we will deal with residuals that compare observed and expected average item scores in groups. We therefore define average item scores in groups defined by exogenous variables

$$A_{gi} = \frac{1}{n_g} \sum_{v:G_v=g} X_{vi} \quad [5.3]$$

by score intervals

$$A_{si} = \frac{1}{n_s} \sum_{v:S_v=s} X_{vi} \quad [5.4]$$

and by raw scores

$$A_{ri} = \frac{1}{n_t} \sum_{v:R_v=r} X_{vi} \quad [5.5]$$

Group residuals compare the observed average scores [5.3]–[5.5] to the expected values $B_{gi} = \frac{1}{n_g} \sum_{v:G_v=g} E_{vi}$, $B_{si} = \frac{1}{n_s} \sum_{v:S_v=s} E_{vi}$ and $B_{ri} = \frac{1}{n_r} \sum_{v:R_v=r} E_{vi}$.

5.2.2. *Individual response residuals: outfits and infits*

The raw residuals are

$$R_{vi} = X_{vi} - E_{vi}$$

Because item and person parameters are unknown, it is a standard statistical practice to use $\hat{E}_{vi}$ instead of E_{vi} for the calculation of residuals. The problems created by this practice during item analysis by Rasch models are discussed below, but for now we disregard these problems and assume that the true expected values are available and define individual response residual statistics in the following way. The standardized residuals are

$$Z_{vi} = \frac{X_{vi} - E_{vi}}{\sqrt{VAR(X_{vi} - E_{vi})}} = \frac{R_{vi}}{\sqrt{VAR(X_{vi})}} \qquad [5.6]$$

The squared standardized residuals are

$$Z_{vi}^2 = \frac{R_{vi}^2}{VAR(X_{vi})} \qquad [5.7]$$

The theory of Rasch models defines two summary item fit statistics called OUTFIT and INFIT based on these residuals:

$$\text{OUTFIT}_i = \frac{1}{n}\sum_{v=1}^{n} Z_{vi}^2 \qquad [5.8]$$

$$\text{INFIT}_i = \frac{\sum_{v=1}^{n} R_{vi}^2}{\sum_{v=1}^{n} VAR(X_{vi})} \qquad [5.9]$$

Because $R_{vi}^2 = VAR(X_{vi})Z_{vi}^2$, we can redefine the infit as a weighted mean of the standardized squared residuals Z_{vi}^2:

$$\text{INFIT}_i = \sum_{v=1}^{n} w_{wi} Z_{vi}^2 \qquad [5.10]$$

where $w_{vi} = VAR(X_{vi}) / \sum_{v=1}^{n} VAR(X_{vi})$.

The range of these statistics consists of non-negative real numbers and they both have expected values equal to one under the Rasch model. Infit or outfit values close to zero or much greater than one are therefore regarded as evidence against the fit of an item to the Rasch model. Exactly when these statistics are too small or too large to be acceptable is, however, a difficult question and the established practice surrounding these fit statistics is infested with a number of misunderstandings and misconceptions. In this chapter, we therefore take a closer look at how to calculate the expected responses when item and person parameters are estimated values and on the distributions of the item outfit and infit under the Rasch model.

5.2.3. *Problem 1: the distribution of outfit and infit test statistics*

Let us take the distribution first. We need to know the distribution of outfit and infit test statistics if we want to assess whether or not the observed outfit and infit test statistics disagree with the Rasch model. It is sometimes claimed [SMI 04] that the standardized residuals Z_{vi} "are distributed as approximate unit normals" and thus Z_{vi}^2 "can be evaluated as a chi-square (χ^2) with one degree of freedom", so that the "sum across the persons to assess the fit of the responses to a particular item ... results in a chi-square".

Unfortunately, these claims are false. This is not a new result [VAN 82], but belief in these claims persists, and widely used computer programs for item analysis by Rasch models implement assessment of the significance of the fit statistics based on these misunderstandings.

It is not difficult to see why the claims are wrong. Recall that item responses X_{vi} are categorical variables with a relatively small number of possible outcomes. Subtracting the expected response from X_{vi} does not change this and the resulting residual statistics, R_{vi}, Z_{vi} and Z_{vi}^2, are therefore also discrete with the same number of potential outcomes as X_{vi}. The standardized residual of a binary variable is, for instance, still a binary variable and therefore as far away from the continuous normal distribution as we can imagine.

We cannot assume that the Z_{vi} variables are identically distributed but the means and variances of these variables are the same. We might therefore hope for a version of the central limit theorem (CLT) to guarantee that the asymptotic distribution of the average of the Z_{vi} variables was normal. Such CLT versions do exist, but they require some additional assumptions concerning the distribution of the Z_{vi} variables are satisfied and it is not clear at all whether the Z_{vi} variables meet these requirements. Transforming the standardized residuals into squared standardized residuals complicates things to a degree where even this hope is unrealistic. It is true that the expected values of Z_{vi}^2 are equal to one, but its standard deviation (which would equal to two if Z_{vi}^2 had a χ^2 distribution with one degree of freedom) depends strongly on E_{vi}. Consider, as an example, two dichotomous items with E_{vi} equal to 0.5 and 0.1, respectively. In the first case, Z_{vi} can be either -1 or $+1$ with probabilities

$$P(Z_{vi} = -1) = P(Z_{vi} = +1) = 0.5$$

so that Z_{vi}^2 always is equal to one, $P(Z_{vi}^2 = 1) = 1$, and $VAR(Z_{vi}^2) = 0$. In the second case, Z_{vi}^2 has one of the two values, $P(Z_{vi}^2 = 0.1111) = 0.9$ and $P(Z_{vi}^2 = 9) = 0.1$ and $VAR(Z_{vi}^2) = 7.1$. Apart from illustrating that $VAR(Z_{vi}^2)$ is very different from two, the example shows that the result of the test of fit of an item would depend strongly on the targeting of the items to the population. If the set of items is well targeted with many persons with probabilities of positive responses that were relatively close to 0.5, it would be extraordinary to find items that did not fit the Rasch model. If items are off target with many persons with low probabilities of positive responses on many items, the opposite would be the case.

According to formula [5.1], there is one expected item score and therefore one residual distribution for each combination of a person and an item. If this statement is taken at face value, there is no easy solution to the problem of finding an appropriate distribution for the outfit and infit test statistics. There is, however, every reason to take a closer look at the way to calculate E_{vi} when person and item parameter estimates are used instead of the unknown parameters, and this will not only lead to better ways to calculate E_{vi} but also to a more viable solution to the distribution problem.

5.2.4. *Problem 2: calculating* E_{vi}

It is easy to find examples – linear regression analysis being the most obvious – of statistical analyses where $\hat{E}_{vi}$ can replace E_{vi} during the analysis of residuals. The reason why this often works in practice is that the analyses use consistent estimates of unknown parameters where bias and standard errors disappear as sample sizes increase toward infinity. These situations are, however, very different from the situation with the individual response residuals in Rasch models. The problem is that $\hat{E}_{vi}$ depend on two types of parameters: item parameters and person parameters where consistent estimates are available for one, but not for both types of parameters. Item parameter estimates can be assumed to be consistent except for the so-called joint estimates that are known to be inconsistent. Person parameter estimates could also be regarded as consistent if the number of items is large, but this is never (or at least very rarely) the case in health-related scales where the typical number of items lies between five and 25.

Recall the discussion of person parameter estimates in Chapter 4 where it has been shown that standard errors can be large for all persons and the bias can be considerable for a large number of persons. If there are no other reasons, it follows that *estimates* of expected values must be expected to be biased with relatively large standard errors. Recall also that the bias of the person parameter estimate depends on the choice of an estimator. Before we calculate $\hat{E}_{vi}$, we have to think carefully about the choice of person parameter estimate: ML, WML, JML or Bayesian. The estimates can be very different – some with more bias and error than others – but since we want to estimate $\hat{E}_{vi}$, we have to select the person parameter estimate that reduces the error and the bias of $\hat{E}_{vi}$, and there are – to our knowledge – no published results about the degree to which the differences between person parameter estimates influence the error and the bias of $\hat{E}_{vi}$. These problems are in themselves reason enough for a cautious attitude toward the application of $\hat{E}_{vi}$, but there is another problem that we also have to take into account: formula [5.2] does not give the correct value because estimates of person locations are used instead of the true values. To see this, we have to take a closer look at what happens during the calculation of the expected values.

Recall first that the Rasch model probabilities are *conditional* probabilities given outcomes on a latent variable. The proper way to write these probabilities is

$$P(X_{vi} = x|\Theta_v = \theta; \bar{\psi}_i) = \frac{\exp(x\theta + \psi_{ix})}{K(\theta; \bar{\psi}_i)} \tag{5.11}$$

where Θ_v is the latent variable, θ is an outcome on this variable and $\bar{\psi}_i$ is the vector of item parameters. Attempting to replace θ by an estimate $\hat{\theta}$ in [5.11] means that we replace the variable Θ_v in [5.11] by a different variable $\hat{\Theta}_v$ with outcomes equal to the estimates $\hat{\theta}$, thus replacing [5.11] by

$$P(X_{vi} = x|\hat{\Theta}_v = \hat{\theta}; \bar{\psi}_i) = \frac{\exp(x\hat{\theta} + \psi_{ix})}{K(\hat{\theta}; \bar{\psi}_i)} \tag{5.12}$$

Next, recall that the total score R is sufficient for θ. From this, it follows that the range of $\hat{\Theta}_v$ consists of $m_. + 1$ values

$$\{\theta^{(0)}, \theta^{(1)}, \ldots, \theta^{(r)}, \ldots, \theta^{(m_.)}\}$$

where $\hat{\Theta}_v = \theta^{(r)}$ if and only if $R_v = r$. Furthermore, the true conditional probability $P(X_{vi} = x|\hat{\Theta}_v = \hat{\theta}; \bar{\psi}_i)$ cannot be equal to the probability in formula [5.12]. The true probability has to be derived from the conditional distribution of X_{vi} given R_v:

$$\begin{aligned} P(X_{vi} = x|\hat{\Theta}_v = \theta_r; \bar{\psi}_i) &= P(X_{vi} = x|R_v = r; \bar{\psi}_i) \\ &= \frac{\exp(\psi_{ix})\gamma_{r-x}\left(\bar{\psi}_1, \ldots, \bar{\psi}_{i-1}, \bar{\psi}_{i+1}, \ldots, \bar{\psi}_k\right)}{\gamma_r(\bar{\psi})} \end{aligned} \tag{5.13}$$

Formula [5.13] defines the correct conditional distribution of X_{vi} given $\hat{\Theta}_v = \theta^{(r)}$ and illustrates the advantages of conditional inference in Rasch models. According to formula [5.13], the conditional probability of X_{vi} given $\hat{\Theta}_v = \theta^{(r)}$ does not depend on the *value* of $\theta^{(r)}$, but only on r. This means that (1) we do not have to be concerned about how person parameters are estimated, (2) $E_{vi} = E(X_{vi}|R_v = r)$ when $\hat{\Theta}_v = \theta^{(r)}$, and (3) formula [5.13] also can be used to derive the conditional probabilities of R_{vi}, Z_{vi}, R^2_{vi} and Z^2_{vi} because these variables are simple functions of X_{vi} and E_{vi}. Finally, formula [5.13] shows that the distributions of X_{vi}, R_{vi}, Z_{vi}, R^2_{vi} and Z^2_{vi} are the same for all persons with the same score (and therefore the same person parameter estimate) so that the CLT can be used to determine the asymptotic distribution of outfit and infit test statistics.

For instance, the outfit test statistic defined in [5.8] can be rewritten as a weighted mean of the average of a number of identically distributed Z^2_{vi} values

$$\text{OUTFIT}_i = \frac{1}{n}\sum_{v=1}^{n} Z^2_{vi} = \frac{1}{n}\sum_{r=1}^{m_.-1}\sum_{v:R_v=r} Z^2_{vi} = \sum_{r=1}^{m_.-1} w_r V_{ri} \tag{5.14}$$

where $w_r = \frac{n_r}{n}$ and

$$V_{ri} = \frac{1}{n_r} \sum_{v:R_v=r} Z_{vi}^2$$

is the average of n_r identically distributed outcomes on Z_{vi}^2. It follows from the CLT that V_r has an asymptotically normal distribution whose mean is equal to one and whose variance depends on the conditional variance of Z_{vi}^2 given $R_v = r$. Since OUTFIT$_i$ is a weighted mean of $m_. - 1$ variables with asymptotically normal distributions, it follows that OUTFIT$_i$ is also asymptotically normal under the Rasch model with a mean that is equal to one and with a variance that is a weighted mean of the variances:

$$VAR(\text{OUTFIT}_i) = \sum_{r=1}^{m_.-1} w_r^2 VAR(V_{ri}) \qquad [5.15]$$

The asymptotic distribution of the item INFIT defined in [5.9] and [5.10] can be derived in the same way.

EXAMPLE 5.1.– We continue the analysis of the items from the disinhibited eating (DE) subscale of the Diabetes Health Profile (DHP) with calculation of outfit and infit tests statistics. Table 5.1 shows the results.

	OUTFIT			INFIT		
Item	Observed	SD	p-value	Observed	SD	p-value
DHP32	1.237	0.107	0.027	1.246	0.108	0.022
DHP34	1.042	0.146	0.772	0.910	0.107	0.400
DHP36	1.260	0.110	0.018	1.190	0.094	0.043
DHP38	0.754	0.125	0.048	0.815	0.128	0.147
DHP39	0.937	0.128	0.624	0.923	0.119	0.517

Table 5.1. *Outfit and infit test statistics for the five items in disinhibited eating (DE) subscale of the Diabetes Health Profile (DHP)*

Significant evidence of misfit was found for three out of five items. However, the evidence provided by p-values greater than 1% is not strong, and adjustment for multiple testing by, for example, the Benjamini–Hochberg procedure [BEN 95] dismisses this evidence. So according to these fit statistics, the DHP–DE items do fit the Rasch model.

5.2.5. *Group residuals*

Group residuals compare the *average* item score in a group A_{gi} to the expected *average* score B_{vi} under the Rasch model. There is a close link between individual residuals and group residuals, but there are also important differences. Before we go into details, it should be noted that the introduction of groups to some extent changes the issue that the item fit statistics try to address. Groups can be defined in three different ways during the analysis of the data-model fit: (1) score groups, (2) score intervals and (3) groups defined by exogenous variables.

The natural groups under Rasch models are the score groups consisting of persons with the same total score because all persons in these groups have the same conditional response probabilities for all items. For large sample sizes, item fit within these groups should be analyzed separately. When this is not the case, we can define groups by score *intervals* instead of separate scores. This complicates things in technical terms, but in principle, there is no difference between the analysis using score groups and the analysis using score intervals. Since low and high scores are associated with low and high values of θ, we could say that the analysis of group residuals defined by the scores on all items tries to do the same as item fit statistics based on individual response residuals, namely testing that items are homogeneous in the sense that they function in the same way at all levels of θ. Groups may also be defined by exogenous variables that are not part of the Rasch model as such. When this happens, analyses of residuals address a completely different and, to some extent, a more fundamental issue, namely the question of whether items function in the same way in different groups. If the groups, for instance, are defined by gender, we summarize residuals calculated for men and women separately to test that there is no differential item functioning (DIF) relative to gender.

Many of the methods used during the analysis of homogeneity are the same as those used during the analysis of DIF, but there are also important differences where methods do not transfer effortlessly from one type of problem to the other. Therefore, we consider the analysis of homogeneity first, and return to a discussion of the analysis of DIF later.

5.2.6. *Group residuals for analysis of homogeneity*

It is easy to see that the group residual is nothing but the average individual residual in the group

$$D_{gi} = A_{gi} - B_{gi} = \frac{1}{n_g} \sum_{v:G_v=g} X_{vi} - \frac{1}{n_g} \sum_{v:G_v=g} E_{vi} = \frac{1}{n_g} \sum_{v:G_v=g} R_{vi} \quad [5.16]$$

The standardized group residual is

$$F_{gi} = \frac{D_{gi}}{\sqrt{VAR(A_{gi})}}$$

where

$$VAR(A_{gi}) = \frac{1}{n_g^2} \sum_{v:G_v=g} VAR(X_{vi})$$

and the squared standardized group residual is

$$F_{gi}^2 = \frac{\left(\sum_{v:G_v=g} R_{vi}\right)^2}{\sum_{v:G_v=g} VAR(X_{vi})} \qquad [5.17]$$

We still assume that E_{vi} is the *conditional* mean of X_{vi}, given $R_v = r$ so that A_{gi} is a weighted mean of the averages of item responses in a number of score groups and that A_{gi} is asymptotically normal. Thus, the asymptotic distribution of F_{gi} is standardized normal and the asymptotic distribution of F_{gi}^2 is a χ^2 distribution with one degree of freedom.

Therefore, we might expect that inference summarizing information on a specific item from several groups should be easier, but this is not the case as illustrated in the following example.

EXAMPLE 5.2.– Consider the results in Table 5.2 concerning group residuals in the score intervals from one to five and six to 15. Each of these score intervals provides evidence for or against the fit of the items to the Rasch model. The item fit statistics appear to agree in the majority of cases; in most cases, the evidence from the different score intervals appears to agree, but there is one item (DHP38) where the conclusions differ and there is another item (DHP32) where the evidence from the two score intervals is insignificant taken separately but where we might expect that an assessment based on a summary of the two residuals also might result in evidence against the item-model fit.

Score 1–5				
		Mean		
Item	n	Obs.	Exp.	F_{gi}
DHP32	85	0.61	0.50	1.73
DHP34	85	0.66	0.71	−0.61
DHP36	85	0.81	0.72	1.07
DHP38	85	0.29	0.43	−2.35
DHP39	85	0.88	0.89	−0.15

Score 6–14				
		Mean		
Item	n	Obs.	Exp.	F_{gi}
DHP32	91	1.13	1.23	−1.29
DHP34	91	2.41	2.36	0.59
DHP36	91	1.79	1.88	−1.00
DHP38	91	1.21	1.08	1.63
DHP39	91	1.61	1.61	0.10

Table 5.2. *Analysis of group residuals comparing observed with expected item scores in two score intervals (F_{gi} is the standardized residual)*

An obvious solution to this problem is to calculate the sum of the squared residuals and to assess the significance according to a χ^2 distribution with degrees of freedom equal to the number of groups. Doing this would be an error similar to the error we would make if we assumed that the sum of the squared individual residuals has a χ^2 distribution, but for a different reason. The reason why one would try to calculate $\sum_{g=1}^{m_G} F_{gi}^2$ is that the CLT guarantees that F_{gi}^2 in itself has an asymptotic χ^2 distribution with one degree of freedom and that the sum of χ^2 distributed variables is known to have a χ^2 distribution. However, this result only applies when the variables are stochastically independent and this requirement is not met by the squared group residuals in Rasch models. To see that this is the case, we only have to note that the observed minus expected item scores in the low-score interval is equal to the expected minus observed item scores in the high-score group (except for rounding error). This is a general result that has to do with the sufficiency of the item margins under the Rasch model and the way item parameters are estimated, and it follows that the squared standardized residuals for the same item in different groups are correlated: we cannot assume that $\sum_{g=1}^{m_G} F_{gi}^2$ has a χ^2 distribution.

The requirement that χ^2 distributed variables have to be independent for the sum to be χ^2 distributed is often forgotten and problems caused by this can be found in many summary fit statistics that are implemented in software for Rasch analysis. We will not go deeper into this issue, but advise the reader to take a careful look at software documentation to ensure that implemented fit statistics is not flawed by this mistake.

5.3. Molenaar's U

We will not make that error here and therefore have to look at other ways to summarize the evidence against items from different groups. One of these is the U statistic proposed by Molenaar [MOL 83] summarizing trends in group residuals calculated in different score groups.

Let F_{ri} be the standardized residual for item i in score group r. Molenaar noticed that the patterns in these residuals often had negative values at one end of the score range and positive values at the other end corresponding to what we would expect if the item discrimination of an item were different from the item discrimination of the other items. To capture such departures from the Rasch model, Molenaar partitioned the score range into three intervals

$$\{1, \ldots, r_1\}, \{r_1 + 1 \ldots, r_2\}, \{r_2 + 1, \ldots, m_. - 1\}$$

with approximately the same number of respondents, he defined his item fit statistic as

$$U_i = \frac{1}{\sqrt{r_1 + (m_. - 1 - r_2)}} \left(\sum_{r=r_2+1}^{m_.} F_{ri} - \sum_{r=1}^{r_1} F_{ri} \right) \qquad [5.18]$$

and showed that it has an asymptotic standardized normal distribution under the Rasch model. Positive or negative values indicate that the discriminations of item i is stronger or weaker, respectively, than what is assumed by the Rasch model.

EXAMPLE 5.3.– Table 5.3 shows the values of Molenaar's U for the five DHP items.

Item	U_i	p-value
DHP32	−1.892	0.059
DHP34	0.170	0.865
DHP36	−1.003	0.316
DHP38	2.026	0.043
DHP39	0.780	0.435

Table 5.3. *Molenaar's U comparing residuals in the 0–3 score interval ($n = 45$) to residuals in the 7–14 score interval ($n = 64$) for the five items from the disinhibited eating (DE) subscale of the Diabetes Health Profile (DHP)*

The value of U_i for item DHP38 is significantly greater than zero, but adjusting for multiple testing once again dismisses the significance so that the conclusion drawn from this statistic is the same as the conclusion drawn from the infit and outfit test statistics in Table 5.1: there is no conclusive evidence against the item-model fit.

Molenaar's U attempts to capture the trend in the residuals (if there is one) relative to the total score and therefore focuses on the extreme ends of the score range. The idea is sound, but we might be concerned about the power of the fit statistic because the coefficient disregards about a third of the sample of persons. In the analysis of the five items from the DE subscale of the DHP, U disregarded item responses from 57 respondents. To include these respondents in the analysis of item fit, Kreiner [KRE 11] proposed another item fit statistic targeting this kind of departures from the Rasch model. This statistic is discussed in the following section.

5.4. Analysis of item-restscore association

Instead of looking at residuals that compare *average* item scores to expected average item scores, Kreiner's fit statistic compares observed and expected response frequencies in different score groups to the expected responses in the score groups.

Recall that n_r denotes the observed number of respondents with $R_v = r$ and let $a^{(i)}_{rx}$ denote the number of respondents with $R_v = r$ and $X_{vi} = x$. Given n_r, the expected number of respondents is

$$b^{(i)}_{rx} = n_r P(X_{vi} = x | R_v = r)$$

The conditional distribution of item responses given the total score is one of the standard distributions from the theory of Rasch models (see Chapter 2). Intuition might suggest that this leads to a simple χ^2 test comparing observed to expected frequencies but this would be wrong for exactly the same reasons that summing squared residuals from different score intervals was wrong. Instead, Kreiner [KRE 11] transforms the observed and expected item by score tables into item by restscore tables.

Let $R_{vi} = R - X_{vi}$ denote the restscore without item i. The observed frequencies of the item–rest score table are

$$o_{rx}^{(i)} = a_{(r-x)x}^{(i)}$$

and the expected frequencies of the item–rest score table are

$$f_{rx}^{(i)} = e_{(r-x)x}^{(i)}$$

so that the expected table is still calculated conditionally given the total score on all items. Kreiner argues that a too strong item discrimination will result in an item–rest score correlation that is larger than expected under the Rasch model and that the result of a too weak item discrimination will be that the observed item–rest score correlation will be less than expected. To test whether this is the case, we may calculate Goodman and Kruskal's γ [GOO 54] measuring the degree of association between the item and the rest score in the observed and expected item–rest score tables together with the standard deviation of γ in the expected table and use this to test whether the observed γ disagrees with what the Rasch model expects.

EXAMPLE 5.4.– The results from an analysis of the DE items are shown in Table 5.4.

Item	Obs. γ	Exp. γ	SD	p-value
DHP32	0.305	0.426	0.068	0.07
DHP34	0.500	0.465	0.060	0.57
DHP36	0.345	0.445	0.062	0.11
DHP38	0.686	0.432	0.072	0.0004
DHP39	0.522	0.470	0.070	0.45

Table 5.4. *Analysis of the item–rest score association in five items from the disinhibited eating (DE) subscale of the Diabetes Health Profile (DHP)*

Note that item–rest score associations are not expected to be exactly the same for all items, rather they are expected to be relatively close. The observed association between DHP38 and the rest score is much stronger than expected and the difference is, according to the γ coefficient, highly significant. The item–rest score association therefore rejects the fit of DHP38 to the Rasch model.

5.5. Group residuals and analysis of DIF

The group residuals that were used for the analysis of homogeneity in Table 5.2 can also be calculated for the analysis of DIF when groups are defined by values of a covariate instead of the total score on items. This is illustrated in the following example.

EXAMPLE 5.5.– Table 5.5 shows the group residuals for men and women.

Men				
		Mean		
Item	n	Obs.	Exp.	F_{gi}
DHP32	91	0.72	0.78	-0.78
DHP34	91	1.33	1.39	-0.67
DHP36	91	1.36	1.18	2.17
DHP38	91	0.56	0.66	-1.52
DHP39	91	1.20	1.16	0.51

Women				
		Mean		
Item	n	Obs.	Exp.	F_{gi}
DHP32	84	1.04	0.98	0.78
DHP34	84	1.80	1.73	0.71
DHP36	84	1.25	1.44	−2.26
DHP38	84	0.96	0.86	1.51
DHP39	84	1.31	1.35	−0.50

Table 5.5. *Analysis of group residuals comparing observed to expected item scores among men and women. F_{gi} is the standardized residual*

In this case, the residuals in both groups agree that one item (DHP36) has a DIF problem. It still would have been convenient if it had been possible to add the squared standardized residual together to get one χ^2 statistic summarizing all the evidence concerning DIF in an item, but this is, of course, also impossible here for exactly the same reasons as before: the separate χ^2 statistics are not independent. So we have to find ways to test for DIF where responses from all groups are summarized and where the asymptotic distribution is known. Two tests are discussed: (1) a conditional likelihood ratio (CLR) test suggested by Kelderman [KEL 84] and (2) a non-parametric test of conditional independence in three-way tables. We regard the first test as the fundamental test of DIF in Rasch models, but note that the second test is very popular and widely used because it is easy to calculate. It is, however, not always recognized by users of this test that the test is a Rasch model test because the conditional independence assumptions are only true under the Rasch model.

5.6. Kelderman's conditional likelihood ratio test of no DIF

Assume that G is an exogenous variable with values $0, \ldots, m_G$ and that there is DIF in item X_i relative to G. We say that DIF is uniform within the Rasch model if the Rasch model fits in all groups defined by G and if the item parameters of all the other items are the same in all groups as illustrated below.

G	X_1	X_2	...	X_{i-1}	X_i	X_{i+1}	...	X_k
0	β_1	β_2	...	β_{i-1}	$\beta_i^{(0)}$	β_{i+1}	...	β_k
1	β_1	β_2	...	β_{i-1}	$\beta_i^{(1)}$	β_{i+1}	...	β_k
$\vdots$	$\vdots$	$\vdots$		$\vdots$	$\vdots$	$\vdots$		$\vdots$
m_G	β_1	β_2	...	β_{i-1}	$\beta_i^{(m_G)}$	β_{i+1}	...	β_k

It is convenient to reparameterize the model by letting

$$\beta_i^{(g)} = (\beta_{i1}^{(g)}, \ldots, \beta_{im}^{(g)})$$

and

$$\beta_i = \beta_{i1}^{(0)}$$

and

$$\delta_{ix}^{(g)} = \beta_{ix}^{(g)} - \beta_{ix}^{(0)}$$

so that $\delta_{ix}^{(0)} = 0$. Replacing the previous parameters by these new parameters yields the structure shown below

G	X_1	X_2	...	X_{i-1}	X_i	X_{i+1}	...	X_k
0	β_1	β_2	...	β_{i-1}	β_i	β_{i+1}	...	β_k
1	β_1	β_2	...	β_{i-1}	$\beta_i + \delta_i^{(1)}$	β_{i+1}	...	β_k
$\vdots$	$\vdots$	$\vdots$		$\vdots$	$\vdots$	$\vdots$		$\vdots$
m_G	β_1	β_2	...	β_{i-1}	$\beta_i + \delta_i^{(m_G)}$	β_{i+1}	...	β_k

The joint distribution of item responses is

$$P(x_1, \ldots, x_k | \theta, G = g) = \frac{\exp\left(\sum_{i=1}^{k}\left(x_i\theta - \sum_{j=1}^{x_i}\beta_{ij}\right) + \delta_{ix_i}^{(g)}\right)}{K(\theta, \beta, \delta)}$$

$$= \frac{\exp\left(r\theta - \sum_{i=1}^{k}\sum_{j=1}^{x_i}\beta_{ij} + \delta_{ix_i}^{(g)}\right)}{K(\theta, \beta, \delta)} \quad [5.19]$$

where $\delta_{ix}^{(g)}$ are log-linear interaction parameters describing the DIF effect that G has on item i and where $r = \sum_{i=1}^{k} r_i$ is sufficient as it was in the original Rasch model. It follows from the sufficiency that conditional inference including CLR tests is also available in Rasch models with uniform DIF items. The conditional distribution of items given the total score and given G is equal to

$$P(x_1, \ldots, x_k | r, G = g) = \frac{\exp\left(-\sum_{i=1}^{k}\sum_{j=1}^{x_i}\beta_{ij} + \delta_{ix_i}^{(g)}\right)}{\gamma_r^g(\beta, \delta)} \quad [5.20]$$

To estimate the item and DIF parameters under the uniform DIF model, we maximize the likelihood function

$$L_1(\beta,\delta) = \prod_{v=1}^{n} P(x_{v1},\ldots,x_{vk}|r_v,g_v)$$

and calculate a CLR test comparing $L_1(\beta,\delta)$ to the likelihood of the Rasch model without DIF

$$L_0(\beta,\delta=0) = \prod_{v=1}^{n} P(x_{v1},\ldots,x_{vk}|r_v,g_v)$$

by

$$\chi^2 = -2\log\left(\frac{L_0}{L_1}\right)$$

The CLR test statistic has an asymptotic χ^2 distribution with $m_G \cdot m_i$ degrees of freedom.

EXAMPLE 5.6.– The CLR tests of DIF relative to gender are shown in Table 5.6.

Item	CLR	df	p-value
DHP32	1.47	3	0.69
DHP34	3.19	3	0.36
DHP36	12.72	3	0.0053
DHP38	5.47	3	0.14
DHP39	4.93	3	0.18

Table 5.6. *CLR tests of DIF with respect to gender for the five items of the disinhibited eating (DE) subscale of the Diabetes Health Profile (DHP)*

According to these tests, DHP36 is the only item with a DIF problem and the evidence is too strong to be dismissed by adjustment for multiple testing.

5.7. Test for conditional independence in three-way tables

A completely different approach to the analysis of DIF is to test for conditional independence of an item and an exogenous variable in three-way tables where the relationship between the item and the covariate is stratified according to the score. When items are dichotomous variables and covariates are binary, such tests are often called Mantel–Haenszel tests, but it is easy to extend such tests to ordinal items and all types of covariates.

Mantel–Haenszel techniques are widely used in all IRT models motivated by the intuition that since the IRT model assumes that the item and the covariate are conditionally independent given the unobserved θ, then it must surely also be true when the total score is used as a proxy for the latent variable. Unfortunately, such an intuition is once again wrong. The only known IRT model where conditional independence between an item and a covariate given the latent θ implies that the item and the covariate are conditionally independent given the total score R is the Rasch model. The hypothesis may be almost true (in some unspecified sense) under other models, but is nevertheless false and it will result in erroneous evidence of DIF in large sample studies where items fit other types of IRT models. In other words, if you have a very large sample and if you do not find any evidence against conditional independence after stratification by the total score, then you have every reason to believe that your items follow something similar to a Rasch model whether or not that was what you aimed for to begin with.

EXAMPLE 5.7.– To illustrate what goes on during such an analysis, we show the relationship between item DHP36 and gender in two score strata (Table 5.7).

Score		0	1	2	3	Total	
6	Male	1	1	4	3	9	
	%	11.1	11.1	44.4	33.3	100.0	
	Female	2	2	4	0	8	
	%	25.0	25.0	50.0	0.0	100.0	
	Total	3	3	8	3	17	$\chi^2 = 3.6$, df $= 3$, $p = 0.305$
	%	17.6	17.6	47.1	17.6	100.0	$\gamma = -0.62$, $p = 0.023$
7	Male	1	4	6	1	12	
	%	8.3	33.3	50.0	8.3	100.0	
	Female	4	3	6	1	14	
	%	28.6	21.4	42.9	7.1	100.0	
	Total	5	7	12	2	26	$\chi^2 = 1.8$, df $= 3$, $p = 0.615$
	%	19.2	26.9	46.2	7.7	100.0	$\gamma = -0.23$, $p = 0.220$

Table 5.7. *Association between DHP and gender in two strata with total score 6 and 7, respectively*

In Table 5.7, the strength of the conditional association between item DHP36 and gender is measured by Goodman and Kruskal's γ because this measure is appropriate for ordinal categorical data. In both tables, males have higher item scores than females, but the difference is only significant in the stratum containing respondents with score 7. To summarize the results over all strata, we use the partial γ coefficient [DAV 67] and use Monte Carlo estimates of exact conditional p-values [KRE 87] to avoid problems with inappropriate asymptotic results in large sparse contingency tables.

The partial γ is -0.32 with $p = 0.01$, confirming the results of Kelderman's CLR test. Gender is a source of DIF for item DHP36.

5.8. Discussion and recommendations

There are several topics that we need to discuss regarding this chapter, including technical problems relating to the choice of item fit statistics and the more fundamental problems concerning what to do, when item fit statistics disclose evidence against the item-model fit.

5.8.1. *Technical issues*

Let us take the technical problem first. A lot of fit statistics for Rasch models have been suggested and several statistics have been implemented in available software for Rasch models. Most, if not all, suggestions are based on sound ideas and on unquestionable knowledge about Rasch measurement (as opposed to Rasch inference), but the implementation of these methods in many cases is limited and based on the lack of understanding of statistical inference, to a degree where we expect that many published results based on these implementations are erroneous. The best advice we can give to the users of Rasch models is that they should search for implementations of methods based on the principles of conditional inference because conditional inference guarantees that results are consistent without bias and less errorneous in large sample studies. Other methods may – it has to be admitted – work almost as well as conditional methods in small sample studies but they are guaranteed to have bias and to inflate the type I error rates as sample sizes increase because implementation of fit statistics that are not based on conditional inference tests hypotheses that at best are almost true, but always false. This, at least, is what statistical theory tells us. If you doubt this and want to see what happens when you analyze data using your favorite Rasch program, we suggest that you simulate data from Rasch models and take special care to see what happens when sample sizes increase. If the program systematically rejects the model as sample sizes increase, you can be sure that your program has a problem.

We have already referred to Glas and Verhelst [GLA 95a, GLA 95b] for an overview of item fit statistics and additional references. We would also like to point out that item fit statistics developed for other IRT models ([GLA 99] is a particular useful reference) are also useful for the assessment of item fit to Rasch models because the Rasch model is a special case of these models.

If we find, for instance, that an item does not agree with the non-parametric IRT model, it follows automatically that it cannot agree with the Rasch model. Christensen and Kreiner [CHR 07] have pursued this point and have found that the power of the Loevinger scalability H coefficient derived from non-parametric IRT models compares favorably to the power of fit statistics developed within the theory of Rasch models.

Given the large number of available item fit statistics, it is common for new users of Rasch models to be confused. We would, of course, always search for the most powerful statistics, but there are few studies comparing the power of item fit statistics in a systematic and comprehensive way. For what it is worth, we can inform the reader that we have performed a number of (unpublished) Monte Carlo studies without finding indisputable evidence that some of the fit statistics are more powerful than others to a degree that makes a difference in practice. So feel free to choose any fit statistic that has captured your attention. However, that does not mean that your choice of item fit statistic should be indiscriminate. It is your responsibility to ensure that the implementation of these methods is up to standard. You will find, when you look into these matters, that many of these methods were developed and implemented in the 1970s and early 1980s based on technology available at that time, but the developments in statistical inference, in general, and psychometric methods, in particular, since then have been ignored. This is regrettable but also common, and there are no reasons to complain to those who at some point have invested time and money in developing these programs. The responsibility solely lies with the user. It is the responsibility of the user to check that the methods have been implemented in ways that guarantee against other errors than those we cannot avoid during statistical analyses because of random variation in data.

5.8.2. *What to do when items do not agree with the Rasch model*

It is important to understand that the item fit statistics targeting the item-model fit and, in particular, the item fits statistics checking the response homogeneity do not question the fundamental assumptions of unidimensionality, local independence and no DIF. The item fit statistics are only concerned about the choice of the probability functions and not about anything else. Evidence against item-model fit may turn up – or rather will turn up – if the fundamental assumptions of IRT and Rasch models are violated. You are therefore required to look into all these issues before you decide to either eliminate an apparently bad item or choose a different probability function – a different IRT model – to obtain a better fit to data. You should be aware, for instance, that local dependence will have the effect that it appears as if items have different item discriminations and that local dependence itself may be caused by multidimensionality and/or DIF relative to observed and unobserved covariates. Evidence of item misfit is therefore often only the first step of a long (and sometimes tedious) journey to find out what is really wrong and what to do about it. Needless to say – but let us say it, nevertheless, to ensure that we do not forget it – that you are also required to take a second look both at the subject matter arguments that lead to the development of your items and the contents and formulations of questions and response categories. You will find – as we have found many times – that items are rejected not because of the content of the items but because of inept, unprofessional and careless item writing. Local response dependence and DIF are typically caused by these reasons, and when this happens, there are only three options: you eliminate the items, rewrite the items or select an IRT model that adjusts for the local dependence and the DIF. In other cases, the lack of item-model fit challenges the subject matter arguments leading to your items. In our experience, this happens less often than because of bad item writing, but it does happen, in particular, in connection with what we could refer to as *ad hoc* scales. When this happens, you must rethink the whole theoretical foundation underlying the items. Exploratory methods searching for multidimensional models providing a better fit to data may be of help here, but they cannot stand alone without serious subject matter considerations. Item analyses by Rasch models and other IRT models are confirmatory analyses, which assume that you know what you are doing but acknowledge that you may be wrong and therefore want to check that you have not made any errors. Turning to exploratory methods when data-model fit fails is the same as admitting that you did not know anything and, therefore, need the computer to sort things out, and that, of course, cannot be true. You do know something, but the lack of fit tells you that you have made some errors. The best solution to that problem is to think again.

5.9. Bibliography

[AND 04] ANDRICH D., "Controversy and the Rasch model: a characteristic of incompatible paradigms?", *Medical Care*, vol. 42, pp. 7–16, 2004.

[BEN 95] BENJAMINI Y., HOCHBERG Y., "Controlling the false discovery rate: a practical and powerful approach to multiple testing", *Journal Royal Statistical Society, Series B*, vol. 27, pp. 313–324, 1995.

[CHR 07] CHRISTENSEN K.B., KREINER S., "A Monte Carlo test approach to unidimensionality testing in polytomous Rasch models", *Applied Psychological Measurement*, vol. 31, pp. 20–30, 2007.

[DAV 67] DAVIS J.A., "A partial coefficient for Goodman and Kruskall's gamma", *Journal of the American Statistical Association*, vol. 69, pp. 37–46, 1967.

[GLA 95a] GLAS C.A.W., VERHELST N.D., "Testing the Rasch model", in FISCHER G.H., MOLENAAR I.W. (eds), *Rasch models: Foundations, Recent Developments, and Applications*, Springer-Verlag, New York, NY, pp. 69–95, 1995.

[GLA 95b] GLAS C.A.W., VERHELST N.D. "Tests of fit for polytomous Rasch models", in FISCHER G.H., MOLENAAR I.W. (eds), *Rasch models: Foundations, Recent Developments, and Applications*, Springer-Verlag, New York, NY, pp. 325–352, 1995.

[GLA 99] GLAS C.A.W., "Modification indices for the 2-pl and the nominal response model", *Psychometrika*, vol. 64, pp. 273–294, 1999.

[GOO 54] GOODMAN L.A., KRUSKAL W.H., "Measures of association for cross classifications", *Journal of the American Statistical Association*, vol. 49, pp. 732–764, 1954.

[KEL 84] KELDERMAN H., "Loglinear Rasch model tests", *Psychometrika*, vol. 49, pp. 223–245, 1984.

[KRE 87] KREINER S., "Analysis of multidimensional contingency tables by exact conditional tests: techniques and strategies", *Scandinavian Journal of Statistics*, vol. 14, pp. 97–112, 1987.

[KRE 11] KREINER S., "A note on item-restscore association in Rasch models", *Applied Psychological Measurement*, vol. 35, pp. 557–561, 2011.

[MOL 83] MOLENAAR I.W., "Some improved diagnostics for failure of the Rasch model", *Psychometrika*, vol. 48, pp. 49–72, 1983.

[SMI 04] SMITH R.M., "Fit analysis in latent trait measurement models", in SMITH E.V., SMITH R.M. (eds) *Introduction to Rasch measurement*, JAM Press, Maple Grove, Minnesota, pp. 73–92, 2004.

[VAN 82] VAN DEN WOLLENBERG A.L., "Two new test statistics for the Rasch model", *Psychometrika*, vol. 47, pp. 123–139, 1982.

Chapter 6

Overall Tests of the Rasch Model

6.1. Introduction

This chapter describes the overall model fit. Overall fit statistics assess the adequacy of the model for a data set as a whole. Such notions are well known in statistics. During the analysis by generalized linear models, the deviance of the model (the likelihood ratio test of the model relative to a saturated model including all main effects and interaction parameters) is such a statistic. A χ^2 test comparing observed counts of a multidimensional contingency table to the expected counts according to the model is a similar example.

Overall tests of fit are also useful for Rasch models, even though their lack of transparency concerning why the model does not fit means that such fit statistics can never stand alone. This chapter describes a test derived by Erling B. Andersen in the early 1970s and illustrates its use on the data on the disinhibited eating (DE) subscale of the Diabetes Health Profile (DHP) described in Chapter 2. Andersen's test represented a major step forward in the theory of Rasch models at the time. Since then, other overall tests have been proposed but Andersen's test is still unsurpassed by the competitors.

6.2. The conditional likelihood ratio test

The conditional likelihood ratio (CLR) test of Andersen [AND 73] is an overall test of fit of data to the model defined within the conditional frame of inference where the unknown person parameters are replaced by the total scores. The CLR test

---

Chapter written by Svend KREINER and Karl Bang CHRISTENSEN.

compares conditional maximum likelihood (CML) estimates of item parameters in different subgroups to the CML estimates for the complete sample of persons. Let η be a vector of item parameters and let

$$L_v(\eta) = L(X_{v1}, \dots, X_{vk}|R_v = r, \eta) = \exp\left(\sum_{i=1}^{k} \beta_{ix_{vi}}\right) / \gamma_r(\eta) \qquad [6.1]$$

be the conditional probabilities of person v's responses to items given the total score. The conditional likelihood function for all persons of a group G is equal to the product of these probabilities

$$L(G, \eta) = \prod_{v \in G} L_v(\eta) \qquad [6.2]$$

The group G in [6.2] can be the complete sample of persons or any subset of persons. To define a CLR test statistic, we assume that the complete sample of respondents can be decomposed into disjoint subset

$$\{1, \dots, n\} = G_1 \cup \dots \cup G_l$$

of respondents. To test the model, calculate CML estimates $\hat{\beta}$ for the complete sample and CML estimates $\hat{\beta}_g$ in each subsample and define CLR test statistic as

$$CLR = -2 \log \left(\frac{L_0(\hat{\beta})}{\prod_{g=1}^{l} L_g(G_g, \hat{\beta}^{(g)})} \right) \qquad [6.3]$$

Andersen shows that the CLR is asymptotically χ^2 distributed with degrees of freedom equal to $(K-1)(l-1)$, where K is the number of item parameters and l is the number of subsamples. The CLR test can be used in two different ways depending on how the groups are defined. If groups are defined by outcomes on the total score on all items, we refer to the test as a test of *homogeneity* because the test assesses the degrees to which item parameters are homogeneous across all levels of θ. If groups are defined by outcomes of an exogenous covariate, a significant test result is evident that item parameters depend to some degree on the covariate. Therefore, we regard such CLR tests as the overall test of no DIF. Significant evidence of DIF from such tests states that some of the item parameters are different, but a significant result on an overall CLR test of no DIF does not imply that all items function differently in different groups. Overall CLR tests of no DIF are therefore either the first check of no DIF that has to be followed by a careful analysis of the nature of DIF and how to deal with it or the final check that the attempt to take care of the DIF has been successful.

The CLR test is not the only overall test of fit, but there is no convincing evidence that alternative tests developed later are more powerful. Also, mathematical arguments prove that the difference between the true distribution of the CLR statistic and the approximating χ^2 distribution disappears as it increases toward infinity, which is not true for many competing overall tests where asymptotic claims are based on heuristic arguments rather than on rigorous mathematical analysis. Finally, the use of the CLR test for an overall test of no DIF appears to be unique in the theory of Rasch models and psychometrics. In all other cases, the DIF relative to a covariate is always addressed as a problem related to single items and not as a problem connected to a set of items.

For the reasons stated above, we regard the CLR test as the preferable overall fit statistic. This does not mean that other overall tests are useless. They have their weaknesses – for example they always reject the model with a large probability in large sample studies – but when you know about them it is better to take these weaknesses into account for deriving the conclusion.

Having acknowledged the usefulness of overall fit statistics, we should also acknowledge that overall tests are destructive tests. They may disclose misfit between observed data and models, but they rarely provide concrete evidence of what is wrong. Item responses can be heterogeneous for many different reasons so that the fact that the CLR test lets us know that responses are not homogeneous does not tell us exactly what is wrong. Also, the fact that the set of items function differently in different populations does not mean that all items have this problem. Rejecting the data–model fit by a significant CLR test is of very little help when it comes to deciding what to do about it. For this purpose, we need the kind of fit statistics targeting specific types of departure from the model that we looked into in Chapter 5 of this book.

EXAMPLE 6.1.– We illustrate the CLR test by tests of homogeneity and no DIF of the DHP items measuring the degree of DE. Despite the fact that the CLR test is used to test two very different requirements of Rasch models, the information provided and assessed during the tests is very similar. For this reason, we only provide the details for the test of homogeneity and restrict ourselves to the summary results of the test of DIF.

The CLR test of homogeneity compares estimates of item parameters in subjects in different score groups. In the example here, we distinguish between low scores and high scores, but score groups can be defined in any way as long as the number in each score group is acceptable. In this case, 13 out of 189 subjects had extreme scores and therefore provided no information on the item parameters. These are consequently disregarded. The remaining 176 subjects are partitioned into two score groups with approximately the same number of subjects: low scores from one to five and high scores from six to 14.

In each of these groups, we estimate the item parameters, compare the observed and expected item scores under the assumption that item responses are homogeneous and calculate the likelihood functions. Table 6.1 shows the CML estimates of the item thresholds in the two score intervals and in the total sample. Note that for the subsample with low scores, the largest observed item score on DHP38 is equal to one and, for this reason, the estimates of the thresholds higher than one are equal to $+\infty$.

Low scores

Item	β_1	β_2	β_3
DHP32	−0.61	0.45	0.88
DHP34	0.02	−0.67	0.83
DHP36	0.03	−1.07	0.80
DHP38	−0.04	$+\infty$	$+\infty$
DHP39	−1.93	1.50	−0.18

High scores

Item	β_1	β_2	β_3
DHP32	−0.49	1.09	1.10
DHP34	0.18	−0.65	−0.87
DHP36	−0.33	−0.63	0.95
DHP38	−1.28	1.91	0.36
DHP39	−2.58	1.37	−0.11

Complete sample

Item	β_1	β_2	β_3
DHP32	−0.72	0.84	1.25
DHP34	−0.07	−0.67	−0.69
DHP36	−0.31	−0.91	0.93
DHP38	−0.65	1.91	0.19
DHP39	−2.23	1.32	−0.18

Table 6.1. *Estimated item parameters in two score intervals and in the complete sample*

Comparing estimates for the two score intervals with each other and with the item parameter estimates for the complete sample, differences appear to be large, but it is difficult to asses the differences in the expected item scores because item parameters are standardized so that the total sum of all item thresholds is equal to zero. In the low-score group, the largest obtained item score on DHP38 is equal to one and, for this reason, the estimates of the thresholds above one are equal to $+\infty$. These thresholds are therefore disregarded when the sum of thresholds is calculated.

A closer look at the rank order of the item thresholds in the different score intervals discloses similarities and differences, but it is still difficult to say anything concretely about systematic differences in item scores between the two groups. Thresholds are also disordered, which makes it even less transparent what we should expect in terms of observed responses. The only thing we can say is that item thresholds appear to be different. To say more needs at least two things. First, a proper test of the differences and, second, a set of item fit statistics that are more informative than the set of threshold estimates in Table 6.1. The second problem has been solved in Chapter 5. To test whether the difference between the two sets of estimated parameters is larger than that we could explain as a random variation, we use the CLR test discussed above.

To calculate the CLR test, the log likelihood in the low- and high-score groups is -245.09 and -319.08, respectively. For the sample as a whole, the logarithm of the likelihood is equal to -577.75. From this, it follows that the CLR test of homogeneity is equal to 27.2. Since the number of degrees of freedom is 14, it follows that the p-value is equal to 0.018. The evidence is, in other words, significant, although – it has to be admitted – not strongly significant.

The test of DIF relative to gender and age also provides little evidence of DIF. The CLR test comparing item parameter estimates in four age groups is clearly insignificant (CLR $= 42.4$, df $= 42$, $p = 0.45$). The CLR test comparing item parameter estimates for men and women suggests that there may be some DIF (CLR $= 23.7$, df $= 14$, $p = 0.0499$). To get a better understanding of the evidence of DIF, we have to look at the kind of item DIF tests that are described in Chapter 5. These fit statistics indicate that the DIF problem relates to a single item (DHP38) that functions differentially relative to gender. To check that this is the case, we calculate the CLR test of no DIF among the remaining four items. Since CLR $= 10.9$, df $= 11$ and $p = 0.45$, we conclude that the only DIF problem relates to DHP38.

6.3. Other overall tests of fit

As mentioned above, there are other overall tests of fit for the Rasch model. None have been shown to have greater power than Andersen's CLR test and some tests are based on less than solid statistical grounding. Among these are all the statistics defined as sums of item fit statistics or other kinds of summary measures of response residuals. We refer the reader to Chapter 5 on item fit statistics and the discussion of how to calculate Rasch model residuals.

6.4. Bibliography

[AND 73] ANDERSEN E.B., "A goodness of fit test for the Rasch model", *Psychometrika*, vol. 38, pp. 123–140, 1973.

Chapter 7

Local Dependence

7.1. Introduction

The unidimensional Rasch model for dichotomous items

$$P(X_{vi} = x_{vi}|\Theta_v = \theta_v) = \frac{\exp(x_{vi}(\theta_v - \beta_i))}{1 + \exp(\theta_v - \beta_i)} \qquad [7.1]$$

and the unidimensional Rasch model for more than two ordered categories

$$P(X_{vi} = x|\Theta = \theta_v) = \frac{\exp(\theta_v x + \psi_{ix})}{\sum_{h=0}^{m_i} \exp(\theta_v h + \psi_{ih})} \qquad [7.2]$$

rely on the assumption of *local independence*:

$$P(\mathbf{X_v} = \mathbf{x}|\theta_v) = \prod_{i=1}^{k} P(X_{vi} = x_i|\theta_v) \qquad [7.3]$$

where $\mathbf{X_v} = (X_{v1}, \ldots, X_{vk})$ and $\mathbf{x} = (x_1, \ldots, x_k)$. This chapter discusses tests of this assumption and the implications of violations of this assumption in data. Local dependence is related to subtest structure and to estimates of reliability, and therefore these topics are reviewed briefly in this introduction.

Chapter written by Ida MARAIS.

7.1.1. *Reduced rank parameterization model for subtests*

David Andrich [AND 85] described an early attempt to address situations where the assumption of local independence is violated. Assume equally spaced thresholds for an item. Then the model of [7.2] can be rewritten as

$$P(X_{vi} = x|\Theta = \theta_v) = \frac{\exp(x(\theta_v - \delta_i) + x(m_i - x)\lambda_i)}{K(\theta_v, \delta_i, \lambda_i)} \qquad [7.4]$$

where δ_i is a location parameter, λ_i is a spread parameter and this parameterization is effectively of reduced rank for polytomous items with $m_i > 2$. On the basis of this parameterization, a model that takes account of dependencies among items in subtests is

$$P(X_{vi} = x|\Theta = \theta_v) = \frac{\exp(x(\theta_v - \delta_k) + x(m_i - x)\lambda_k)}{K(\theta_v, \delta_k, \lambda_k)} \qquad [7.5]$$

for items in subtest $k = 1, 2, \ldots$ has been proposed [AND 85]. The spread parameter for each subtest can be used to confirm the presence of response dependence.

It characterizes the spread or dispersion of the responses in subtest k. The greater the value, the smaller is the spread of responses, that is, the greater is the proportion of responses in the middle response category, and the greater is the spread of the corresponding thresholds. The smaller the value of the spread parameter, the greater is the spread of responses, that is, the greater is the proportion of responses in the extreme categories, and the smaller is the spread of the threshold values. The dispersion of responses reflects dependence and this parameter provides a way of detecting dependence in a data set. Local dependence implies that, when one item in a subtest is local answered in a specified way, then there is increased probability, over and above that accounted for by θ, of answering other items in the subtest in the same way. Therefore, the greater the dependence, the greater is the prevalence of responses in the extreme categories. Andrich [AND 85] provides values below which there is likely to be local dependence in the set of items.

7.1.2. *Reliability indices*

Local dependence in data impacts estimates of reliability. The traditional index of reliability used in classical test theory is Cronbach's coefficient α [CRO 51], but an index constructed with Rasch measurement, the Person Separation Index (PSI), also exists. The PSI is based on the traditional true score reliability formula [GUL 50], where reliability is a function of both the variance of the observed estimates $\hat{\sigma}^2_{\hat{\beta}}$ and the error of measurement $\hat{\sigma}^2_{\hat{e}}$. The PSI is given by

$$r_{\beta\beta} = \frac{\sigma^2_\beta}{\sigma^2_\beta + \sigma^2_e} = \frac{\hat{\sigma}^2_{\hat{\beta}} - \hat{\sigma}^2_{\hat{e}}}{\hat{\sigma}^2_{\hat{\beta}}}$$

where $\hat{\sigma}_{\hat{\beta}}^2$ is the estimated variance of the locations of the persons and $\hat{\sigma}_{\hat{e}}^2$ is the average squared standard error of measurement for each person. The PSI is a function of both the variance of the estimates of the person locations and the error of measurement variance. Under the conditions where the distribution of the total score R is not artificially skewed because of floor and ceiling effects so that the relationship between R and θ is close to linear, the values of this index and Cronbach's α are virtually identical [AND 82].

7.2. Local dependence in Rasch models

The term *local* refers to the idea that all the variation among responses to an item is accounted for by the person parameter θ, and therefore that for the same value of θ, there is no further relationship among responses [AND 91, LAZ 68].

In the Rasch models, the person parameter θ_v, which is the source of dependence among item responses, can be eliminated by sufficiency and conditioning arguments because it can be shown that two items from a Rasch model are conditionally independent, given the rest score without one of the two items [TJU 82, KRE 04]. With the person parameter eliminated in this way, there should be no more dependence among items. The entire correlation between items has to be captured by the latent trait (i.e. the person parameter θ). Correlations between items not captured by the latent trait are indicative of local dependence.

Local independence in Rasch models as defined here can be violated in several generic ways. Two of these have been formalized algebraically by Marais and Andrich [MAR 08a]. First, there may be person parameters other than θ that are involved in the response. This condition is a violation of unidimensionality and hence of statistical independence relative to the unidimensional Rasch model. This type of violation is addressed in Chapter 9 on multidimensionality.

Second, for the same person and therefore the same value of θ, the response to one item might depend on the response to a previous item. This condition is clearly a violation of statistical independence. To distinguish this latter violation from violations of unidimensionality, Marais and Andrich have referred to it as *response dependence* [MAR 08a, MAR 08b]. This type of violation of Rasch models is the subject of this chapter.

7.2.1. *Response dependence*

Response dependence occurs when a person's response to an item depends on the response to a previous item. For valid sums from sets of items, each item in the set needs to provide related but independent information, or relevant but not redundant information. An extreme case of response dependence occurs when the responses of each person to the two items are identical, thus making one item completely redundant.

An example of response dependence is found in the physical functioning subscale of the SF-36. The SF-36 is a widely used rating scale in health research [WAR 93]. It has eight subscales: physical functioning, role-physical, bodily pain, general health, vitality, social functioning, role-emotional, and mental health. Kreiner and Christensen showed that, in the physical functioning subscale, the items *climbing one flight of stairs* and *climbing several flights of stairs* are response dependent and that the items *walking one block, walking several blocks* and *walking more than a mile* are response dependent [KRE 07].

Response dependence can be also found in patient satisfaction questionnaires, with an item requesting an *overall* level of satisfaction following several other satisfaction items. The response to an overall level of satisfaction item is often dependent on the responses to the other satisfaction items. Response dependence is also found when a person's *overall* quality of life (QOL) is assessed in a question following several other, more specific, QOL questions, for example in the Parkinson's Disease Questionnaire (PDQ-39) question, *Everything taken together, how do you perceive your overall quality of life?* Response dependence can also be found when one item is made a negative of the other, for example, *I feel people like me* and *I don't feel people like me* [HAG 09].

Response dependence is also often found where raters make judgments on a set of criteria. Patients are sometimes assessed by others using a rating scale consisting of a number of criteria. The use of ratings by different raters rests on the assumption that raters can make an independent judgment on each criterion. However, it has been shown that, despite training, raters sometimes assign ratings on the different criteria, which are more similar than they would be if rated independently [MYF 04]. Such a rater fails to distinguish between distinct aspects of the person's proficiency or health outcome to the degree that would be found, for example, if different raters each judged all persons by one criterion only. This phenomenon is called a "halo effect" and is a violation of the assumption of independence. It leads to an artificial consistency between the ratings of a rater. Criteria become redundant because they do not provide information independent of other criteria.

7.3. Effects of response dependence on measurement

Until fairly recently, response dependence was rarely addressed in Rasch analyses in health outcome studies. If accurate person measurement is the goal, this type of violation of the assumption of independence cannot be ignored.

Of those who have studied the various effects of response dependence on measurement by the Rasch model [MAR 08a, MAR 08b, SMI 05], some have concluded that it did not have a significant effect on estimates [SMI 05], whereas others have found the effects to be large and of concern [MAR 08a, MAR 08b]. It is well known that positive local response dependence inflates measures of reliability in Rasch models and other congeneric measurement models [LUC 05].

Marais and Andrich varied the *magnitude* of dependence among selected items, rather than having only an extreme magnitude of dependence [MAR 08b]. They formalized the dependence of a dichotomous item j on a dichotomous item i by

$$P(X_{vj} = x_j | X_{vi} = x_i) = \frac{\exp(x_j(\theta_v - \beta_j - (1 - 2x_i)d))}{1 + \exp(x_j(\theta_v - \beta_j - (1 - 2x_i)d))} \qquad [7.6]$$

If a person's response to item i is $x_{vi} = 1$, then the difficulty of the dependent item j changes from β_j to $\beta_j - d$ for that person. Hence, the dependent item becomes easier to endorse, thus also increasing the probability of a response of $x_{vj} = 1$. Conversely, if a person's response to item i is $x_{vi} = 0$ then the location of the dependent item changes to $\beta_j + d$ for that person, consequently increasing the probability of a response $x_{vj} = 0$. The value d quantifies the *magnitude* of response dependence. They found that as the magnitude of dependence increases, the similarity of the responses of persons across items increases, so fit statistics and parameters showed increasing discrepancies from their theoretical values as a function of the magnitude of dependence. The also found that indices of reliability and the standard deviation (SD) of the distribution of the person parameter estimates under the Rasch model increased with increasing magnitude of dependence.

Andrich, Humphry and Marais formalized dependence between two polytomous items in a different way. In the case of a polytomous item j dependent on a polytomous item i with the same number of categories they formalized the dependence as a change in the location of thresholds separating adjacent categories in item j caused by its dependence on item i [AND 12]

Both the traditional index of reliability, Cronbach's coefficient α, and the PSI constructed with Rasch measurement, are increased in the presence of positive response dependence. The increase in the SD of the distribution of person estimates and PSI due to local response dependency gives an impression of improvement with increasing dependence, and these statistics appear more favorable than they really are. These are favorable in the sense that they indicate that persons have been separated by measures of the latent trait. However, reliability in the presence of response dependence is inflated. This inflation is an example of a situation where higher reliability does not mean better measurement. These effects can be predicted by the attenuation paradox of traditional test theory, which states that, up to a point, reliability and validity increase together, but any further increase in reliability decreases validity.

With increasing response dependence, a reliability index systematically increases as a result of an increase in similarity of responses among items. If responses for all items are identical for all persons, the reliability reaches its maximum, but the validity is that of only one item.

In addition to the magnitude of dependence, Marais and Andrich also varied the difficulties of the item on which others depended and the number of items that were dependent on any one item. The effects of the statistics were different for these different patterns of dependence. When items were dependent on an easily endorsed item, the person location mean increased and the person distribution was skewed and unimodal. When items were dependent on an item with an average item location parameter, the person location mean did not increase significantly and the person distribution was bimodal.

To illustrate the effect of disregarding local response dependence, Figure 7.1 shows the estimated person–item distributions for a simulated data set with no dependence (top), and for a data set simulated according to the same specifications but with all items dependent on an easily endorsed item (low β_i, middle) and for a data simulated according to the same specifications but with items dependent on an item with an average value of β_i (bottom). Dependence was simulated according to [7.6] with $d = 1$. Data were simulated for $N = 1{,}000$ persons and $I = 30$ items. All items were *dichotomous* and were analyzed with the dichotomous Rasch model using RUMM2030 [AND 10b].

What is evident from the figure is the increased person SD in the cases with dependence relative to the case with no dependence. With no dependence, the SD was 1.102, close to the simulated value of one. In the case of dependence on an easily endorsed item, the SD increased to 1.344. The shape of the person location distribution changed from matching the simulation source, which was normal, in the case of no dependence, to being positively skewed in the case of dependence on an easily endorsed item. The reason for this skew shift is that there is a high probability of a response of one on the conditioning item i. It follows that the dependent items will also have a high probability of a response of one. Hence, many persons will be scoring one on items resulting in higher person estimates.

In the case of dependence on an item with an average location parameter, the SD was 1.794 and the person location distribution changes to being bimodal. If a person scores one on the conditioning item, then as a result of dependence the person will tend to score one on the majority of the dependent items too. Likewise, if a person scores zero on the conditioning item, then as a result of dependence the person will tend to score zero on the majority of the dependent items too. Because the item has an average location parameter, approximately half of the persons will score one on the conditioning item and the other half will score 0 on it. These two halves are separated by the conditioning, which results in the bimodal structure of the distribution.

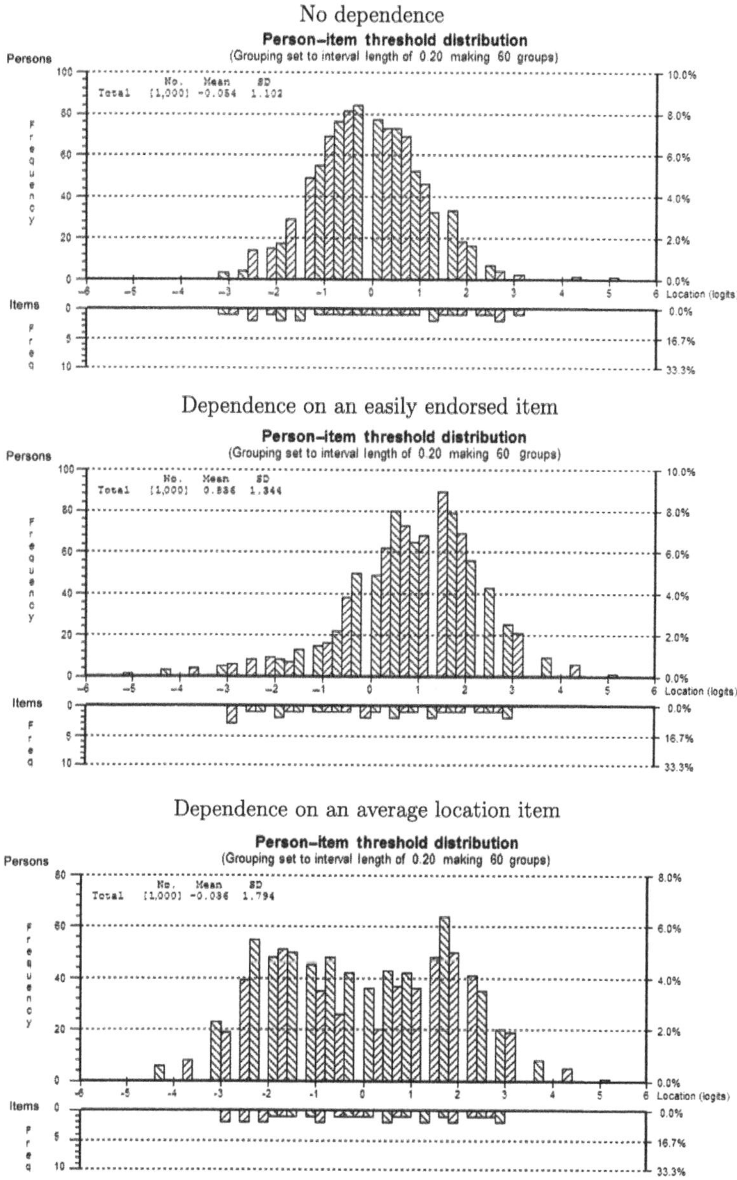

Figure 7.1. *Person and item location distributions for a data set with no dependence (top), data simulated according to the same specifications but with items dependent on an easily endorsed item (middle) and data simulated according to the same specifications but with items dependent on a item with an average location parameter (bottom)*

With the variance of person estimates affected by dependence, it is easy to see how the PSI is also affected. The PSI is a function of both the variance of person estimates and of the error of measurement. Report of an inflated reliability of an instrument is misleading and gives a false impression of the accuracy and precision of estimates.

Change scores may be affected, if calculated by using person estimates from data with dependence. When response dependence is present, which results in an increased person SD and a comparable or diminished $\hat{\sigma}_{\hat{e}}^2$, there may be an increased risk of a type one error during tests comparing repeated measurements. A minor change in the conditioning item may be associated with exaggerated signals arising from the dependent items.

7.4. Diagnosing and detecting response dependence

The Rasch models, with their assumption of local independence of responses, are a formal representation and definition of measurement. Hence, an analysis according to a Rasch model will reveal a violation of the assumption of independence as an anomaly [AND 04].

7.4.1. *Item fit*

Response dependence will be reflected in the fit of data to the model. Response dependence increases the similarity of the responses of persons across items and responses are then more Guttman-like than they should be under no dependence. Fit can be assessed *for each item* by assigning the persons into class intervals according to their locations on the measured construct. The degree of accordance between class interval responses and model expectations, represented by the item characteristic curve (ICC), is then studied graphically as well as statistically. Positive local response dependence will generate evidence of overdiscrimination and evidence that items are overdiscriminating often indicates response dependence. Kreiner gives an example on this situation on data measuring mobility among the older adults [KRE 11]. However, response dependence is not the only reason for overdiscriminating items. Other reasons include, for example, effects of the unit of measurement [HUM 08].

Whereas response dependence increases the similarity of the responses of persons across items and generates responses that are more Guttman-like than they should be under no dependence, multidimensionality acts as an extra source of variation (noise) in the data, and the responses are less Guttman-like than they should be under no dependence. This then results in items underdiscriminating. Figure 7.2 shows the ICCs for an item that fits reasonably well (top), an overdiscriminating item (middle) and an underdiscriminating item (bottom).

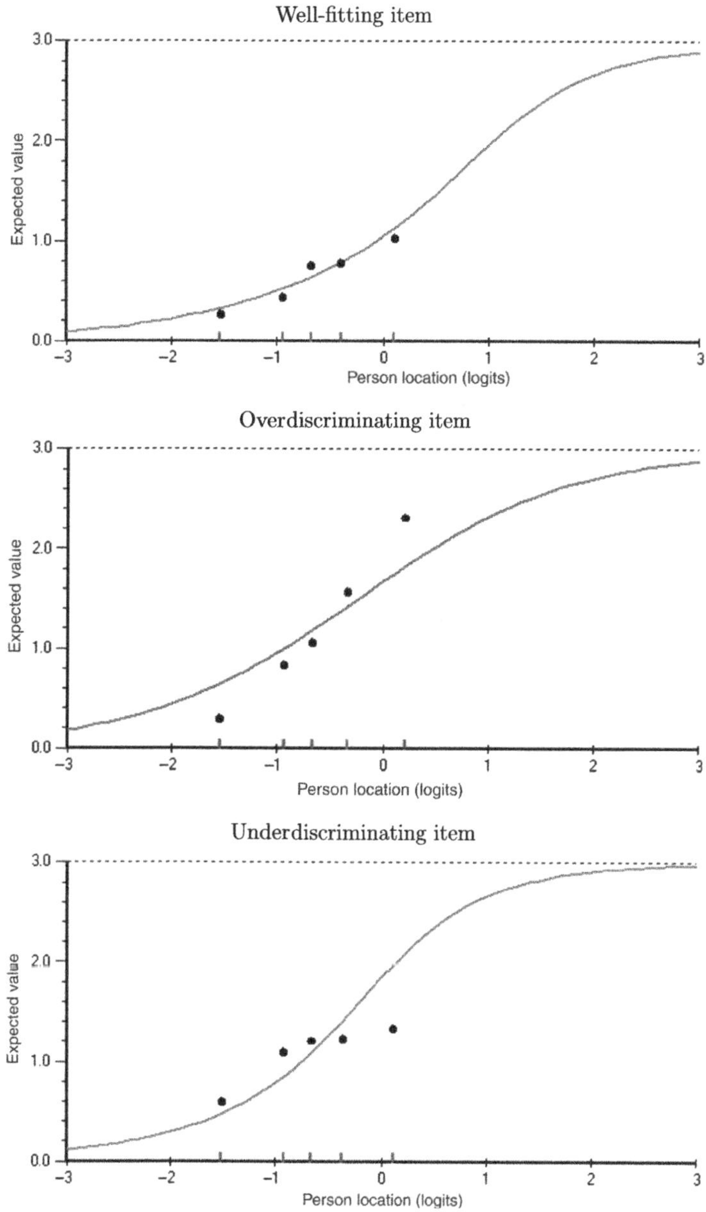

Figure 7.2. *ICCs for an item that fits reasonably well (top), an overdiscriminating item (middle) and an underdiscriminating item (bottom)*

7.4.2. *Item residual correlations*

Response dependence can be detected by examining the item residual correlations. Residuals are person–item differences between the observed data and what is expected by the model for each person's response to each item. Therefore, the *standardized residual* is given by

$$Z_{vi} = \frac{X_{vi} - E[X_{vi}]}{\sqrt{V[X_{vi}]}} \qquad [7.7]$$

where X_{vi} is the observed response, $E[X_{vi}]$ the expected response of person v to item i and $V[X_{vi}]$ the variance of the observed responses for all persons to item i as calculated under the Rasch model.

If the data fit the model, then over a reasonably large number of persons and items, the residuals for any pair of items should not be correlated with each other, but be generally close to 0. High correlations between standardized item residuals indicate a violation of the assumption of local independence by the corresponding pair of items. If the observed correlation is relatively large, it suggests that the pair of items have something more in common than all of the items have in common with each other. The larger the number of items, the more easily interpretable are the residual correlations, and perhaps at least 20 items should be present before observed residual correlations are interpreted confidently. In addition, the correlations should also always be considered *relative to overall set of correlations*.

Positive local response dependence between two items may create spurious evidence of negative local dependence among items that are independent. This evidence will be very pronounced if the number of items is small, for example five or six.

This is illustrated in Table 7.1, which shows the item residual correlations for the first five items of three simulated data sets with five, 15 and 25 polytomous items, respectively. Because of space restrictions, only the correlations amongst the first five items are shown, and these are sufficient to illustrate the point. The simulation specifications for the three data sets were identical, except for the number of items. All items have four response categories. Item three was simulated to be dependent on item one, with the same magnitude of dependence in all three sets and dependence in polytomous items was simulated according to the same principle as in the dichotomous case, by adjusting the location of the dependent item by a constant, $d = 1$. No other items were simulated to be dependent.

It is clear from the table that the magnitude of the residual correlation between items one and three depends on the number of items in the data set. With only five items, the correlation is 0.087, with 15 items it increases to 0.172 and with 25 items it increases to 0.317. Unfortunately, the sampling properties of the correlations among residuals are unknown. It is therefore not possible to use these statistics for formal tests of local independence. Instead, item pairs with item residual correlations above a cutoff of 0.3 are often considered as being response dependent. If a cutoff of 0.3 was used, the dependence in the data sets with five and 15 items would go undetected, even though it is of the same magnitude as the dependence in the 25-item data set.

5 items	1	2	3	4	5	
1	1					
2	−0.337	1				
3	**0.087**	−0.276	1			
4	−0.207	−0.201	−0.235	1		
5	−0.122	−0.125	−0.160	−0.154	1	**average: −0.173**
15 items	1	2	3	4	5	
1	1					
2	−0.025	1				
3	**0.172**	−0.069	1			
4	−0.060	−0.100	−0.106	1		
5	−0.125	−0.053	−0.073	−0.089	1	**average: −0.053**
25 items	1	2	3	4	5	
1	1					
2	−0.057	1				
3	**0.317**	−0.033	1			
4	−0.057	−0.041	−0.081	1		
5	−0.108	−0.076	−0.087	−0.034	1	**average: −0.026**

Table 7.1. *First five item residual correlations for three data sets with five, 15 and 25 items*

Such cut points should be used carefully. If we examine the *relative magnitude* of the item residual correlations, the dependence can be detected in all three data sets. Compared to the average item residual correlation of −0.173 in the five-item data set, the correlation between items one and three of 0.087 is relatively large and is the only positive correlation. Compared to the average item residual correlation of −0.053 in the 15-item data set, the correlation between items one and three of 0.172 is relatively large and is the only positive correlation. (The average of only the first five items is used for illustrative purposes and this average is representative of the overall average.) Compared to the average item residual correlation of −0.026 in the 25-item data set, the correlation between items one and three of 0.317 is relatively large and is the only positive correlation. The conclusion is that, in diagnosing response dependence, item residual correlations should be considered relative to each other and in the light of the number of items.

7.4.3. *Subtests and reliability*

Another way of detecting response dependence is by comparing reliability estimates from two separate analyses of the data [AND 85, ZEN 02]. The first estimate uses the original items and assumes that all items are statistically independent. In a second analysis, items hypothesized to be dependent are combined into higher-order polytomous items and the data reanalyzed as polytomous items. If the reliability estimate from this analysis is lower than the reliability estimate from the first analysis, the case for the hypothesis of response dependence is strengthened. In RUMM2030, such higher-order polytomous items made up of other items are called *subtests*. Reduced reliability in the second analysis in the presence of dependence occurs for both Cronbach α and the PSI, and this reduced reliability should be taken as the more valid description of the data.

7.4.4. *Estimating the magnitude of response dependence*

Marais and Andrich [MAR 08a] described the response dependence of two dichotomous items by the model [7.6] where d is a measure of the strength of the dependence of the items. The estimation of d is described in [AND 10a] where d is interpreted as a change in the location of the second item because of its dependence on the first item. In other words, the estimate is a value, in logits, of how much the dependence on item i has changed the location of item j on the measurement continuum. In [AND 12], the focus is on dependence between two dichotomous items, but it has been generalized to polytomous items. In the case of response dependence between two polytomous items, the magnitude can be estimated as a change in the location of thresholds separating adjacent categories in the dependent item. Log-linear Rasch models [KEL 84] add interaction terms to the joint distribution of items, which can also be interpreted as changes in location due to responses on other items, but there are subtle differences between the model of Andrich and Kreiner [AND 10a] and Kelderman's log-linear Rasch model [KEL 84]. One of these is that the total score over dependent items is distributed as a partial credit item under the Kelderman's model. The same is not true under the model discussed by Andrich and Kreiner. In this sense, we could argue that it is the Kelderman model that lies behind the analysis of reliability and subtests described above.

7.4.5. *Illustration*

To illustrate the aforementioned methods of detecting and diagnosing response dependence, two data sets were simulated. The data were simulated according to exactly the same specifications, including the same magnitude of dependence. The only difference was the number of items in each data set. One data set had 10 dichotomous items (data set A) and the other had 20 dichotomous items (data set B).

Items two and three were simulated to be dependent on item one according to [7.6] using $d = 1$. Each data set contained responses for 1,000 persons. The data were analyzed using RUMM2030 [AND 10b].

Data set A: 10 items					
Item	β (SE)	FitResid	χ^2	df	p-value
I0001	−0.07 (0.08)	−3.87	59.39	6	0.00
I0002	−0.13 (0.08)	−3.84	44.99	6	0.00
I0003	0.09 (0.08)	−3.27	29.51	6	0.00
I0004	−3.36 (0.14)	−1.04	8.65	6	0.19
I0005	−1.88 (0.09)	0.62	16.85	6	0.01
I0006	−0.97 (0.08)	−0.88	14.30	6	0.03
I0007	0.04 (0.08)	0.92	12.35	6	0.05
I0008	1.06 (0.08)	0.67	10.97	6	0.09
I0009	2.04 (0.09)	−0.13	13.94	6	0.03
I0010	3.19 (0.13)	−0.65	11.61	6	0.07
Data set B: 20 items					
Item	β (SE)	FitResid	χ^2	df	p-value
I0001	0.06 (0.07)	−3.58	29.07	9	0.00
I0002	0.05 (0.07)	−4.00	39.60	9	0.00
I0003	0.07 (0.07)	−3.47	28.74	9	0.00
I0004	−3.12 (0.13)	−0.91	5.77	9	0.76
I0005	−2.38 (0.10)	0.56	18.29	9	0.03
I0006	−2.23 (0.10)	−0.11	12.26	9	0.20
I0007	−1.95 (0.09)	−1.18	6.56	9	0.68
I0008	−1.62 (0.08)	−0.19	12.94	9	0.17
I0009	−1.07 (0.08)	1.66	8.16	9	0.52
I0010	−0.74 (0.07)	−1.03	10.18	9	0.34
I0011	−0.32 (0.07)	0.25	6.04	9	0.74
I0012	0.02 (0.07)	−0.67	13.13	9	0.16
I0013	0.25 (0.07)	1.58	9.08	9	0.43
I0014	0.67 (0.07)	1.19	4.61	9	0.87
I0015	1.18 (0.08)	−0.18	4.70	9	0.86
I0016	1.58 (0.09)	0.37	3.76	9	0.93
I0017	1.79 (0.09)	−0.80	4.25	9	0.89
I0018	2.40 (0.10)	−1.03	4.33	9	0.89
I0019	2.48 (0.11)	0.04	15.98	9	0.07
I0020	2.88 (0.12)	0.26	9.18	9	0.42

Table 7.2. *Item locations and fit statistics for data set A and B*

The first diagnostic that indicated misfit to the model was item fit. Table 7.2 shows the item locations (with standard errors (s.e.)), the average of the standardized response residuals (FitResid) with degrees of freedom (df) and χ^2 fit statistic, for both data sets, as shown by using RUMM2030. Items one, two and three overdiscriminated in both data sets. This inference is indicated by the relatively large negative fit residual statistic. The misfit is statistically significant. The ICCs for items one, two and three for data set A, are shown in Figure 7.3, clearly show the misfit. In these figures, Locn is the location of the item, FitResid is the average standardized response residuals and ChiSqu is the p-value of the χ^2 fit statistic.

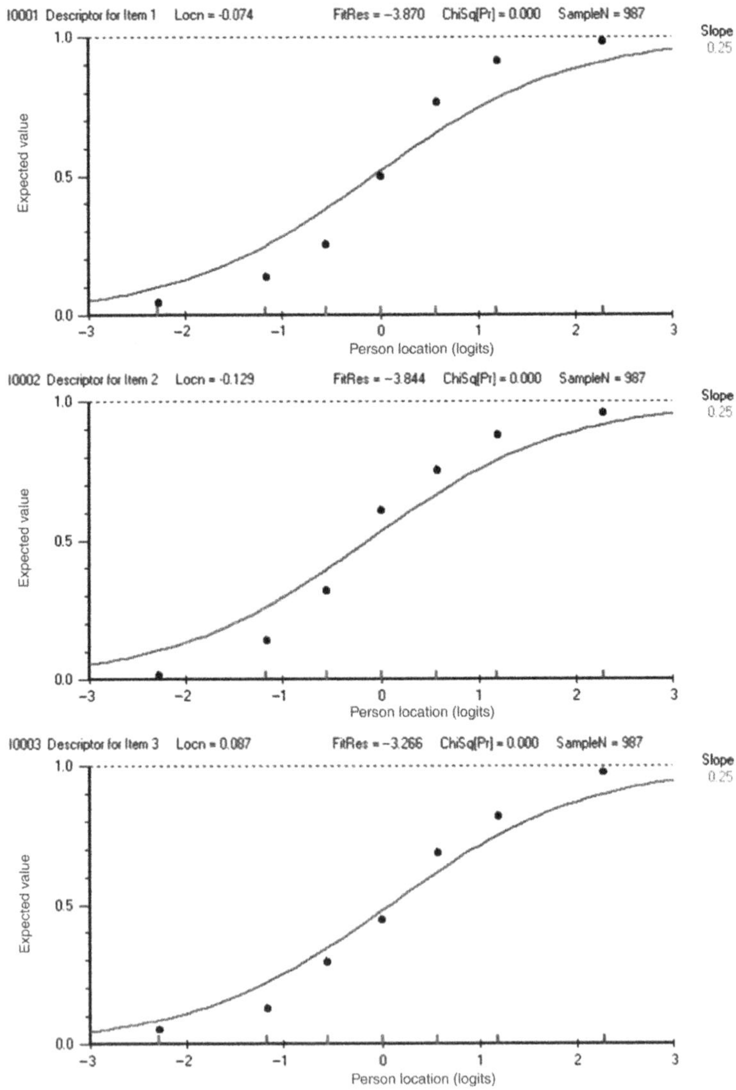

Figure 7.3. *Item characteristic curves (ICCs) for items one, two and three from data set A. Black dots are observed proportions*

The first diagnostic indicating response dependence involved the item residual correlations. Table 7.3 shows these values, with only correlations between items in the first set of 10 shown for data set B due to space restrictions.

Data set A: 10 items

Item	1	2	3	4	5	6	7	8	9	10
1	1									
2	**0.192**	1								
3	**0.204**	−0.061	1							
4	−0.141	−0.077	−0.081	1						
5	−0.171	−0.162	−0.172	−0.050	1					
6	−0.176	−0.201	−0.169	−0.019	−0.065	1				
7	−0.256	−0.126	−0.211	−0.089	−0.110	−0.094	1			
8	−0.203	−0.204	−0.183	−0.062	−0.038	−0.160	−0.063	1		
9	−0.165	−0.127	−0.131	−0.051	−0.075	−0.050	−0.073	−0.075	1	
10	−0.116	−0.106	−0.094	0.025	−0.092	−0.035	−0.046	−0.055	−0.063	1
									Average:	**−0.095**

Data set B: 20 items

Item	1	2	3	4	5	6	7	8	9	10
1	1									
2	**0.360**	1								
3	**0.284**	0.069	1							
4	−0.060	−0.040	−0.110	1						
5	−0.063	−0.025	−0.043	−0.042	1					
6	−0.090	−0.101	−0.046	0.031	0.015	1				
7	−0.091	−0.073	−0.060	−0.077	−0.043	−0.035	1			
8	−0.109	−0.031	−0.089	−0.055	0.006	0.012	−0.030	1		
9	−0.140	−0.036	−0.105	−0.035	0.026	−0.032	−0.020	−0.008	1	
10	−0.065	−0.083	−0.054	−0.040	−0.009	−0.056	−0.062	−0.055	−0.042	1
									Average:	**−0.030**

Table 7.3. *Item residual correlations for data sets A and B*

It is clear from the table that, even though simulated with the same magnitude of dependence, the item residual correlations between the dependent items of data set A (0.192 and 0.204) are lower than the corresponding correlations of data set B (0.360 and 0.284). However, relative to the other correlations (average correlation of −0.095) of item pairs in data set A, the positive correlations between items one and two and items one and three are large.

The second diagnostic that indicated response dependence was the decrease in reliability when the dependent items were summed into a subtest. Table 7.4 shows, for both data sets, $\hat{\sigma}^2_{\hat{\beta}}$ and $\hat{\sigma}^2_{\hat{e}}$, and the PSI for the first analysis and the subtest analysis wherein items one, two and three were summed into one subtest. For data set A, the PSI decreased from 0.65 to 0.60. This evidence strengthens the case for the hypothesis of response dependence. For data set B, the PSI decreased from 0.74 to 0.72. Even though this decrease does not seem large, it is consistent with evidence for response dependence from the other diagnostics and therefore strengthens the case for dependence. The PSIs from the first analyses were inflated whereas the PSIs from the subtest analyses were more realistic.

Data set A: 10 items			
Analysis	$\hat{\sigma}^2_{\hat{\beta}}$	$\hat{\sigma}^2_{\hat{e}}$	PSI
First (before subtest)	2.217	0.774	0.651
Subtest	1.765	0.700	0.603
Data set B: 20 items			
Analysis	$\hat{\sigma}^2_{\hat{\beta}}$	$\hat{\sigma}^2_{\hat{e}}$	PSI
First (before subtest)	1.349	0.352	0.739
Subtest	1.158	0.329	0.716

Table 7.4. *The values $\hat{\sigma}^2_{\hat{\beta}}$, $\hat{\sigma}^2_{\hat{e}}$, and the Person Separation Index (PSI) before and after the subtest analyses for data sets A and B*

Table 7.5 shows the estimated values of the spread parameters λ_k; see [7.5] for subtests $k = 1, 2, 3$ for data sets A and B. As mentioned above, subtest one consisted of the summed responses of the dependent items one, two and three. Subtests two and three were each created by combining three non-dependent items drawn randomly from the remaining items. The RUMM2030 output also shows the location and slope estimate calculated as the slope of the ICC for the subtest at the point on the curves where the expected score equals the person location.

Data set A: 10 items						
Subtest	Location	SE	Slope	SE	Spread	SE
1	−0.61	0.04	1.25	0.03	0.00	0.035
2	−2.29	0.05	0.77	0.03	0.52	0.036
3	0.40	0.04	0.69	0.02	0.63	0.035
Data set B: 20 items						
Subtest	Location	SE	Slope	SE	Spread	SE
1	−0.40	0.03	1.31	0.03	−0.06	0.03
2	−3.00	0.06	0.67	0.03	0.66	0.04
3	0.24	0.04	0.74	0.03	0.56	0.03

Table 7.5. *Location, slope and spread (λ_k) parameters for three subtests.*

For data set A, the value of the spread parameter for the first subtest was 0.00, well below the cutoff value of 0.55 suggested for subtests with a maximum score of 3 [AND 85]. The values 0.52 and 0.63 were considerably higher. For data set B, the value was -0.06, again well below the cutoff value of 0.55. The values 0.66 and 0.56, respectively, were considerably higher.

The fourth diagnostic that confirmed response dependence and gave an indication of its magnitude involved the values of d, calculated according to Andrich and Kreiner [AND 10a]. Table 7.6 shows the location values of items two and three after they had been resolved on the basis of the persons' responses to item one. Item 2S0 contains the responses to item two of those persons who responded zero to item one. Item 2S1 contains the responses to item two of those persons who responded one to item one. For data set A, the item locations for items 2S0 and 2S1 are 0.82 and -1.06, respectively. That is, when persons scored zero on item one, item two was more difficult to endorse than it would otherwise have been. In contrast, when persons scored one on item one, item two was easier for them to endorse than it would otherwise have been.

Table 7.6 also shows the calculated values of d, the magnitude of dependence, according to Andrich and Kreiner [AND 10a]. The calculated values of d (0.939 and 0.923 for data set A and 1.104 and 0.957 for data set B) were all close to the simulated value of d=1. This output shows that the magnitude of dependence was the same for data sets A and B, even though the item residual correlations were smaller for data set A than for data set B. It shows, once again, that the residual correlations need to be examined relative to all correlations in the matrix, and taking into consideration the number of items. Furthermore, we see that a model-based analysis estimating the phenomenon in question gives a clearer picture than heuristic fit statistics.

Data set A: 10 items			
Item	Location	SE	
2S0	0.82	0.12	
2S1	-1.06	0.12	$d = (0.82 - 1.06)/2 = 0.939$
3S0	1.03	0.12	
3S1	-0.82	0.11	$d = (1.03 - 0.82)/2 = 0.923$
Data set B: 20 items			
Item	Location	SE	
2S0	1.15	0.12	
2S1	-1.06	0.12	$d = (1.15 - 1.06)/2 = 1.104$
3S0	1.00	0.11	
3S1	-0.91	0.11	$d = (1.00 - 0.91)/2 = 0.957$

Table 7.6. *Resolved item locations and values of d*

7.5. Summary

In this chapter, some examples of response dependence in health outcome scales were given. The effects of response dependence on estimates were outlined, using evidence from simulation studies. Different ways by which response dependence can be detected and diagnosed were discussed and illustrated.

The methods discussed in this chapter are not the only approaches to detecting and diagnosing response dependence. Another approach to detecting violations of independence is through graphical log-linear Rasch models (GLLRMs). These models are visual diagrams illustrating the structure of Rasch models, allowing the use of graphical model theory [KRE 04]. Items are presented by nodes and nodes are disconnected if items are conditionally independent. Hence, the properties of Rasch models, and violations of these properties, are encoded in a graphical representation. Dependence parameters, partial gamma coefficients, are estimated and describe the interactions between two items (e.g. [KRE 04, KRE 07]).

Lawson and Brailovsky describe the impact of dependence on structured clinical chiropractic examination ratings and suggest the use of the multifaceted Rasch model to account for dependence [LAW 06].

The Rasch models, with their assumption of local independence of responses, are a formal representation and definition of measurement. Hence, an analysis according to a Rasch model will reveal a violation of this assumption as an anomaly [AND 04]. Andrich describes two approaches that can be taken when there is a data-model misfit, as is the case with dependence in the data. In the traditional approach, a model that better fits the data is sought whenever there is a misfit. In the Rasch approach, misfit reveals anomalies. Ideally, items are modified and new data without the anomalies are collected so that measurements conform better to the measurement model and also enhance the validity of the assessment.

7.6. Bibliography

[AND 82] ANDRICH D., "A two parameter extension of the Rasch model for ratings", *Psychometrika*, vol. 47, pp. 105–113, 1982.

[AND 85] ANDRICH D., "A latent trait model for items with response dependencies: Implications for instrument construction and analysis", in EMBRETSON S. (ed.), *Test Design: Contributions from Psychology, Education and Psychometrics*, Academic Press, New York, pp. 245–273, 1985.

[AND 91] ANDRICH D., "Essay. Review of Rolf Langeheine and Jurgen Rost, Latent Trait and Latent Class Analysis, New York, 1988", *Psychometrika*, vol. 56, pp. 155–168, 1991.

[AND 04] ANDRICH D., "Controversy and the Rasch model: a characteristic of incompatible paradigms?" *Medical Care*, vol. 42, pp. 1–15, 2004.

[AND 10a] ANDRICH D., KREINER S., "Quantifying response dependence between two dichotomous items using the Rasch model", *Applied Psychological Measurement*, vol. 34, pp. 181–192, 2010.

[AND 10b] ANDRICH D., SHERIDAN B., LUO G., RUMM2030, computer software and manual, RUMM Laboratory, Perth, Australia, 2010.

[AND 12] ANDRICH D., HUMPHRY S.M., MARAIS I., "Quantifying local, response dependence between two polytomous items using the Rasch model", *Applied Psychological Measurement*, vol. 36, pp. 309–324, 2012.

[CRO 51] CRONBACH L.J., "Coefficient alpha and the internal structure of tests", *Psychometrika*, vol. 16, pp. 297–334, 1951.

[GUL 50] GULLIKSEN H., *Theory of Mental Tests*, Wiley, New York, NY, 1950.

[HAG 09] HAGQUIST C., BRUCE M., GUSTAVSSON J.P., "Using the Rasch model in nursing research: an introduction and illustrative example", *International Journal of Nursing Studies*, vol. 46, pp. 380–393, 2009.

[HUM 08] HUMPHRY S.M., ANDRICH D., "Understanding the unit in the Rasch model", *Journal of Applied Measurement*, vol. 9, pp. 249–264, 2008.

[KEL 84] KELDERMAN H., "Loglinear Rasch model tests", *Psychometrika*, vol. 49, pp. 223–245, 1984.

[KRE 04] KREINER S., CHRISTENSEN K.B., "Analysis of local dependence and multidimensionality in graphical loglinear models", *Communications in Statistics – Theory and Methods*, vol. 33, pp. 1239–1276, 2004.

[KRE 07] KREINER S., CHRISTENSEN K.B., "Validity and objectivity in health related scales: analysis by graphical loglinear Rasch models", in VON DAVIER M., CARSTENSEN C.H. (eds), *Multivariate and Mixture Distribution Rasch Models: Extensions and Applications*, Springer, New York, pp. 329–346, 2007.

[KRE 11] KREINER S., "A Note on item-restscore association in Rasch models", *Applied Psychological Measurement*, vol. 35, pp. 557–561, 2011.

[LAW 06] LAWSON D.M., BRAILOVSKY C., "The presence and impact of local item dependence on objective structured clinical examinations scores and the potential use of the polytomous, many-facet Rasch model", *Journal of Manipulative and Physiological Therapeutics*, vol. 29, pp. 651–657, 2006.

[LAZ 68] LAZARSFELD P.F., HENRY N.W., *Latent Structure Analysis*, Houghton Mifflin, Boston, 1968.

[LUC 05] LUCKE J.F., "Rassling the hog: the influence of correlated item error on internal consistency, classical reliability, and congeneric reliability", *Applied Psychological Measurement*, vol. 29, pp. 106–125, 2005.

[MAR 08a] MARAIS I., ANDRICH D., "Formalising dimension and response violations of local independence in the unidimensional Rasch model", *Journal of Applied Measurement*, vol. 9, pp. 1–16, 2008.

[MAR 08b] MARAIS I., ANDRICH D., "Effects of varying magnitude and patterns of response dependence in the unidimensional Rasch model", *Journal of Applied Measurement*, vol. 9, pp. 1 20, 2008.

[MYF 04] MYFORD C.M., WOLFE E.W., "Detecting and measuring rater effects using many-facet Rasch measurement: part II", in SMITH E.V. JR., SMITH R.M. (eds), *Introduction to Rasch Measurement*, Jam Press, Maple Grove, MN, pp. 518–574, 2004.

[SMI 05] SMITH E., "Effect of item redundancy on Rasch item and person estimates", *Journal of Applied Measurement*, vol. 6, pp. 147–163, 2005.

[TJU 82] TJUR T., "A connection between Rasch's item analysis model and a multiplicative Poisson model", *Scandinavian Journal of Statistics*, vol. 9, pp. 23–30, 1982.

[WAR 93] WARE J.E. JR., SNOW K.K., KOSINSKI M., GANDEK B., SF-36 health survey. Manual and interpretation guide, The Health institute, New England Medical Center, Boston, 1993.

[ZEN 02] ZENISKY A.L., HAMBLETON R.K., SIRECI S.G., "Identification and evaluation of local item dependencies in the medical college admissions test", *Journal of Educational Measurement*, vol. 39, pp. 291–309, 2002.

Chapter 8

Two Tests of Local Independence

8.1. Introduction

Local response dependency has been a challenge to Rasch models (and other IRT models) from the days of their conception and it is not unfair to say that even today the assumption of local independence in many application is treated as an assumption of convenience that cannot be tested. Calculation of correlation among person residuals as described in Chapter 7 and implemented in RUMM2030 [AND 10] represents a step toward the solution of this problem, but the solution is hampered by the fact that the distributions of these coefficients under the Rasch model are not known and the assessment of these coefficients relies on informal subjective evaluation of the size of these coefficients together with arbitrary cut points defining correlations that appear to be stronger than what the Rasch model expects. Fortunately, the theory of Rasch models contains two relatively simple test statistics addressing the hypothesis of local independence that are statistically sound.

The first test is the conditional likelihood ratio (CLR) test proposed by Henk Kelderman in his seminal paper on log-linear Rasch models [KEL 84]. The second test is a simple non-parametric test that does not require specialized Rasch software. This test was first proposed by Kreiner [KRE 93] and later was elaborated by Kreiner and Christensen [KRE 04]. This chapter discusses how these tests work and how the simple approach proposed by Kreiner and Christensen addresses the issue of local response dependence in a way equivalent to Kelderman's approach.

Chapter written by Svend KREINER and Karl Bang CHRISTENSEN.

8.2. Kelderman's conditional likelihood ratio test of local independence

As in previous chapters, we assume that $X_1, \ldots, X_k$ are items from a Rasch model depending on a latent variable θ and that $R = \sum_{i=1}^k X_i$ is the total score. The joint conditional distributions of the item responses are given by

$$P(X_1 = x_1, \ldots, X_k = x_k | \theta) = \frac{\exp(r\theta + \sum_{i=1}^k \psi_{ix_i})}{K(\theta, \bar{\psi}_1, \ldots, \bar{\psi}_k)} \qquad [8.1]$$

where $\bar{\psi}_i = (\psi_{i1}, \ldots, \psi_{im_i})$ are the item parameters in the exponential representation of the Rasch model for polytomous items. Assume that we are concerned about the local dependence between X_a and X_b and want to define a proper statistical test of the hypothesis that X_a and X_b are conditionally independent given θ

$$X_a \perp X_b | \theta$$

Kelderman's suggestion was to add log-linear interaction parameters to formula [8.1] which had the effect that the assumption of local independence was satisfied if and only if these parameters were equal to zero and so that a statistical test of the hypothesis that these parameters were equal to zero could be regarded as a test of local independence. Kelderman's alternative to local independence is shown in formula [8.2], where $\lambda^{ab}_{x_a, x_b}$ represents the local dependence

$$P(X_1 = x_1, \ldots, X_k = x_k | \theta) = \frac{\exp(r\theta + \sum_{i=1}^k \psi_{ix_i} + \lambda^{ab}_{x_a, x_b})}{K(\theta, \bar{\psi}_1, \ldots, \bar{\psi}_k, \bar{\lambda})} \qquad [8.2]$$

To better understand Kelderman's approach, it is convenient to rewrite [8.2] as follows:

$$\log P(X_1 = x_1, \ldots, X_k = x_k | \theta) = \lambda_0 + \sum_{i=1}^k (x_i\theta + \psi_{ix_i}) + \lambda^{ab}_{x_a, x_b} \qquad [8.3]$$

where $\lambda_0 = -\log K(\theta, \bar{\psi}_1, \ldots, \bar{\psi}_k, \bar{\lambda})$ because this formulation shows that the joint distribution of item response, conditionally, given a specific value of θ, is a standard log-linear model [BIS 75] with main effects $x_i\theta + \psi_{ix_i}$ depending on θ and an interaction between X_a and X_b that does not depend on θ. We refer to the model defined by [8.2] and [8.3] as a log-linear Rasch model because formula [8.2] shows that R is sufficient for θ in exactly the way it is in the Rasch model [8.1]. From this, it follows that conditional inference is also feasible under the log-linear Rasch model [8.2] and that it is possible to calculate conditional maximum likelihood parameters of $\lambda^{ab}_{x_a, x_b}$ and a CLR test of the hypothesis

$$H_0 : \lambda^{ab}_{x_a, x_b} = 0$$

We refer to [KEL 84] for the technical details concerning the estimation and testing in log-linear Rasch models.

EXAMPLE 8.1.– We illustrate the methods of the data about the disinhibited eating (DE) subscale of the Diabetes Health Profile (DHP) described in Chapter 2. This scale includes two items:

– DHP34: "How likely are you to eat something extra when you feel bored or fed up?"

– DHP38: "Do you have problems keeping to your diet because you eat to cheer yourself up?"

These two items are so closely related that we should be concerned about the assumption of local independence. To test the claim of the Rasch model that items are locally independent, we first calculate CML estimates of the item parameters under the Rasch model and CML estimates of the item parameters and the interaction parameters under the log-linear Rasch model and then calculate the CLR test of the hypothesis that the interaction parameters are equal to zero. The end result is a CLR test equal to 41.3. The degrees of freedom are equal to the product of numbers of response categories minus one for each of the items, that is df $= 9$ and $p < 0.00005$. Kelderman's CLR test therefore provides very strong evidence against local independence of the two items.

8.3. Simple conditional independence tests

There is a more direct and much simpler way to test the local independence in Rasch models that does not require specialized software. To understand this test, recall that local independence of X_a and X_b means that the two items are *conditionally* independent given θ:

$$X_a \perp X_b | \theta$$

Because conditional independence between two variables, given a third variable, implies that the *partial* correlation between the two variables controlled for the third has to be equal to zero, it follows intuitively that we should be able to use the partial correlation between items controlled for an appropriate proxy of the latent variable as a test statistic expecting this correlation to be zero under the Rasch model.

To develop such a test, we have to address three problems: (1) we have to select an appropriate proxy for θ, (2) we have to select an appropriate measure of partial correlation and (3) we have to find the distribution of the partial correlation under the hypothesis of conditional independence in order to evaluate the significance of the observed partial correlation.

Fortunately, there are various ways to solve these problems. The first problem may appear to be an easy one because of the sufficiency of the total score R under the Rasch model. Intuition may therefore suggest that conditional independence of X_a

and X_b should be tested given R, because this procedure works fine for tests of no DIF in Rasch models. Another equally attractive option might be to subtract both items X_a and X_b from R and test the conditional independence of X_a and X_b given $R - X_a - X_b$. Both of these solutions have been proposed for IRT models and should therefore also be attractive under the Rasch model. It can, however, be shown that intuition plays a trick upon us if we try this because the hypotheses $X_a \perp X_b | R$ and $X_a \perp X_b | R - X_a - X_b$ are almost, but not exactly, true under both IRT and Rasch models. In terms of the partial correlations between X_a and X_b, the departure from conditional independence follows from the fact that the partial correlation is known to be negative when we control R and positive when we control $R - X_a - X_b$. For large sample sizes, test of these hypotheses will have a type I risk much larger than 5%. In general IRT models, there is no easy solution to this problem, but in Rasch models there exists a solution because of the following result, the proof of which can be found in [KRE 93]:

Rasch items X_a and X_b are conditionally independent given rest scores without one of the two items:

$$X_a \perp X_b | R - X_a \qquad X_a \perp X_b | R - X_b \qquad [8.4]$$

This result can be proved in several ways, but it is not difficult to grasp why it must be true. Assume, for instance, that all items fit the Rasch model. If this is true, then it is also true for the subset of items without X_a and thus $R - X_a$ is sufficient for θ and all covariates are conditionally independent of items given $R - X_a$. Again note that X_a is an exogenous covariate relative to the subscore. The conditional independence of items and exogenous variables given $R - X_a$ therefore also applies to X_a, as stated in [8.4]. Seen from such a point of view, formula [8.4] transforms the local independence assumption into an assumption about absence of DIF. From this, it follows that all techniques developed for the analysis of DIF can be applied for the analysis of local dependence.

Returning to the question of measuring the partial correlation among items, it follows from [8.4] that the partial correlation between items controlling $R - X_a$ and/or $R - X_b$ is an appropriate test of local independence. The choice of a partial correlation coefficient is simple in the sense that any partial correlation coefficient can be applied as long as it is possible to derive the distribution of the test statistic under the Rasch model. In our examples, we use the partial γ coefficient [DAV 67] because item responses are assumed to be ordinal, but we make no claim that this partial correlation coefficient is more powerful than other coefficients. If items had been dichotomous items, we could also use the Mantel–Haentzel procedure. The distribution of the partial γ coefficient is known to be asymptotically normal, and experience suggests that the approximation by the normal distribution is fairly accurate also in connection with moderate sample sizes. If we are concerned about the approximation by the normal distribution, we can use a Monte Carlo test procedure [KRE 87] to provide an unbiased estimate of the true p-values under the hypothesis of conditional independence.

EXAMPLE 8.2.– We illustrate this method using the same items (DHP34 and DHP38) as before. We calculate partial γ coefficients controlling rest scores without one of the two items. The partial γ is equal to 0.60 ($p < 0.0001$) when we control the rest score without DHP34 and equal to 0.33 ($p = 0.019$) when we control the rest score without DHP38, thus providing strong evidence of local dependence.

It is not surprising that the two tests agree with the result of Kelderman's CLR test. The differences between the two tests do not mean that there are no similarities. Underneath the partial γ is a three-dimensional contingency table. The natural parametric model for such a table is a log-linear model [BIS 75] where the question of conditional independence of items is a question of whether all interaction parameters relating to the two items are equal to zero. The situation is complicated because the table contains structural zeros, but it still follows that the test for conditional independence reduces to a simple exercise in log-linear modeling. A likelihood ratio test of conditional independence of items against a saturated alternative for the three-way table partitions naturally into a test of no three-way interaction and a test of no two-way interaction against an alternative without three-way interactions where both tests should be accepted if the items are locally independent. It can also be shown that there can be no three-factor interaction in the table under Kelderman's log-linear Rasch model. A log-linear analysis of this table can therefore provide a test of uniform local dependence by a test of no three-factor interaction, estimates of the $\bar{\lambda}$ parameters and a test of local independence against uniform local dependence that is equivalent to Kelderman's CLR test.

8.4. Discussion and recommendations

The purpose of this chapter was to show that testing for local dependence in Rasch models using formal statistical tests is not only possible but also (in principle at least) relatively simple. In this connection, analysis of partial correlation is particularly attractive because such tests only require software for analysis of three-dimensional contingency tables. It may be argued that partial γ coefficients are not available in all statistical programs. In such cases, Mantel–Haenszel techniques analyzing the association between dichotomized versions of the items could be used as long as the controlling variable is a rest score defined by the original polytomous items.

The main difference between Kelderman's CLR test and the analysis by partial γ coefficients is that the CLR test does not take the ordering of response categories into account. Therefore, it is possible that the power of the partial γ coefficients could be larger than the power of the CLR test despite the fact that the partial γ is a non-parametric measure of conditional association whereas the CLR test is a parametric test. Therefore, we suggest that both tests should be applied during the analysis of local dependence.

8.5. Bibliography

[AND 10] ANDRICH D., SHERIDAN B., LUO G., RUMM2030, Computer software and manual, RUMM Laboratory, Perth, Australia, 2010.

[BIS 75] BISHOP Y.M.M., FEINBERG S.E., HOLLAND P.W., *Discrete Multivariate Analysis: Theory and Practice*, MIT press, Cambridge, MA, 1975.

[DAV 67] DAVIS J.A., "A partial coefficient for Goodman and Kruskalls gamma", *Journal of the American Statistical Association*, vol. 69, pp. 37–46, 1967.

[KEL 84] KELDERMAN H., "Loglinear Rasch model tests", *Psychometrika*, vol. 49, pp. 223–245, 1984.

[KRE 87] KREINER S., "Analysis of multidimensional contingency tables by exact conditional tests: techniques and strategies", *Scandinavian Journal of Statistics*, vol. 14, pp. 97–112, 1987.

[KRE 93] KREINER S., "Validation of index scales for analysis of survey data: the symptom index", in DEAN K. (ed.), *Population Health Research. Linking Theory and Method*, Sage Publications, pp. 116–144, 1993.

[KRE 04] KREINER S., CHRISTENSEN K.B., "Analysis of local dependence and multidimensionality in graphical loglinear models", *Communications in Statistics – Theory and Methods*, vol. 33, pp. 1239–1276, 2004.

Chapter 9

Dimensionality

9.1. Introduction

The Rasch model assumes that the underlying variable is unidimensional and it is crucial that this assumption is tested before attempts at interpreting the results of a Rasch analysis are made. Many tests of the Rasch model, including tests of the overall fit of data to the model and tests of the specific assumptions of the Rasch model, have been proposed [GLA 95], but relatively few of these are specifically aimed at disclosing multidimensionality. Smith recognized that despite unidimensionality being a necessary requirement to interpret Rasch models, the primary sources on Rasch measurement have been vague about this requirement, and about providing recommendations as to its assessment [SMI 96]. Therefore, in many cases unidimensionality of an item set is merely assumed, without being explicitly tested.

When the majority of items measure one dimension, item fit statistics are able to indicate the minority items as misfitting. When the different dimensions have equal number of items contributing to them, item fit statistics may be insensitive to multidimensionality, but analyzing patterns in the residuals are able to detect multidimensionality [SMI 02]. It is to be expected that evidence of local dependence will turn up, if there is more than one underlying dimension. However, evidence of local dependence should not automatically be interpreted as evidence of multidimensionality. Similarly, it is unreasonable to claim that there is only one underlying dimension based solely on item fit statistics.

Chapter written by Mike HORTON, Ida MARAIS and Karl Bang CHRISTENSEN.

This chapter offers a discussion of multidimensionality in health outcome scales and describes methods that can help indicate if there is multidimensionality in a data set. Two different situations are considered: confirmatory analysis where an *a priori* hypothesis is tested regarding which items measure what latent construct, and exploratory analysis where no such hypotheses exist.

9.1.1. *Background*

The idea that useful measurement only ever measures one thing was conceived by Thurstone [THU 31], who stated:

> *The measurement of any object or entity describes only one attribute of the object measured. This is a universal characteristic of all measurement.*

This thought was echoed by [MCN 46], who recognized that:

> *Measurement implies that one characteristic at a time is being quantified. The scores on an attitude scale are most meaningful when it is known that only one continuum is involved.*

This view was further supported by Stout [STO 87], who stated that there are at least three important reasons why it is essential that a test should be unidimensional. First, an assessment that purports to measure the level of a construct should not be significantly influenced by varying levels of one or more other constructs. Second, for an assessment to be used in identifying individual differences, the assessment must measure a unidimensional construct in order for two individuals with the same score to be considered similar. Third, unidimensionality must hold before a total score is calculated, otherwise item or person parameters may not be valid.

In order to make a direct comparison between two entities, it is required that this comparison is based on a measurement of only one attribute. In other words, it is a requirement that the comparison is based on a unidimensional measurement. It is important that the assumption of unidimensionality is tested before attempts at interpreting the results of a Rasch analysis are made. This view is shared by [SMI 02], who stated:

> *...prior to evaluating the impact of multidimensionality, methods for assessing the degree to which a set of data represents a unidimensional construct must be employed.*

The strict mathematical assumption of unidimensionality in IRT models is seldom fully met in practice, but even if unidimensionality is recognized to be relative, the construction of a set of items measuring a unidimensional latent variable requires subject-matter knowledge. Stout defined the concept of essential unidimensionality, where a dominant dimension coexists with one or more minor dimensions, the dominant dimension being so strong that estimates of this dimension are not affected by the presence of the minor dimensions [STO 87]. In this framework, it has been proposed that responses satisfy essential unidimensionality when the average between-item residual covariance, after fitting a unidimensional model, approaches zero as the number of items increase. Smith, in a similar vein, viewed unidimensionality not as a dichotomous "yes" or "no" decision, but rather a continuum, where rather than asking whether a scale is unidimensional or not, it may be more appropriate to pose the question: "At what point on the continuum does multidimensionality threaten the interpretation of item and person estimates?" [SMI 02].

9.1.2. *Multidimensionality in health outcome scales*

Patient-reported outcome scales typically tap various physical, mental and social aspects of health, thus broadly operationalizing the World Health Organization (WHO) definition of health.

In practice, violations of unidimensionality are found in many such scales that are constructed to measure a single variable, but are composed of subsets of items that measure somewhat different aspects of the variable.

The Functional Independence Measure (FIM™) contains 18 items and was originally intended as a unidimensional measure of functional independence [KEI 87], but later analyses using the Rasch model showed that items grouped into a 13-item motor subscale and a five-item cognitive subscale [LIN 94]. Since then, the FIM items have largely been used as two measures of functional independence based on these subscales. However, the motor scale's 13 items range from eating to bladder management to climbing stairs and can be further grouped into subsets. Although the presence of subsets captures better the complexity of the variable and increases its validity, it compromises its unidimensionality. When subscales are analyzed separately, items often do not fit the Rasch model, for example Chang *et al.* found that the items *bladder management* and *climbing stairs* do not fit a unidimensional Rasch model [CHA 97]. In fact, the FIM™ has been assessed using Rasch methods numerous times in numerous different ways. A historic summary of all of these analyses is presented in a paper by [LUN 11].

Another scale where violations of unidimensionality have been found is the 39-item Parkinson's Disease Questionnaire (PDQ-39); one of the most widely used disease-specific patient completed health status questionnaires [FRA 08]. The 39 items of the PDQ are usually grouped into eight subscales and sum scores are calculated for each subscale: mobility, activities of daily living, emotional well-being, stigma, social support, cognitions, communication and bodily discomfort. An evaluation of each subscale with a Rasch analysis found that eight items in four of the scales did not fit a unidimensional Rasch model [HAG 03]. Lack of confirmation for the eight subscale structures has also been found in other studies [HAG 07].

Exploratory factor analysis, qualitative clinical evidence or a combination of both has traditionally been used to determine the dimensional structure of many health outcome scales and to compose the subscales. For example, exploratory factor analysis was used to compose the initial eight subscale structures of PDQ-39 [PET 95]. However, items sometimes cluster together in factor analysis due to being similar in their "difficulty to endorse", reflecting endorsement patterns rather than dimensionality [NUN 94]. This could explain why Rasch analyses have not always confirmed the factor structures determined by factor analysis. Another reason may be the inappropriate use of ordinal data within parametric techniques such as factor analysis, which assume at least an interval scale of measurement.

9.1.3. *Consequences of multidimensionality*

Violation of the requirement of unidimensionality will result in misleading statistical analysis, so care must be taken that the variable measured is unidimensional at a reasonable level of precision. Furthermore, failure to disclose multidimensionality will invalidate fit tests, and can thus lead to incorrect conclusions about item discrimination, local dependence or differential item functioning.

A simulation study indicated that analyzing multidimensional data using the Rasch model yielded reduced variation in the person location estimates and a reduction in reliability indices [MAR 08]. The latter effect of multidimensionality was observed for the traditional reliability index Cronbach's coefficient α [CRO 51] used in classical test theory, and the Person Separation Index (PSI) suggested by Andrich [AND 82].

9.1.4. *Motivating example: the HADS data*

The Hospital Anxiety and Depression Scale (HADS) is a brief instrument used to assess symptoms of anxiety and depression [ZIG 83, BJE 02]. It is a 14-item scale often scored as two seven-item subscales of anxiety and depression. Pallant and Tennant studied this scale by analyzing patterns in the residuals using a principal components analysis (PCA) and the analysis confirmed the two subscales, with the exception of an anxiety item (item seven) loading with the depression items [PAL 07]. The HADS data set, as analyzed by Pallant and Tennant in their study, is used for illustration throughout the chapter. "Depression" items are the even numbered items, and "anxiety" items are the odd numbered items and four setups are considered.

In order to compare methods for item sets of varying size, we not only reanalyze the 14-item scale but also consider analyses of the first six items and analyses of the first 12 items. In all three cases, two analyses are considered: (1) analyses where depression items and anxiety items are mixed within hypothesized subscales (i.e. a random/arbitrary-based selection) and (2) analyses where each hypothesized subscale contains only one type of item (i.e. a conceptual/theory-based selection).

9.2. Multidimensional models

One way of testing unidimensionality is to formulate multidimensional models and test the unidimensional model against them. Item parameters are estimated using either a marginal maximum likelihood (MML) approach or a conditional maximum likelihood (CML) approach. The MML approach assumes a parametric (typically normal) distribution for the latent trait, which in turn is integrated out of the likelihood. The CML approach is based on the conditional likelihood of the vector of item responses given a sufficient statistic. Multidimensional Rasch models have been proposed in the MML framework [ADA 97, BRI 03] as well as in the CML framework [KEL 94].

Formulation of two-dimensional alternatives can be done using both marginal and conditional techniques, by assuming a bivariate normal latent distribution or considering conditional distributions of item responses given subscores for each of the latent dimensions. In either case, it is possible to test the assumptions of the Rasch model for each of the latent dimensions. In what follows, two-dimensional Rasch models are described, but all results can be generalized for more dimensions. For a vector $\mathbf{X_v} = (X_{v1}, \ldots, X_{vk})$ of polytomous items, assume without loss of generality that $\mathbf{X_v^{(1)}} = (X_{v1}, \ldots, X_{vl})$ measures one latent variable $\Theta^{(1)}$ and that $\mathbf{X_v^{(2)}} = (X_{v,l+1}, \ldots, X_{vk})$ measures another latent variable $\Theta^{(2)}$. We will use the notation $P(\cdot|\theta_d) = P(\cdot|\Theta_v^{(d)} = \theta_d)$, and $P(\cdot|\theta_1, \theta_2) = P(\cdot|\Theta_v^{(1)} = \theta_1, \Theta_v^{(2)} = \theta_2)$ where convenient. As before items take the values $x_{vi} = 0, 1, \ldots, m_i$ and the conditional probability of observing the response vector $\mathbf{x_v} = (\mathbf{x_v^{(1)}}, \mathbf{x_v^{(2)}})$ given $(\theta^{(1)}, \theta^{(2)})$ is

$$P(\mathbf{X_v} = \mathbf{x_v}|\theta_v^{(1)}, \theta_v^{(2)}) = P(\mathbf{X_v^{(1)}} = \mathbf{x_v^{(1)}}|\theta_v^{(1)})P(\mathbf{X_v^{(2)}} = \mathbf{x_v^{(2)}}|\theta_v^{(2)}) \quad [9.1]$$

where, for each dimension, $d = 1, 2$,

$$P(\mathbf{X_v^{(d)}} = \mathbf{x_v^{(d)}}|\Theta_v^{(d)} = \theta^{(d)}) \quad [9.2]$$

are probabilities from a polytomous Rasch model. Note that this implies that answers to items in the subgroup d depend only on $\theta^{(d)}$. This is sometimes referred to as *between-item multidimensionality*.

9.2.1. *Marginal likelihood function*

The two-dimensional marginal likelihood function can be written as

$$L_M^{(1,2)}(\psi_1, \ldots, \psi_k, \mu, \mathbf{\Sigma}) = \prod_{v=1}^{n} \int\int P(\mathbf{X_v} = \mathbf{x_v}|\theta^{(1)}, \theta^{(2)})\varphi_{\mu,\mathbf{\Sigma}}(\theta^{(1)}, \theta^{(2)})d\theta^{(1)}d\theta^{(2)} \quad [9.3]$$

where $\varphi_{\mu,\mathbf{\Sigma}}$ is the density of a two-dimensional normal distribution with mean vector and covariance given by

$$\mu = \begin{bmatrix} \mu_1 \\ \mu_2 \end{bmatrix} \qquad \mathbf{\Sigma} = \begin{bmatrix} \sigma_1^2 & \sigma_{12} \\ \sigma_{21} & \sigma_2^2 \end{bmatrix}$$

This multidimensional model is a special case of the multidimensional random coefficients logit models of Adams, Wilson, and Wang [ADA 97].

9.2.2. *Conditional likelihood function*

The two subscores $(R_v^{(1)}, R_v^{(2)}) = (\sum_{i=1}^{l} X_{vi}, \sum_{i=l+1}^{k} X_{vi})$ are sufficient for $(\theta_v^{(1)}, \theta_v^{(2)})$ and the *two-dimensional conditional likelihood function* is

$$L_C^{(1,2)}(\psi_1, \ldots, \psi_k) = L_C^{(1)}(\psi_1, \ldots, \psi_l)L_C^{(2)}(\psi_{l+1}, \ldots, \psi_k) \quad [9.4]$$

where, for $d = 1, 2$,

$$L_C^{(d)} = \prod_{v=1}^{n} P(\mathbf{X_v^{(d)}} = \mathbf{x_v^{(d)}}|R_v^{(d)})$$

like before this does not depend on the values of the latent variables. An alternative model is the *two-dimensional extended likelihood function*

$$L_E^{(1,2)}(\psi_1, \ldots, \psi_k, \nu) = L_C^{(1,2)}(\psi_1, \ldots, \psi_k) \prod_{v=1}^{n} \nu_{\mathbf{r_v^{(1)}}, \mathbf{r_v^{(2)}}}$$

where the probabilities $\nu_{\mathbf{r}^{(1)}, \mathbf{r}^{(2)}} = P(R_v^{(1)} = r^{(1)}, R_v^{(2)} = r^{(2)})$ are used as unrestricted parameters. This two-dimensional likelihood function generalizes the extended likelihood function proposed by Tjur [TJU 82].

9.3. Diagnostics for detection of multidimensionality

There is an abundance of tests of the Rasch model [GLA 95], but relatively few of these are aimed directly at disclosing multidimensionality. When item fit statistics do not show significant misfit, the conclusion should not automatically be that the data fit the Rasch model. Similarly, Cronbach's coefficient α can be quite high for multidimensional data [COR 93].

9.3.1. *Analysis of residuals*

Residuals are standardized differences $(X_{vi} - E_{vi})/\sqrt{V_{vi}}$ between the observed item responses X_{vi} and the model expected responses

$$E_{vi} = E(X_{vi}) = \sum_{h=1}^{m_i} hP(X_{vi} = h|\theta_v)$$

standardized with the square root of the variance

$$V_{vi} = V(X_{vi}) = \sum_{h=1}^{m_i} h^2 P(X_{vi} = h|\theta_v) - [E_{vi}]^2$$

As was noted in Chapter 5 on item fit statistics, calculation of the expected value is complicated.

Calculating these residuals for each person's response to each item and performing a PCA detects patterns among the residuals. If data fit a unidimensional Rasch model, there should be no discernible pattern in the residuals and PCA will show whether subsets of items have more in common than is accounted for by a single latent variable. For example, groupings of items may be observed within the loadings (either positive or negative loading) of the first principal component of the residuals. A number of studies have compared the effectiveness of this method with other methods of assessing unidimensionality [SMI 96, SMI 02, SMI 94].

Analyzing items one–six from the HADS data set in this way confirms the two subscales, while analyzing items one–12 in this way finds a single anxiety item (item seven) loading with depression items. This result is identical to the one obtained in the full 14-item analysis [PAL 07].

9.3.2. *Observed and expected counts*

When items are partitioned into two subgroups, the table of subscore combinations is considered. Let

$$O_{r_1,r_2} = \sum_{v=1}^{n} 1_{(R_v^{(1)}=r_1)} 1_{(R_v^{(2)}=r_2)} \qquad [9.5]$$

denote the observed number of persons with each score combination and let $N_r = \sum_{v=1}^{n} 1_{(R_v=r)}$ denote the number of persons with total score r. Under the assumption of one common dimension behind both subscales and the distribution of the score, it follows that the joint distribution of the subscores is

$$P(R_v^{(1)} = r_1, R_v^{(2)} = r_2|\theta) = \frac{\gamma_{r_1}^{(1)} \exp(r_1\theta)\gamma_{r_2}^{(2)} \exp(r_2\theta)}{\prod_{i=1}^{k} K_i} \qquad [9.6]$$

where $\psi_i = (\psi_{i1}, \ldots, \psi_{im_i})$ is the vector of item parameters for item i, $\gamma^{(1)}_{r_1} = \gamma_{r_1}(\psi_1, \ldots, \psi_l)$ and $\gamma^{(2)}_{r_2} = \gamma_{r_2}(\psi_{l+1}, \ldots, \psi_k)$. The conditional probability given the total score is

$$P(R_v^{(1)} = r_1, R_v^{(2)} = r_2 | R_v^{(1)} + R_v^{(2)} = r_1 + r_2, \theta) = \frac{\gamma^{(1)}_{r_1}\gamma^{(2)}_{r_2}}{\gamma_{r_1+r_2}}$$

that is independent of the latent variable. Inserting item parameter estimates then makes it possible to calculate the expected numbers $E_{r_1,r_2} = E(N_{r_1,r_2})$ as

$$n_{r_1+r_2} P(R_v^{(1)} = r_1, R_v^{(2)} = r_2 | R_v^{(1)} + R_v^{(2)} = r_1 + r_2)$$

and the table of the standardized residuals

$$\left(\frac{O_{r_1,r_2} - E_{r_1,r_2}}{\sqrt{VAR(N_{r_1,r_2})}} \right)$$

Comparing observed and expected counts, focusing on those with low scores on one of the subscales and high scores on the other is a useful diagnostic technique for identifying deviations from unidimensionality.

Using this methodology for the first six items in the HADS data yields a table with 100 residuals (because there are 10 possible subscore values $0, 1, \ldots, 9$). For $R_v^{(1)} = X_{v1} + X_{v3} + X_{v5}$ and $R_v^{(2)} = X_{v2} + X_{v4} + X_{v6}$ (i.e. subscales selected on a conceptual basis), we find a total of 11 residuals to be outside the interval [−1.96, 1.96].

				3.03		**2.20**	**5.11**		
									19.94
3.24						**2.15**			
									2.46
					−2.21				
		4.93	**4.83**						
							3.66		

Figure 9.1. *Residuals: subscales $R_v^{(1)} = X_{v1} + X_{v3} + X_{v5}$ and $R_v^{(2)} = X_{v2} + X_{v4} + X_{v6}$ selected on a conceptual basis*

Approximately, half of these are observed for high scores on one subscale and low scores on the other. For $R_v^{(1)} = X_{v1} + X_{v2} + X_{v3}$ and $R_v^{(2)} = X_{v4} + X_{v5} + X_{v6}$ (i.e. subscales selected on an arbitrary basis), we find 10 residuals were outside the interval [−1.96, 1.96].

While this also constitutes evidence against the model, none of these are observed for high scores on one subscale and low scores on the other. Using this methodology for 12 HADS items yields a table with $19^2 = 361$ residuals (because there are 19 possible values for each subscore). For $R_v^{(1)} = X_{v1} + X_{v3} + \cdots + X_{v11}$ and $R_v^{(2)} = X_{v2} + X_{v4} + \cdots + X_{v,12}$ (i.e. subsets selected on a conceptual basis), 25 residuals were outside of the interval $[-1.96, 1.96]$ and six of these were observed for high scores on one subscale and low scores on the other. For $R_v^{(1)} = X_{v1} + \cdots + X_{v6}$ and $R_v^{(2)} = X_{v8} + \cdots + X_{v,13}$ (i.e. subsets selected on an arbitrary basis), only eight residuals (less than 5%) are outside the interval $[-1.96, 1.96]$.

				2.38	**2.02**				
		–2.13							
			2.39						
						2.33			
						2.39	**2.23**	**-2.04**	
						3.01			
						4.42			

Figure 9.2. *Residuals: subscales $R_v^{(1)} = X_{v1} + X_{v2} + X_{v3}$ and $R_v^{(2)} = X_{v4} + X_{v5} + X_{v6}$ selected on an arbitrary basis*

Using all 14 HADS items yields a table with $22^2 = 484$ residuals (because there are 22 possible values for each subscore). For $R_v^{(1)} = X_{v1} + X_{v3} + \cdots + X_{v,13}$ and $R_v^{(2)} = X_{v2} + X_{v4} + \cdots + X_{v,14}$ (i.e. subsets selected on a conceptual basis), 26 residuals were outside of the interval $[-1.96, 1.96]$, 11 observed for high scores on one subscale and low scores on the other. For $R_v^{(1)} = X_{v1} + \cdots + X_{v7}$ and $R_v^{(2)} = X_{v8} + \cdots + X_{v,14}$ (i.e. subsets selected on an arbitrary basis), only five residuals (less than 5%) are outside the interval $[-1.96, 1.96]$, that is this test does not indicate problems for the arbitrarily selected subscales.

9.3.3. *Observed and expected correlations*

A similar approach to diagnosing multidimensionality uses the observed and expected correlation between the subscores $R_v^{(1)}$ and $R_v^{(2)}$. The correlation between subscales measuring different traits will be weaker than the expected correlation between subscales measuring the same unidimensional trait. Because the subscores are ordinal discrete variables, Goodman and Kruskal's γ coefficient is an appropriate measure of the correlation [GOO 54]. Let γ_{OBS} denote the coefficient calculated in the observed table (O_{r_1,r_2}) and let γ_{EXP} denote the coefficient calculated in the expected table (E_{r_1,r_2}). Using the asymptotic standard error $s.e.(\gamma_{EXP})$, these can be compared.

For the conceptual subscales $R_v^{(1)} = X_{v1} + X_{v3} + X_{v5}$ by $R_v^{(2)} = X_{v2} + X_{v4} + X_{v6}$, we observe $\gamma_{OBS} = 0.51$ and this is much smaller than the expected value $\gamma_{EXP} = 0.61 \quad (s.e. = 0.02)$. For $R_v^{(1)} = X_{v1} + X_{v2} + X_{v3}$ and $R_v^{(2)} = X_{v4} + X_{v5} + X_{v6}$ (i.e. arbitrary subsets), $\gamma_{OBS} = 0.65$ and $\gamma_{EXP} = 0.61 \quad (s.e. = 0.03)$ do not differ much.

The table of conceptual subscales $R_v^{(1)} = X_{v1} + X_{v3} + \cdots + X_{v,11}$ and $R_v^{(2)} = X_{v2} + X_{v4} + \cdots + X_{v,12}$ yields $\gamma_{OBS} = 0.53$ and $\gamma_{EXP} = 0.67 \quad (s.e. = 0.03)$, the observed association being much lower than the expected. For the arbitrary subsets $R_v^{(1)} = X_{v1} + \cdots + X_{v6}$ by $R_v^{(2)} = X_{v7} + \cdots + X_{v,12}$, the difference is much smaller: $\gamma_{OBS} = 0.71$ and $\gamma_{EXP} = 0.67 \quad (s.e. = 0.02)$. Once again results suggest that, for arbitrarily selected subscales, multidimensionality is not disclosed.

For the full HADS data, the conceptual subsets $R_v^{(1)} = X_{v1} + X_{v3} + \cdots + X_{v,13}$ and $R_v^{(2)} = X_{v2} + X_{v4} + \cdots + X_{v,14}$ yield $\gamma_{OBS} = 0.53$ and $\gamma_{EXP} = 0.69 \quad (s.e. = 0.03)$, while for the arbitrary subsets $R_v^{(1)} = X_{v1} + \cdots + X_{v7}$ and $R_v^{(2)} = X_{v8} + \cdots + X_{v,14}$, the difference is much smaller: $\gamma_{OBS} = 0.74$ and $\gamma_{EXP} = 0.69 \quad (s.e. = 0.02)$.

9.3.4. *The t-test approach*

Testing the equivalence of person estimates from two subsets of items has been suggested as a way of detecting multidimensionality by [SMI 02]. This involves taking two item subsets, estimating person locations based on each of these subsets, and then, after converting the estimates to the same metric, testing if they are statistically equivalent for each person. For two item subsets, let $\hat{\theta}_v^{(1)}$ and $\hat{\theta}_v^{(2)}$ denote the resulting estimates of the location of person v, and let the standard errors of these be denoted by $\hat{\sigma}_v^{(d)} = s.e.(\hat{\theta}_v^{(d)})$, $d = 1, 2$. These estimates are from independent subsets of items, and the two estimates can be compared using the standard formula:

$$t_v = \frac{\hat{\theta}_v^{(1)} - \hat{\theta}_v^{(2)}}{\sqrt{[\hat{\sigma}_v^{(1)}]^2 + [\hat{\sigma}_v^{(2)}]^2}}$$

In situations where the distribution of the person location estimates is approximately normal, a value outside the interval $[-1.96, 1.96]$ is to be considered significant and if the proportion of significant results is much larger than 5%, this is evidence against unidimensionality. The originally proposed approach compared individual person estimates generated on subsets of items to the individual person estimate derived from the complete item set. However, in this situation, the subset person estimates and the complete scale person estimates are not independent. This was identified by Tennant and Conaghan [TEN 07], who also proposed an amended approach. This amended approach compares estimates from independent subsets of items, but ensures that these estimates are anchored to the same underlying scale.

Recall, however, that estimates of person locations for high and low scores are biased and non-normal and a cautious approach is therefore recommended. This is especially important when the distribution of scores is skewed (i.e. in situations with poor targeting).

This methodology can be extended by applying a binomial confidence interval to the proportion of significant test results, where the lower bound must overlap 5% to confirm acceptable unidimensionality. Sometimes, the proportion of tests that are significant at the 1% level is also reported.

In their assessment of the nursing self-efficacy scale (NSE), Hagquist and colleagues divided the items into two subscales: one comprising the items with negative item residual correlations and one comprising the items with positive item residual correlations. The t-test indicated that the estimates from the two subscales were significantly different for approximately 7% of the persons. Because it only just exceeded the critical value of 5%, it was considered a minor violation of unidimensionality [HAG 09].

In our example, the conceptual subsets showed that estimated person locations based on X_{v1}, X_{v3}, X_{v5} differed from estimated person locations based on X_{v2}, X_{v4}, X_{v6} for less than 4.4% of the persons. For the arbitrary subsets, comparing estimated person locations based on X_{v1}, X_{v2}, X_{v3} and X_{v4}, X_{v5}, X_{v6}, respectively, also did not show evidence of multidimensionality. However, with the larger item set, the conceptual subsets showed that the estimated person locations based on X_{v1}, X_{v3}, ..., X_{v11} differed from estimated person locations based on X_{v2}, X_{v4}, ..., X_{v12} for 10.5% of the persons, while the arbitrary subsets showed that estimated person locations based on X_{v1}, ..., X_{v6} and estimated person locations based on X_{v7}, ..., $X_{v,12}$ were significantly different for less than 5% of the persons. This was even more pronounced for the complete 14-item analysis where estimates based on X_{v1}, X_{v3}, ..., $X_{v,13}$ and estimates based on X_{v2}, X_{v4}, ..., $X_{v,12}$ differed for 13.3% of the persons, while estimates based on $X_{v1}, \dots, X_{v7}$ and estimates based on X_{v8}, ..., $X_{v,14}$ differed for 3.1% of the persons.

Once again evidence against unidimensionality was disclosed for conceptual subsets only.

9.3.5. *Using reliability estimates as diagnostics of multidimensionality*

Another way to detect multidimensionality is by comparing reliability estimates from two separate analyses of the data [AND 85, ZEN 02]. The first estimate uses the original items and assumes local independence. In the second analysis, the items of each hypothesized subdimension are combined into a single polytomous item with as many response categories as there are possible subscores. Since multidimensionality decreases Cronbach's coefficient α as well as the PSI, both of these reliability measures can be used.

If the reliability estimates from the second analysis is lower than the reliability estimate from the first analysis, the case for the hypothesis of multidimensionality is strengthened. These groups of items hypothesized to be dependent have been called subtests [AND 85], item bundles [ROS 88] or testlets [WAN 02].

It has also been suggested to use backward Cronbach's α curves (BCAC) as a diagnostic [CUR 97, HAR 07, MES 10] technique. This entails calculating α for all items and then, successively, removing the item that leaves the remaining set with the highest α until only two items remain. The BCAC is the plot of α against the number of remaining items and since α increases with the number of items when certain requirements are met, the non-monotonous curve can be taken as evidence that not all of these requirements are met. However, unidimensionality is only one of these requirements.

It has been suggested that this curve can be used to quickly find a unidimensional set of items, followed by goodness of fit tests of the Rasch model to confirm the unidimensionality of the identified set of items. It is important to remember, however, that Cronbach's coefficient α is valid only under certain conditions, for example when distributions are not artificially skewed due to floor and ceiling effects.

For the first six HADS items, α is 0.81. For the scale with the two subscales $R_v^{(1)} = X_{v1} + X_{v3} + X_{v5}$ and $R_v^{(2)} = X_{v2} + X_{v4} + X_{v6}$ as items, the value decreases to 0.73, while for the scale using $X_{v1} + X_{v2} + X_{v3}$ and $X_{v4} + X_{v5} + X_{v6}$ as items, α does not decrease.

For the first 12 HADS items, α is 0.88. For the scale with the two subscales $R_v^{(1)} = X_{v1} + X_{v3} + \cdots + X_{v,11}$ and $R_v^{(2)} = X_{v2} + X_{v4} + \cdots + X_{v,12}$ as items, α drops to 0.80, while for the scale using $X_{v1} + \ldots + X_{v6}$ and $X_{v7} + \ldots + X_{v12}$ as items, α does not decrease.

For all the 14 HADS items α is 0.89 while for the scale with the two subscales $R_v^{(1)} = X_{v1} + X_{v3} + \cdots + X_{v,13}$ and $R_v^{(2)} = X_{v2} + X_{v4} + \cdots + X_{v,14}$ as items α is 0.80. Again the α value does not decrease using two arbitrarily defined subscales as items.

9.4. Tests of unidimensionality

This section studies confirmatory tests, where a unidimensional model is tested against a specified alternative, given by a partition of the items into subgroups that are believed to measure different latent variables.

9.4.1. *Tests based on diagnostics*

Many of the diagnostics can be used to construct tests. The observed and expected number of persons with each subscore combination (r_1, r_2) can also be used as the basis for a formal test, for example by comparing O_{r_1,r_2} and E_{r_1,r_2} with a Pearson-type test statistic

$$\sum_{r_1,r_2} (O_{r_1,r_2} - E_{r_1,r_2})^2 / E_{r_1,r_2} \qquad [9.7]$$

This test statistic will be asymptotically chi-squared distributed. The observed and expected correlation between the two subscores can also be used for a test statistic

$$(\gamma_{OBS} - \gamma_{EXP}) / s.e.(\gamma_{EXP})$$

which will be asymptotically normally distributed.

As mentioned previously, in the t-test approach, a binomial confidence interval for the proportion of significant test results can be calculated and the lower bound must overlap 5%. Furthermore, an informal test statistic can be derived by squaring and summing the t-test for each person v

$$\sum_{v=1}^{n} t^2 = \sum_{v=1}^{n} \left[\frac{\hat{\theta}_v^{(1)} - \hat{\theta}_v^{(2)}}{\sqrt{[\hat{\sigma}_v^{(1)}]^2 + [\hat{\sigma}_v^{(2)}]^2}} \right]^2 \qquad [9.8]$$

Assuming that the standardized differences are normally distributed, this sum of squared standardized differences can be compared to a chi-squared distribution with $n-1$ degrees of freedom.

9.4.2. *Likelihood tests*

Likelihood ratio tests can also be calculated. For the two-dimensional marginal likelihood function $L_M(\psi_1, \ldots, \psi_k, \mu, \Sigma)$, the null hypothesis of unidimensionality can be represented as $L_M(\psi_1, \ldots, \psi_k, \mu_0, \Sigma_0)$ with mean vector and covariance given by

$$\mu_0 = \begin{bmatrix} \mu \\ \mu \end{bmatrix}, \qquad \Sigma_0 = \begin{bmatrix} \sigma^2 & \sigma^2 \\ \sigma^2 & \sigma^2 \end{bmatrix}$$

and a likelihood test can be calculated using

$$-2\log(L_M^{(1,2)}(\psi_1,\ldots,\psi_k,\mu,\Sigma)-\log(L_M(\psi_1,\ldots,\psi_k,\mu_0,\Sigma_0))$$

However, since Σ_0 is located on the boundary of the parameter space, ordinary asymptotic theory does not apply. For the two-dimensional extended likelihood function

$$L_E^{(1,2)}(\psi_1,\ldots,\psi_k,\nu)=L_C^{(1,2)}(\psi_1,\ldots,\psi_k)\prod_{v=1}^{n}\nu_{r_v^{(1)},r_v^{(2)}}$$

the null hypothesis of unidimensionality can be represented by using the probabilities $\kappa_r = P(R_v = r)$ as unrestricted parameters

$$L_E(\psi_1,\ldots,\psi_k,\kappa)=L_C(\psi_1,\ldots,\psi_k)\prod_{v=1}^{n}\kappa_{r_v^{(1)}+r_v^{(2)}}$$

The family of extended likelihood functions is thus nested within the family of two-dimensional extended likelihood functions and the likelihood ratio test

$$-2[l_C^{(1,2)}-l_C]-2\left[\sum_{v=1}^{n}\log\left(\nu_{r_v^{(1)},r_v^{(2)}}\right)-\sum_{v=1}^{n}\log\left(\kappa_{r_v^{(1)}+r_v^{(2)}}\right)\right]$$

(using the short notation $l_C^{(1,2)} = \log L_C^{(1,2)}(\psi_1,\ldots,\psi_k)$ and $l_C = \log L_C(\psi_1,\ldots,\psi_k)$) is the Martin-Löf test of unidimensionality [MAR 70, CHR 02]. In order to calculate the Martin-Löf test statistic, parameters ν_{r_1,r_2} must be estimated for each combination of subscores. The null distribution is known to deviate from the asymptotic chi-square distribution unless the sample size is very large [VER 01, CHR 02], and a better procedure for calculating p-values can be obtained from a bootstrap approach. Using the extended likelihood function proposed by Tjur [TJU 82], a sampling procedure without reference to the underlying distribution of the latent variable can be implemented using well-known recursion formulae for calculation of symmetrical polynomials [CHR 07].

Returning to the HADS example, considering conceptual subscales $R_v^{(1)} = X_{v1} + X_{v3} + X_{v5}$ and $R_v^{(2)} = X_{v2} + X_{v4} + X_{v6}$, the Pearson test statistic is 110.5, which, with 99 degrees of freedom, is insignificant. The observed correlation is significantly lower than the expected correlation:

$$(\gamma_{OBS}-\gamma_{EXP})/s.e.(\gamma_{EXP})=(0.51-0.61)/0.033=-3.03$$

yielding $p < 0.01$. The sum of squared standardized differences $\sum_{v=1}^{n} t_v^2$ is 285.7, which is insignificant and the Martin-Löf test statistic is 102.4 with 80 degrees of freedom ($p = 0.05$). For arbitrary subsets $R_v^{(1)} = X_{v1} + X_{v2} + X_{v3}$ and

$R_v^{(2)} = X_{v4} + X_{v5} + X_{v6}$, the Pearson test statistic is 122.3 (df=99, $p = 0.06$); the test based on observed and expected correlation is

$$(\gamma_{OBS} - \gamma_{EXP})/s.e.(\gamma_{EXP}) = (0.66 - 0.61)/0.033 = 1.52$$

yielding $p = 0.13$. The sum of squared standardized $\sum_{v=1}^{n} t_v^2$ differences is insignificant ($\sum_{v=1}^{n} t_v^2 = 220.3$), but the Martin-Löf test statistic 109.4 is significant (df $= 80$, $p = 0.02$).

For subsets $R_v^{(1)} = X_{v1} + X_{v3} + \cdots + X_{v,11}$ and $R_v^{(2)} = X_{v2} + X_{v4} + \cdots + X_{v,12}$, the value of the Pearson test statistic is 282.2, but with $19^2 - 1 = 360$ degrees of freedom, this is not significant. The observed correlation is significantly lower than the expected

$$(\gamma_{OBS} - \gamma_{EXP})/s.e.(\gamma_{EXP}) = (0.53 - 0.67)/0.025 = -5.60$$

($p < 0.01$). The sum of squared standardized differences is $\sum_{v=1}^{n} t_v^2 = 432.3$ ($p < 0.01$) and the Martin-Löf test statistic is 283.1 ($p = 0.91$).

For the extended arbitrary subsets $R_v^{(1)} = X_{v1} + \cdots + X_{v6}$ and $R_v^{(2)} = X_{v7} + \cdots + X_{v,12}$, the Pearson test statistic is 135.4 and again shows no evidence of multidimensionality. The observed correlation does not differ significantly from the expected

$$(\gamma_{OBS} - \gamma_{EXP})/s.e.(\gamma_{EXP}) = (0.71 - 0.67)/0.025 = 1.60$$

($p = 0.11$). The sum of squared standardized differences is insignificant as is the Martin-Löf test.

For $R_v^{(1)} = X_{v1} + X_{v3} + \cdots + X_{v,13}$ and $R_v^{(2)} = X_{v2} + X_{v4} + \cdots + X_{v,14}$, the Pearson test statistic is again insignificant. The observed correlation is significantly lower than the expected

$$(\gamma_{OBS} - \gamma_{EXP})/s.e.(\gamma_{EXP}) = (0.53 - 0.69)/0.023 = -6.96$$

which is again highly significant. The sum of squared standardized differences is $\sum_{v=1}^{n} t_v^2 = 479.9$ ($p < 0.01$) and the Martin-Löf test statistic is 342.5 ($p = 0.99$).

For the arbitrary subsets $R_v^{(1)} = X_{v1} + \cdots + X_{v7}$ and $R_v^{(2)} = X_{v8} + \cdots + X_{v,14}$, the Pearson test statistic is also insignificant and the observed correlation is not smaller than the observed correlation. The sum of squared standardized differences is insignificant, as is the Martin-Löf test.

As observed in section 9.3 on diagnostics, the tests of unidimensionality disclose evidence for the theoretically derived subscales, but not for the arbitrarily chosen subscales.

9.5. Estimating the magnitude of multidimensionality

Based on the formulation of multidimensionality presented by Marais and Andrich [MAR 08], we can consider a scale composed of two subsets, $d = 1, 2$, and assume the structure

$$\theta_{vd} = \theta_v + c_d\theta'_{vd}$$

where θ_v is the common value of the latent trait for person v and θ'_{vd} is the *distinct* trait for subset d assumed to be uncorrelated with θ_v. The numbers $c_1, c_2 > 0$, characterize the *magnitude* of the variable of subset s relative to the common variable among subsets. Using this formulation, Andrich described a way of estimating the magnitude of multidimensionality [AND 09]. A way of estimating the theoretical correlation between the traits of two items in different subsets then also follows. This is effectively the summary correlation among all pairs of subscales corrected for attenuation because of a random error. A value substantially less than one indicates multidimensionality.

9.6. Implementation

The t-test approach and the approach described to estimate the magnitude of multidimensionality have been implemented in the RUMM2030 computer program [AND 10], while the Martin-Löf test is implemented in the computer programs MULTIRA [CAR 01] and DIGRAM [KRE 03], as well as in SAS macros [CHR 03]. The test based on observed and expected association measures is also implemented in DIGRAM.

9.7. Summary

The chapter gives some examples of multidimensionality in health outcome scales, discusses its effects and outlines some ways to detect multidimensionality.

Residuals are standardized differences between observed data and expected values. If data fits the Rasch model and expected values are correctly calculated, there should be no structure in these and any kind of model misfit will result in some pattern in the residuals. PCA can sometimes help disclose multidimensionality, typically when the first principal component of the residuals shows a number of items with large positive loadings and another number with large negative loadings. Calculation of residuals is sometimes referred to as "extracting the Rasch factor". The two analyses of HADS items managed to confirm the two dimensions of anxiety and depression, with the exception of a single anxiety item loading with depression items. This result is identical to the result obtained in the complete 14-item analysis [PAL 07]. Further analyses are warranted in order to find out whether there is a general problem with this item.

Comparison of observed and expected counts yields a relatively small number of residuals where it is possible to get an overview. Large positive residuals corresponding to high scores on one subscale and low scores on the other indicate multidimensionality. In both analyses of HADS data, this pattern was seen when splitting data into hypothesized anxiety items and hypothesized depression items. The disclosed patterns were similar to those seen in the paper where the residuals were originally proposed [CHR 02, p. 572].

Squaring the residuals and calculating the Pearson-type test statistic yield insignificant results for all HADS analyses; it is most likely that very large sample sizes would be needed for a test of this kind to have any power.

The test based on observed and expected association measures is perhaps the most simple and intuitive method discussed in this chapter. It also has the advantage of being a test with one degree of freedom. Applying this test to the HADS data clearly rejected unidimensionality when items were split into anxiety and depression. When splitting into mixed subsets, the observed correlation did not differ significantly from the expected.

The t-test approach to dimensionality assessment suggested by Smith [SMI 02] and amended by Tennant and Conaghan [TEN 07] is based on the fact that when data fit the Rasch model, all subsets of items should produce equivalent person measurements. The approach can be supplemented with calculation of a binomial confidence interval for the proportion of significant tests or by calculation of the sum of squared standardized differences. Estimated person locations differed for less than 5% of the persons when analyzing 6 HADS items, but the 12-item analysis did indicate multidimensionality with significantly different locations for 10.5% of the sample when dividing items into anxiety and depression subscales. The lower bound of the binomial confidence interval was 8.10% and the sum of squared standardized differences was signifiant. Estimated person locations based on the first six items were significantly different from estimated person locations based on the last six for less than 5% of the persons.

The Martin-Löf test is a likelihood ratio test for unidimensionality. First used for dichotomous responses divided into two subscales [MAR 70, GUS 80, GLA 95], it has been generalized to polytomous items divided into two or more subscales [CHR 02]. For small sample sizes, the distribution deviates from the asymptotic chi-squared distribution; this has been noted by many authors [VER 01, CHR 02] and this was also seen in the HADS data application. Using the critical value from the empirical distribution rather than critical value from the chi-squared distribution dramatically increases the power [CHR 02, Table 1]. This approach has been formalized by Christensen and Kreiner [CHR 07].

The Martin-Löf test and the test based on observed and expected gamma coefficients require specification of hypotheses in advance, while other tests of unidimensionality in the Rasch model use residual covariance between pairs of items, yielding a more exploratory approach in which multiple testing problems are inherent.

It is uncertain when methods have enough power to detect multidimensionality. The analyses of the HADS data indicate that some of the methods may have a problem when the number of items is small and the Pearson-type test statistic and the Martin-Löf test have low power unless the sample size is very large.

Beyond sample size, the amount of thresholds estimated within each item subset, the correlation between the two hypothesized latent variables and targeting should also be considered carefully.

The qualitative judgment as to whether a scale is unidimensional enough for its purpose should always rest on a collection of evidence, both quantitative and qualitative. The way the scale is used in terms of the specific circumstances and goals of its administration should always be taken into account. The construction of a set of items measuring a unidimensional latent variable requires subject-matter knowledge, and the importance of this subject-matter knowledge should not be dismissed in favour of blind dimensionality testing.

9.8. Bibliography

[ADA 97] ADAMS R.J., WILSON M.R., WANG W.C., "The multidimensional random coefficients multinomial logit model", *Applied Psychological Measurement*, vol. 21, pp. 1–24, 1997.

[AND 82] ANDRICH D., "An index of person separation in latent trait theory, the traditional KR20 index, and the Guttman scale response pattern", *Education Research and Perspectives*, vol. 9, pp. 95–104, 1982.

[AND 85] ANDRICH D., "A latent trait model for items with response dependencies: implications for test construction and analysis", in EMBRETSON S.E. (ed.), *Test Design*, Academic Press, New York, pp. 245–275, 1985.

[AND 09] ANDRICH D., *Interpreting RUMM2030 Part IV. Multidimensionality and subtests in RUMM*, RUMM Laboratory, Perth, Australia, 2009.

[AND 10] ANDRICH D., SHERIDAN B., LUO G., RUMM2030, Computer software and manual, RUMM Laboratory, Perth, Australia, 2010.

[BJE 02] BJELLAND I., DAHL A.A., HAUGH T.T., NECKELMANN D., "The validity of the hospital anxiety and depression scale: an updated literature review", *Journal of Psychosomatic Research*, vol. 52, pp. 69–77, 2002.

[BRI 03] BRIGGS D.C., WILSON M., "An introduction to multidimensional measurement using Rasch models", *Journal of Applied Measurement*, vol. 4, pp. 87–100, 2003.

[CAR 01] CARSTENSEN C.H., ROST J., MULTIRA (Version 1.65), Computer software and manual. Retrieved from http://www.multira.de.

[CHA 97] CHANG W., SLAUGHTER S., CARTWRIGHT D., CHAN C., "Evaluating the FONE FIM: Part I. construct validity", *Journal of Outcome Measurement*, vol. 1, pp. 192–218, 1997.

[CHR 02] CHRISTENSEN K.B., BJORNER J.B., KREINER S., PETERSEN J.H., "Testing unidimensionality in polytomous Rasch models", *Psychometrika*, vol. 67, pp. 563–574, 2002.

[CHR 03] CHRISTENSEN K.B., BJORNER J.B., SAS macros for Rasch based latent variable modelling, Research Report 13, Department of Biostatistics, University of Copenhagen, 2003.

[CHR 07] CHRISTENSEN K.B., KREINER S., "A Monte Carlo approach to unidimensionality testing in polytomous Rasch models", *Applied Psychological Measurement*, vol. 3, pp. 20–30, 2007.

[COR 93] CORTINA J.M., "What is coefficient alpha? An examination of theory and applications", *Journal of Applied Psychology*, vol. 78, pp. 98–104, 1993.

[CRO 51] CRONBACH L.J., "Coefficient alpha and the internal structure of tests", *Psychometrika*, vol. 16, pp. 297–334, 1951.

[CUR 97] CURT F., MESBAH M., LELLOUCH J., DELLATOLAS G., "Handedness scale: how many and which items?", *Laterality*, vol. 2, pp. 137–154, 1997.

[FRA 08] FRANCHIGNONI F., GIORDANI A., FERRIERO G., "Rasch analysis of the short form 8-item Parkinson's Disease Questionnaire (PDQ-8)", *Quality of Life Research*, vol. 17, pp. 541–548, 2008.

[GLA 95] GLAS C.A.W., VERHELST N.D., "Testing the Rasch model", in FISCHER G.H., MOLENAAR I.W. (eds), *Rasch Models – Foundations, Recent Developments, and Applications*, Springer-Verlag, Berlin, pp. 69–95, 1995.

[GOO 54] GOODMAN L.A., KRUSKAL W.H., "Measures of association for cross classifications", *Journal of the American Statistical Association*, vol. 49, pp. 732–764, 1954.

[GUS 80] GUSTAFSSON J.E., "Testing and obtaining fit of data to the Rasch model", *British Journal of Mathematical and Statistical Psychology*, vol. 33, pp. 205–233, 1980.

[HAG 03] HAGELL P., WHALLEY D., MCKENNA S.P., LINDVALL O., "Health status measurement in Parkinson's disease: validity of the PDQ-39 and Nottingham Health Profile", *Movement Disorders*, vol. 18, pp. 773–783, 2003.

[HAG 07] HAGELL P., NYGREN C., "The 39 item Parkinson's disease questionnaire (PDQ-39) revisited: implications for evidence based medicine", *Journal of Neurology, Neurosurgery, and Psychiatry*, vol. 78, pp. 1191–1198, 2007.

[HAG 09] HAGQUIST C., BRUCE M., GUSTAVSON J.P., "Using the Rasch model in nursing research: an introduction and illustrative example", *International Journal of Nursing Studies*, vol. 46, pp. 380–393, 2009.

[HAR 07] HARDOUIN J.B., MESBAH M., "The SAS macro-program %AnaQol to estimate the parameters of item response theory models", *Communications in Statistics – Simulation and Computation*, vol. 36, pp. 437–453, 2007.

[KEI 87] KEITH R.A., GRANGER C.V., HAMILTON B.B., SHERWIN F.S., "The functional independence measure: a new tool for rehabilitation", in EISENBERG M.G., GRZESIAK R.C. (eds), *Advances in Clinical Rehabilitation*, vol. 1, Springer Publishing Co., New York, pp. 6–18, 1987.

[KEL 94] KELDERMAN H., RIJKES C.P.M., "Loglinear multidimensional IRT models for polytomously scored items", *Psychometrika*, vol. 59, pp. 149–176, 1994.

[KRE 03] KREINER S., Introduction to DIGRAM, Research report 03/10, Department of Biostatistics, University of Copenhagen, Copenhagen, 2003.

[LIN 94] LINACRE J.M., HEINEMANN A.W., WRIGHT B.D., GRANGER C.V., HAMILTON B.D., "The structure and stability of the functional independence measure", *Archives of Physical Medicine and Rehabilitation*, vol. 75, pp. 127–132, 1994.

[LUN 11] LUNDGREN NILSSON Å., TENNANT A., "Past and present issues in Rasch analysis: the Functional Independence Measure (FIM) revisited", *Journal of Rehabilitation Medicine*, vol. 43, pp. 884–891, 2011.

[MAR 70] MARTIN-LÖF P., Statistiska modeller. Anteckninger från seminarier läsåret 1969–70 [Statistical models. Notes from the academic year 1969–70], Institut för försäkringsmatematik och matematisk statistik, Stockholm, 1970.

[MAR 08] MARAIS I., ANDRICH D., "Formalising dimension and response violations of local independence in the unidimensional Rasch model", *Journal of Applied Measurement*, vol. 9, pp. 1–16, 2008.

[MCN 46] MCNEMAR Q., "Opinion-attitude methodology", *Psychological Bulletin*, vol. 43, pp. 289–374, 1946.

[MES 10] MESBAH M., "Statistical quality of life", in BALAKRISHNAN N. (ed.), *Method and Applications of Statistics in the Life and Health Sciences*, Wiley, pp. 839–864, 2010.

[NUN 94] NUNNALLY J.C., BERNSTEIN I.H., *Psychometric Theory*, McGraw-Hill, Inc., New York, 1994.

[PAL 07] PALLANT J.F., TENNANT A., "An introduction to the Rasch measurement model: an example using the Hospital Anxiety and Depression Scale (HADS)", *British Journal of Clinical Psychology*, vol. 46, pp. 1–17, 2007.

[PET 95] PETO V., JENKINSON C., FITZPATRICK R., GREENHALL R., "The development and validation of a short measure of functioning and well being for individuals with Parkinson's disease", *Quality of Life Research*, vol. 3, pp. 241–248, 1995.

[ROS 88] ROSENBAUM P.R., "Item bundles", *Psychometrika*, vol. 53, pp. 349–359, 1988.

[SMI 94] SMITH R.M., MIAO C.Y., "Assessing unidimensionality for Rasch measurement", in WILSON M. (ed.), *Objective Measurement: Theory into Practice*, vol. 2, Ablex, Norwood, NJ, pp. 316–327, 1994.

[SMI 96] SMITH R.M., "A comparison of methods for determining dimensionality in Rasch measurement", *Structural Equation Modeling*, vol. 3, pp. 25–40, 1996.

[SMI 02] SMITH E., "Detecting and evaluating the impact of multidimensionality using item fit statistics and principal component analysis of residuals", *Journal of Applied Measurement*, vol. 3, pp. 205–231, 2002.

[STO 87] STOUT W., "A nonparametric approach for assessing latent trait unidimensionality", *Psychometrika*, vol. 52, pp. 589–617, 1987.

[TEN 07] TENNANT A., CONAGHAN P.G., "The Rasch measurement model in rheumatology: What is it and why use it? When should it be applied, and what should one look for in a Rasch paper?", *Arthritis Care & Research*, vol. 57, pp. 1358–1362, 2007.

[THU 31] THURSTONE L.L., "Measurement of social attitudes", *Journal of Abnormal and Social Psychology*, vol. 26, pp. 249–269, 1931.

[TJU 82] TJUR T., "A Connection between Rasch's item analysis model and a multiplicative Poisson model", *Scandinavian Journal of Statistics*, vol. 9, pp. 23–30, 1982.

[VER 01] VERHELST N., "Testing the unidimensionality assumption of the Rasch model", *Methods of Psychological Research Online*, vol. 6, pp. 232–271, 2001.

[WAN 02] WANG X., BRADLOW E.T., WAINER H., "A general Bayesian model for testlets: Theory and applications", *Applied Psychological Measurement*, vol. 26, pp. 109–128, 2002.

[ZEN 02] ZENISKY A.L., HAMBLETON R.K., SIRECI S.G., "Identification and evaluation of local item dependencies in the medical college admissions test", *Journal of Educational Measurement*, vol. 39, pp. 291–309, 2002.

[ZIG 83] ZIGMOND A.S., SNAITH R.P., "The Hospital Anxiety and Depression Scale", *Acta Psychiatrica Scandinavica*, vol. 67, pp. 361–370, 1983.

PART 4

Applying the Rasch Model

Introduction

By far, the most common application of the Rasch model is validation of scales, but the model can also be used for other purposes. This part describes applications of the Rasch model for equating different scales, for studying the rater agreement, and shows how very general models containing the underlying latent variables can be created based on the Rasch model.

Chapter 10

The Polytomous Rasch Model and the Equating of Two Instruments

10.1. Introduction

This chapter describes the application of the polytomous Rasch model (PRM) in equating two instruments intended to assess the same trait using only the total scores on the instruments. The data collection design has one group of persons responding to both instruments. The distinctive feature of the Rasch model for this application is that in estimating the instrument parameters, the person parameters can be eliminated by conditioning on each person's total score. The advantage of the approach is that the relationship between the two instruments is established through the structure of the responses of each instrument rather than through the distribution of the person parameters, about which no assumption needs to be made. The chapter shows the rationale for conducting a test of fit of responses to the model conditional on the total scores. It also shows two approaches to forming an equivalence relationship between the scores from the two instruments, the first using only the total scores on the two instruments and the second using person estimates for each total score on the two instruments. The equating of two instruments, one composed of four items from the WhoQol BREF scale [SKE 04] and the other composed of seven items from the

---

Chapter written by David ANDRICH.
The research reported in this paper was supported in part by the Australian Research Council Linkage Grants with The Curriculum Council of Western Australia, and Pearson plc as industry partners. The Australian National Ministerial Council on Employment, Education, Training and Youth Affairs' Performance Measurement and Reporting Task Force also provided support. Tim Dunne made valuable suggestions. Permission to use data was provided by Mounir Mesbah.

SF12 scale [WAR 96], which are considered to assess the same trait, is provided as an illustration.

Equating different instruments that assess the same trait is an integral task of modern psychometrics. There exists a number of methods for this purpose, including simple equipercentile scaling, linear scaling, and more modern methods summarized as the kernel method [VON 04]. These authors also summarize the key principles and assumptions required for equating two instruments, a major one being that the instruments assess the same trait. We will not canvas all these features in this chapter.

Instead, the purpose of this chapter is to focus on one of the designs articulated by [VON 04] and to show an application of the unidimensional PRM for purpose of equating two instruments that have no items in common. The design is termed the single group design in which the two instruments to be equated are administered to the same group of persons from some relevant population. Because the PRM involves a single person parameter across the two instruments, which implies the assumption that the two instruments assess the same trait, the PRM is relevant for the purpose of equating the two instruments from such a design.

The PRM is usually applied to items of an instrument in which the items generally have a range of scores of the order of zero to four or zero to five. In some cases, a subset of items of the two instruments might be common. In those cases, the instruments can be equated through the common items that are then termed link items. In this chapter, we consider the case where all persons respond to all items of two instruments, where there are no link items, and where we consider only the summed scores of persons on each of the instruments. In this case of the application of the PRM, the scores on the instruments take the role of scores on the items, and the two instruments are equated directly through their total scores across persons rather than through the scores on their constituent items. The advantage of such equating is that it takes account of any local dependence among items within each of the instruments [AND 85].

In the PRM, there is a parameter associated with each total score of an instrument. The range of scores for instruments is usually substantially greater than that for items, and as a result, two complications can arise in the estimation of the PRM parameters of the instruments. First, with so many score parameters, the estimates may be unstable, especially in the extremes of the distribution of scores of each instrument where the frequencies of scores might be low. Second, some total scores, usually high or low scores, will have zero frequencies. Such scores are said to be *null* [LUO 05, WIL 93]. If approached directly, the parameters associated with such null scores will not be finite. These complications are accommodated in the procedure described in this chapter.

The rest of the chapter is structured as follows. Section 10.2 describes the PRM, and section 10.3 a reparameterization of each instrument's parameters. This reparameterization overcomes both estimation complications summarized above – it reduces the number of independent parameters, relative to the maximum possible, that are to be estimated, and it can handle null scores provided there are not too many of them. Section 10.4 describes the conditional statistical test of fit between the data and the model and two graphical tests of fit; section 10.5 summarizes two possible procedures for equating two instruments from a PRM analysis; and section 10.6 provides an example describing which instruments have relatively large maximum scores and which have null scores.

10.2. The Polytomous Rasch Model

For this chapter, the PRM [RAS 61, AND 77, AND 78, WRI 82] is written in the form

$$P((X_{vj} = x_j|(\psi_j), \theta_v) = \frac{1}{\gamma_{vj}} \exp(\psi_{jx} + x_j\theta_v) \qquad [10.1]$$

where (1), $X_{vj} = x_j \in \{0, 1, \ldots, m_j\}$ is the integer random response variable when person v encounters instrument j, (2) θ_v is the location of person v on the trait, (3) $(\psi_{jx})_{x=0,1,\ldots,m_j}$ is a vector of score coefficients, and (4) $\gamma_{vj} = \sum_{k=0}^{m_j} \exp(\psi_{kj} + k\theta_v)$ is a normalizing constant.

The coefficients ψ_j are defined according to

$$\psi_{jx} = -\sum_{k=0}^{x} \beta_{jk} \quad \beta_{j0} \equiv 0 \quad \psi_{j0} \equiv 0 \qquad [10.2]$$

where $(\beta_{jx})_{x=1,\ldots,m_j}$ are m_j thresholds on the continuum between successive scores at which the probabilities of the two successive scores are identical. Thus, for $\theta = \beta_{jx}$, $P((X_{vj} = x - 1) = P((X_{vj} = x)$. The parameter β_{j0} does not exist, and defined as $\delta_{j0} \equiv 0$, it is introduced for notational and algebraic convenience.

10.2.1. *Conditional probabilities*

Suppose that each person v also responds to a second instrument i. If no factors other than the person location parameter θ_v and the instrument parameters

$\{(\psi_j), (\psi_i)\}$ govern the responses according to [10.1], then the responses (x_{nj}, x_{ni}) are assumed to be conditionally independent given θ. This independence is generally termed *local independence*. The joint probability of the two responses is given by

$$P(X_{vj} = x_{vj}, X_{vi} = x_{vi}|\theta_v) = \left[\frac{\exp(\psi_{jx_{vj}} + x_{vj}\theta_v)}{\gamma_{vj}}\right]\left[\frac{\exp(\psi_{ix_{vi}} + x_{vi}\theta_v)}{\gamma_{vi}}\right]$$

$$= \frac{\exp(\psi_{jx_{vj}} + \psi_{ix_{vi}} + (x_{vj} + x_{vi})\theta_v)}{\gamma_{vj}\gamma_{vi}}$$

$$= \frac{\exp(\psi_{jx_{vj}} + \psi_{ix_{vi}} + r_v\theta_v)}{\gamma_{vj}\gamma_{vi}} \qquad [10.3]$$

where $r_v = x_{vj} + x_{vi}$ is the total score of person v on the two instruments j and i. The probability of a total score r_v is given by the sum of the probabilities of all the possible ways that the score can occur. There is only one way that $r_v = 0$ can occur, and only one way that $r_v = m_j + m_i$ can occur. Therefore, these scores are not considered in the conditional equations. Thus, the total scores that can be used are $r_v = 1, 2, \ldots, R$ where $R = m_j + m_i - 1$. This notation will prove convenient in the expressions of conditional probability equation.

To obtain the probability of each score $r_v = 1, 2, \ldots, R$, and subsequently the conditional probability of a pair of responses given the total score r_v, we focus on the instrument j and let $x_{vj} = x$. Then, $x_{vi} = r_v - x$. For convenience, we also drop the subscript v from r_v and let $r_v = r$. For emphasis or clarity, in some expressions, we retain the subscripts in x_{vj} and r_v. Further, for a specified total score of r, the range of values for the two instruments is constrained.

Let $L(r) = \max(0, r - m_i)$ and $U(r) = \min(m_j, r)$. Then, $[L(r), U(r)]$ is the range of possible scores on instrument j when the total score is r. We can then write

$$P(r_v = r|\theta_v) = \sum_{x=L(r)}^{U(r)} \frac{\exp(\psi_{jx} + \psi_{i(r-x)} + r\theta_v)}{\gamma_{vj}\gamma_{vi}} \qquad [10.4]$$

The conditional probability of the responses $(x, r - x)$ of person v to the two instruments, given the person's total score r, is then given by the ratio of [10.3] and [10.4]. On simplification,

$$P(X_{vj} = x, X_{vi} = r - x)|r) = \frac{\exp(\psi_{jx} + \psi_{i(r-x)})}{\Gamma_r} \qquad [10.5]$$

where

$$\Gamma_r = \sum_{k=L(r)}^{U(r)} \exp(\psi_{jk} + \psi_{i(r-k)})$$

is a normalizing factor of all possible response pairs (k_j, k_i) with a total score of $r = k_i + k_j$.

From [10.5], which is independent of the parameter θ_v, it is evident that the total score r_v is a sufficient statistic for θ_v. The elimination of θ_v by conditioning on its sufficient statistic is the defining characteristic of the Rasch class of models [RAS 61]. This elimination of the person parameter by conditioning implies that no assumption needs to be made regarding the distributions of the persons. Clearly, for effective equating, some differences in the total scores among persons are required and the locations of the persons need to be relatively well aligned to the threshold parameters of the instruments. With the elimination of the person parameters, the relationship between the instruments is based on the structure of the responses, within each instrument and not on the distribution of the persons.

10.2.2. *Conditional estimates of the instrument parameters*

In order to estimate the set of parameters $(\psi_j), (\psi_i)$, the likelihood L from the conditional probability of the responses of all $v = 1, \ldots, N$ persons is formed. First, consider the joint probability of the responses of all persons with a score of r.

Let $f_x(r)$ be the number of persons with the score x on instrument j and a total score of r and let

$$F(r) = \sum_{x=L(r)}^{U(r)} f_x(r)$$

be the total number of persons with a score of r. Note, then, that $f_{r-x}(r)$ i must be equal to the number of persons with score x on instrument i and a total score of r; these respectively are the number of times that the scores $x_j = x$ and $x_i = r - x$ appear. Then, the joint probability of their responses is given by

$$\prod_{F(r)} \frac{\exp(\psi_{jx} + \psi_{i(r-x)})}{\Gamma_r} = \frac{\exp[\sum_{F(r)} \psi_{jx} + \sum_{F(r)} \psi_{i(r-x)}]}{\Gamma_r^{F(r)}}$$

$$= \left(\exp\left[\sum_{x=L(r)}^{U(r)} f_x(r)\psi_{jx} + \sum_{x=L(r)}^{U(r)} f_{r-x}(r)\psi_{i(r-x)} \right] \right) / \Gamma_r^{F(r)} \quad [10.6]$$

The likelihood L, which is the conditional probability of the responses of persons across all scores $r = 1, \ldots, R$, is given by

$$L = \prod_{r=1}^{R} \frac{\exp\left[\sum_{x=L(r)}^{U(r)} f_x(r)\psi_{jx} + \sum_{x=L(r)}^{U(r)} f_{r-x}(r)\psi_{i(r-x)}\right]}{\Gamma_r^{F(r)}}$$

$$= \exp\left[\sum_{r=1}^{R}\sum_{x=L(r)}^{U(r)} f_x(r)\psi_{jx} + \sum_{r=1}^{R}\sum_{x=L(r)}^{U(r)} f_{r-x}(r)\psi_{i(r-x)}\right]\left(\prod_{r=1}^{R}\Gamma_r^{F(r)}\right)^{-1}$$

[10.7]

To emphasize the coefficient $\psi_{i(r-x)}$ in its own right, we may notate it as $\psi_{ix'}$ and its frequency as $\sum_{r=1}^{R} f_{x'}(r)$ where $x' = r - x$. The maximum likelihood estimate resulting from this is the conditional maximum likelihood (CML) estimate obtained in the usual way [AND 72]. For completeness, the derivation of the MLE is summarized below. From [10.7],

$$\log L = \sum_{r=1}^{R}\sum_{x=L(r)}^{U(r)} f_x(r)\psi_{jx} + \sum_{r=1}^{R}\sum_{x=L(r)}^{U(r)} f_{r-x}(r)\psi_{i(r-x)} - \sum_{r=1}^{R} F(r)\log(\Gamma_r)$$

[10.8]

and

$$\frac{\partial \log L}{\partial \psi_{jx}} = \sum_{r=1}^{R}\sum_{x=L(r)}^{U(r)} f_x(r) - \sum_{r=1}^{R} F(r)P((x, r-x)|r) \qquad [10.9]$$

$$\frac{\partial \log L}{\partial \psi_{ix'}} = \sum_{r=1}^{R}\sum_{r-x=L(r)}^{U(r)} f_{r-x}(r) - \sum_{r=1}^{R} F(r)P((r-x, x)|r) \qquad [10.10]$$

The MLE for each parameter is given by setting each of these derivatives equal to zero yielding implicit equations that need to be satisfied simultaneously. The common algorithm for finding the solutions to these equations is the Newton–Raphson algorithm. In this algorithm, the equations are solved sequentially and iterations are continued across the equations until all estimates converge simultaneously to a specified level of precision. There are three identifying constraints required, the first two, $\psi_{j0} = \psi_{i0} \equiv 0$ defined in [10.2], are implied in the equations and the third is simply that the sum of the threshold parameters is zero, that is $\sum_{x=1}^{m_j} \beta_{jx} + \sum_{x=1}^{m_i} \beta_{ix} = 0$. From the definition in [10.2], this is equivalent to the constraint $\psi_{jm_j} + \psi_{im_i} \equiv 0$. Thus, the effective number of independent parameters that can be estimated is $m_j + 1 + m_i + 1 - 3 = m_j + m_i - 1$.

It is evident from [10.7] that the vectors of frequencies

$$\left(\sum_{r=1}^{R} f_x(r)\right)_{x=1,\ldots,m_j} \quad \text{and} \quad \left(\sum_{r=1}^{R} f_{r-x}(r)\right)_{x=1,\ldots,m_i}$$

are sufficient statistics for the parameter vectors $(\psi_j), (\psi_i)$. Note that these are just the margins and that we may also notate these frequencies as $(f(\psi_{jx}))_{x=1,\ldots,m_j}$ and $(f(\psi_{ix}))_{x=1,\ldots,m_i}$. With this observation regarding the frequencies, the equations resulting from setting the derivatives [10.9] and [10.10] equal to zero may be written as

$$f(\psi_{jx}) - \sum_{r=1}^{R} F(r)P((r-x,x)|r) = 0$$

$$f(\psi_{ix'}) - \sum_{r=1}^{R} F(r)P((r-x,x)|r) = 0 \qquad [10.11]$$

It is now also evident from [10.11] that if any score x or x' is null, that is, $f(\psi_{jx}) = 0$ or $f(\psi_{ix'}) = 0$, then because the conditional probabilities are required to be zero, the respective estimates of ψ_{jx} and $\psi_{ix'}$ will not be finite – they need to be $-\infty$.

10.2.3. *An illustrative small example*

For illustrative purposes, consider the small example in Table 10.1 in which $x_j \in \{0, 1, 2, 3\}$ and $x_i \in \{0, 1, 2\}$.

Person v	1	2	3	4	5	6	7	8	9	10
$x_j \in \{0,1,2,3\}$	0	0	1	1	1	1	2	2	1	2
$x_i \in \{0,1,2\}$	1	1	0	0	1	2	1	1	2	2
r	1	1	1	1	2	3	3	3	3	4

Table 10.1. *Illustrative small example: 10 persons responding to two instruments*

Table 10.2 shows the same data in terms of frequencies in a two-way contingency table.

The total scores of the persons in the cells are in parentheses. The distribution of the person is $F(1) = 4$, $F(2) = 1$, $F(3) = 4$ and $F(4) = 1$. For a given total score r, the range of instrument j is given by $[L(r), U(r)]$. These values are shown in Table 10.3.

	$x_i = 0$	$x_i = 1$	$x_i = 2$
$x_j = 0$		2 (1)	0 (2)
$x_j = 1$	2 (1)	1 (2)	2 (3)
$x_j = 2$	0 (2)	2 (3)	1 (4)
$x_j = 3$	0 (3)	0 (4)	

Table 10.2. *Illustrative small example. Frequencies of pairs of responses on two instruments. In each cell, the total score is in parentheses*

	$r = 1$	$r = 2$	$r = 3$	$r = 4$
$L(r)$	0	0	1	2
$U(r)$	1	2	3	3

Table 10.3. *Illustrative small example. The range of possible scores on instrument j*

Table 10.4 shows the data rearranged to highlight the frequencies, $f_x(r)$, conditional on the total score $r = 1, 2, 3, 4$. In this small example, although $x_j \in \{0, 1, 2, 3\}$, there is no response $x_{vj} = 3$ and therefore, the coefficient ψ_{j3} has a zero frequency: $\sum_{r=1}^{R} f_3(r) = f(\psi_{j3}) = 0$.

x	$r = 1$	$r = 2$	$r = 3$	$r = 4$	$\sum_{r=1}^{R} f_x(r) = f(\psi_{jx})$
0	2	0			2
1	2	1	2		5
2		0	2	1	3
3			0	0	0
$F(r) = \sum_{x=L(r)}^{U(r)} f_x(r)$	4	1	4	1	10

Table 10.4. *Illustrative small example: Frequencies of responses on the first instrument conditional on the total score $f_x(r)$*

Note that the last column contains the sufficient margins for the score parameters of instrument j. Because $f(\psi_{3j}) = 0$, the solution in [10.11] for ψ_{3j} is

$$0 - \sum_{r=1}^{R} F(r)P((x, r - x)|r) = 0 \qquad x = 3$$

We note that for $r = 1, 2$, x_j cannot have the value 3 – it is evident from Table 10.4 that the limits of x are 0 to 1 and 0 to 2, respectively. Expanding the solution equation for ψ_{j3} gives the following successive expressions.

$$0 - \sum_{r=1}^{R} F(r) \frac{\exp(\psi_{j3} + \psi_{i(r-3)})}{\Gamma_r} =$$

$$0 - \left[F(3) \frac{\exp(\psi_{j3} + \psi_{i0})}{\Gamma_3} + F(4) \frac{\exp(\psi_{j3} + \psi_{i1})}{\Gamma_4} \right] =$$

$$0 - \left[4 \cdot \frac{\exp(\psi_{j3} + \psi_{i0})}{\Gamma_3} + 1 \cdot \frac{\exp(\psi_{j3} + \psi_{i1})}{\Gamma_4} \right] = 0$$

For this solution equation to hold, it is evident that $\psi_{j3} = -\infty$ is a non-finite solution. The presence of null categories is overcome in the estimation by a reparameterization of the thresholds described in the following section.

10.3. Reparameterization of the thresholds

Instead of estimating all $m_j + 1$ coefficients for instrument j, of which m_j are effectively independent, it is possible to reparameterize them to a reduced number of parameters. We begin by illustrating the reparameterization with just two parameters for each instrument.

10.3.1. *Thresholds reparameterized to two parameters for each instrument*

The thresholds may be reparameterized explicitly in terms of only the first two moments of the thresholds given by

$$\psi_{jx} = -x\delta_j + x(m_j - x)\lambda_j \qquad [10.12]$$

where the first parameter $\delta_j = \frac{1}{m_j} \sum_{k=0}^{m_j} \beta_{jk}$ is the mean of the thresholds, and where the second parameter $\lambda_j = (\delta_{jx} - \delta_{j,x-1})/2$ is the average half distance between successive thresholds of instrument j [AND 82]. This reparameterization imposes the constraint that the successive thresholds within each instrumental are equal. With $m_j > 3$, the parameterization of [10.12] is effectively of reduced rank relative to the maximum rank m_j. It is evident that the first term has a linear function of x as the coefficient of δ_j and that the second term has a quadratic function of x as the coefficient of λ_j. The parameters δ_j and λ_j, respectively, characterize the location and spread of the thresholds $(\beta_{jk})_{k=1,\ldots,m_j}$.

With this reparameterization, [10.1] takes the form

$$P(X_{vj} = x_j) = \exp(-x_j\delta_j + x_j(m_j - x_j)\lambda_j + x_j\theta_v)/\gamma_{vj} \qquad [10.13]$$

and the conditional probability [10.5] takes the form

$$\begin{aligned} P(X_{vj} = x, X_{vi} = r - x|r) = \exp(&-x\delta_j \\ &+ x(m_j - x)\lambda_j \\ &- (r - x)\delta_i \\ &+ (r - x)(m_i + x - r)\lambda_i)/\Gamma_r \end{aligned} \qquad [10.14]$$

where

$$\Gamma_r = \sum_{k=L(r)}^{U(r)} \exp(-k\delta_j + k(m_j - k)\lambda_j - (r - k)\delta_i + (r - k)(m_i + k - r)\lambda_i) \qquad [10.15]$$

This reparameterization has two effects relevant for estimation. First, it reduces the number of parameters to be estimated. Second, instead of using [10.7] and frequencies of responses directly in a one-to-one correspondence with each threshold as the relevant statistics in the estimation, the sufficient statistics employed using [10.14] are *functions* of the frequencies of the scores, and not the frequencies of the scores themselves. Therefore, having some null scores is not an impediment to implementing the algorithm. However, there are two conditions in which finite estimates cannot be found for an instrument. First, if all scores of instrument j are either 0 or m_j, then an estimate of the corresponding parameter is not finite. In this case, however, the scores are so pathological that there is no equating to be carried out. Second, if every person on instrument j has a lesser score than on instrument i, or if every person has a greater score on instrument j than on instrument i, then it is not possible to obtain parameter estimates of the instruments using this reparameterization. This case, too, is unusual and it would indicate the problem of estimation is a symptom of the very poor alignment between at least one of the instruments with the location of the sample of persons.

With the above reparameterization, the identifying constraint generally imposed is $\hat{\delta}_j + \hat{\delta}_i = 0$. Therefore, in the above reparameterization, the number of independent parameters estimated is just three, two for each instrument, $(\delta_j, \lambda_j; \delta_i, \lambda_i)$ with the one identifying constraint $\hat{\delta}_j + \hat{\delta}_i = 0$. This is a substantial reduction of rank. The derivation of the estimation equations is summarized below. First, the likelihood L, in parallel to [10.7], is given by

$$L = \prod_{r=1}^{R} \prod_{F(r)} \frac{\exp(\psi_{jx} + \psi_{i(r-x)})}{\Gamma_r}$$

$$= \exp \left[\sum_{r=1}^{R} \sum_{x=L(r)}^{U(r)} f_x(r)x(-\delta_j) \right.$$

$$+ \sum_{r=1}^{R} \sum_{x=L(r)}^{U(r)} f_x(r)x(m_j - x)\lambda_j$$

$$+ \sum_{r=1}^{R} \sum_{x=L(r)}^{U(r)} f_x(r - x)(-\delta_i)$$

$$\left. + \sum_{r=1}^{R} \sum_{x=L(r)}^{U(r)} (r - x)(m_j + x - r) f_x(r - x)\lambda_j \right] / \Gamma_r^{F(r)} \qquad [10.16]$$

Then, the log likelihood is

$$\log L = (-\delta_j) \sum_{r=1}^{R} \sum_{x=L(r)}^{U(r)} x f_x(r) + \lambda_j \sum_{r=1}^{R} \sum_{x=L(r)}^{U} x(m_j - x) f_x(r)$$

$$+ (-\delta_i) \sum_{r=1}^{R} \sum_{x=L(r)}^{U(r)} (r - x) f_{r-x}$$

$$+ \lambda_i \sum_{r=1}^{R} \sum_{x=L(r)}^{U} + f_x(r)(r - x)(m_j + x - r) - \sum_{r=1}^{R} F(r) \log(\Gamma_r)$$

It can be shown readily from [10.15] that

$$\frac{\partial \log \Gamma_r}{\partial \delta_j} = \sum_{x=L(r)}^{U(r)} -xP((x, r - x)|r)$$

$$\frac{\partial \log \Gamma_r}{\partial \lambda_j} = \sum_{x=L(r)}^{U(r)} x(m_j - x)P((x, r-x)|r)$$

$$\frac{\partial \log \Gamma_r}{\partial \delta_i} = \sum_{x=L(r)}^{U(r)} -(r-x)P((x, r-x)|r)$$

$$\frac{\partial \log \Gamma_r}{\partial \lambda_i} = \sum_{x=L(r)}^{U(r)} (r-x)(m_i - r + x)P((x, r-x)|r)$$

Differentiating with respect to each of the four parameters gives the following solution equation for δ_j

$$-\sum_{r=1}^{R} \sum_{x=L(r)}^{U(r)} x f_x(r) + \sum_{r=1}^{R} F(r) \sum_{x=L(r)}^{U(r)} x P((x, r-x)|r) = 0 \qquad [10.17]$$

For λ_j, the solution equation is

$$\sum_{r=1}^{R} \sum_{x=L(r)}^{U(r)} x(m_j - x) f_x(r) - \sum_{r=1}^{R} F(r) \sum_{x=L(r)}^{U(r)} x(m_j - x) P((x, r-x)|r) = 0$$

$$[10.18]$$

For δ_i, the solution equation is

$$-\sum_{r=1}^{R} \sum_{x=L(r)}^{U(r)} (r-x) f_{r-x}(r) + \sum_{r=1}^{R} F(r) \sum_{x=L(r)}^{U(r)} (r-x) P((x, r-x)|r) = 0$$

$$[10.19]$$

and for λ_i, the solution equation is

$$\sum_{r=1}^{R} \sum_{x=L(r)}^{U(r)} (r-x)(m_i + x - r) f_{r-x}(r)$$

$$-\sum_{r=1}^{R} F(r) \sum_{x=L(r)}^{U(r)} (r-x)(m_i - r + x) P((x, r-x)|r) = 0$$

In these equations, the sufficient statistics for the respective parameters are the left-hand terms of the equations. As is evident, they are not frequencies of any response, but functions of these frequencies. As a consequence, some null categories do not force parameter estimates to be undefined. For example, consider again the small example of Table 10.1. The respective terms of the equations are shown in Table 10.5 along with the estimates of the parameters. That $\hat{\lambda}_j = \hat{\lambda}_i$ to three decimal places is a coincidence. That $\hat{\delta}_j = -\hat{\delta}_i$ is not a coincidence – it arises from the constraint imposed. Although the sufficient statistic, 11, for these parameters is the same for both instruments, instrument j and i have respective maximum scores of three and two, resulting in the former instrument being relatively more difficult.

Parameter	Sufficient statistic	Estimate
δ_j	$\sum_{r=1}^{R}\sum_{x=L(r)}^{U(r)} x f_x(r) = 11$	$\hat{\delta}_j = 1.728$
λ_j	$\sum_{r=1}^{R}\sum_{x=L(r)}^{U(r)} x(m_j - x) f_x(r) = 16$	$\hat{\lambda}_j = 3.455$
δ_i	$\sum_{r=1}^{R}\sum_{x=L(r)}^{U(r)} (r - x) f_{r-x}(r) = 11$	$\hat{\delta}_i = -1.728$
λ_i	$\sum_{r=1}^{R}\sum_{x=L(r)}^{U(r)} (r - x)(m_i + x - r) f_{r-x}(r) = 5$	$\hat{\lambda}_i = 3.455$

Table 10.5. *Illustrative small example: sufficient statistics and estimates for the instrument parameters*

10.3.2. *Thresholds reparameterized with more than two parameters*

In principle, the score coefficients ψ_{jx} can be reparameterized in terms of up to m_j successive polynomials of increasing order. For example, Andrich and Luo express the coefficients by up to four moments where the third and fourth moments are, respectively, cubic and quadratic functions of respective parameters of the thresholds [AND 03]. Just as the first two functions and their respective parameters characterize the location and spread of the thresholds, the third and fourth functions and their respective parameters characterize the skewness and the kurtosis of the thresholds. In the example of section 10.6, one analysis is conducted under the parameterization with four moments for each instrument, the other with just two moments. If M_j and M_i are the number of parameters estimated for each instrument, with $M_j < m_j$ and $M_i < m_i$, then the number of independent parameters estimated is $M_j + M_i - 1$, after imposing the constraint $\hat{\delta}_j + \hat{\delta}_i = 0$.

10.3.3. *A reparameterization with four parameters*

Let the first four successive terms of the reparameterized thresholds be defined by $(\varphi_{lj})_{l=1,2,3,4}$, and the first four successive polynomial functions of the responses be defined by $(g_{lj}(x))_{l=1,2,3,4}$. Then from [10.12], the first two terms and two functions are, respectively, $\varphi_{1j} = -\delta_j; \varphi_{2j} = \lambda_j$ and $g_{1j}(x), -x; g_{2j}(x), x(m_j - x)$. The remaining two functions [AND 03] are $g_{3j}(x) = x(m_j - x)(2x - m_j)$ and

$g_{4j}(x) = x(m_j - x)(5x^2 - 5xm_j + m_j^2 + 1)$. Then, the general category coefficient ψ_{xj} is given by

$$\psi_{xj} = \sum_{l=1}^{M_j} g_{lj}(x)\varphi_{lj} \qquad [10.20]$$

where $M_j \leq m_j$. The successive terms $(\varphi_{lj})_{l=1,2,3,4}$ characterize the location, spread, skewness and kurtosis of the thresholds. The maximum value that M_j can take in the software RUMM2030 [AND 10] is $M_j = 4$. In principle, m_j can take any value $m_j \geq 1$.

Equation [10.1] can be written in the general, reparameterized form, as

$$P((X_{vj} = x_j|\theta_v) = \frac{1}{\gamma_{vj}} \exp\left(\sum_{l=1}^{M_j} g_{lj}(x)\varphi_{lj} + x_j\theta_v\right) \qquad [10.21]$$

Then, the parameters (φ_{lj}) are estimated using conditional equations that eliminate the person parameters θ_v, of which [10.17]–[10.20] are special cases. From these estimates, estimates of the vector of category coefficients (ψ_j) can be calculated from [10.20]. Thus, the category coefficients are not estimated directly from the conditional (10.7), but indirectly by first estimating (φ_{lj}). Moreover, the number of moments can be specified in advance without destroying the structure of the model. If the threshold estimates themselves are required, then they are readily obtained from [10.2] according to

$$\beta_{jx} = \psi_{jx-1} - \psi_{jx} = -\sum_{k=0}^{x-1} \delta_{jk} - \left(-\sum_{k=0}^{x} \delta_{jk}\right) \qquad [10.22]$$

In the illustrative small example, and based on the estimates shown in Table 10.5, the estimates for the successive thresholds in instruments j and i are, respectively, $\{-5.182, 1.728, 8.637\}$ and $\{-5.182, 1.727\}$.

10.3.3.1. *A solution algorithm*

The software RUMM2030 that implements the solution equation based on the likelihood in [10.7], but with the coefficients reparameterized, was used in the example. The estimation algorithm was summarized above and is described in further detail in [AND 03].

10.3.3.2. *Leunbach's precedent*

Using [10.5] with two instruments assessing the same proficiency administered to a single group, where the maximum scores of the instruments was of the order of 20, Leunbach [LEU 76] estimated all the score coefficients, with a required constraint for each of the two instruments. Leunbach used the power series representation of the model and for that reason, it was not a problem that a score on one instrument was null. He noticed that each vector of estimates $\hat{\psi}_j, \hat{\psi}_i$ took the shape of a quadratic function. Accordingly, he reparameterized the scoring parameters of each instrument to be such functions each with two terms. This reduced the number of parameters estimated to $m_j + m_i - 1 = 3$. He concluded that the data he was looking at fitted this special case of the model and therefore that the model could be used to equate the two instruments. Rather than estimating the maximum number of parameters, and then summarizing these estimates with less than the maximum number, in the approach described in this chapter, the reparameterization of [10.12] immediately reduces the number of independent parameters for the instruments to many less than the maximum number. Leunbach's conclusion was that the data fitted a parameterization similar to [10.12] for both the instruments.

10.4. Tests of fit

Following the estimation of the parameters of the instruments, some tests of fit between the data and the model are described, one numerical and two graphical. The numerical test takes the observed and expected frequencies under the model, conditional on each total score, for *each cell* of the two-way data matrix of responses and a Pearson χ^2 statistic is formed. The first graphical test estimates the expected value and the confidence interval of the score for each instrument, conditional on each total score. It then shows the plot of the observed mean score of an instrument relative to these confidence intervals. The second graphical test of fit calculates the expected value of the score of each test as a function of the values on the latent continuum, and then compares the means of persons in class intervals with their expected value.

10.4.1. *The conditional test of fit based on cell frequencies*

Given the estimates of the parameters $(\hat{\psi}_j, \hat{\psi}_i)$, obtained from [10.20], we can obtain $\hat{P}((x, r-x)|r)$ for each pair of scores $(x, r-x)$. The Pearson χ^2 statistic is then given by

$$\chi^2 = \sum_{r=1}^{R} \sum_{x=L(r)}^{U(r)} \frac{[f_x(r) - F(r)\hat{P}((x, r-x)|r)]^2}{F(r)\hat{P}((x, r-x)|r)} \qquad [10.23]$$

where we recall that $f_x(r)$ is the number of persons with a score of r who have the pair of scores $(x, r-x)$, and $F(r)$ is the number of persons with a score of r. In this equation, $F(r)\hat{P}((x, r-x)|r)$ is the expected frequency according to the model given the parameter estimates.

10.4.1.1. *Degrees of freedom for the conditional test of fit based on cell frequencies*

Given that the maximum scores for the two instruments j, i are m_j, m_i respectively, the number of cells in the data matrix is $(m_j + 1)(m_i + 1)$. However, total scores zero and $m_j + m_i$ arise from a unique pattern each, and therefore are excluded from any test of fit. Therefore, the number of cells available for the test of fit is $(m_j+1)(m_i+1)-2$. In addition, there is a constraint that the sum of the conditional probabilities of each possible response pattern, given each total score, is one. That is,

$$\sum_{x=L(r)}^{U(r)} P((x, r-x)|r) = 1 \tag{10.24}$$

implying one constraint for each possible total score within the number of independent cells. If cells with scores zero and $m_j + m_i$ from the matrix are not included, the remaining number of possible total scores with relevant cells is $m_j + m_i - 1$, each with a constraint according to [10.24]. Thus, the total effective number of independent cells is

$$\begin{aligned} &(m_j + 1)(m_i + 1) - 2 - (m_j + m_i - 1) \\ &= m_j m_i + m_j + m_i + 1 - 2 - m_j - m_i + 1 \\ &= m_j m_i \end{aligned} \tag{10.25}$$

If a parameter is estimated for each threshold of each instrument, then there are $m_j + m_i$ parameters estimated with one constraint, giving $m_j + m_i - 1$ independent parameters estimated. Thus, the total degrees of freedom for a test of fit based on the observed and conditional expected frequency of each cell in the $(m_j + 1)$ by $(m_i + 1)$ table is

$$m_j m_i - (m_j + m_i - 1) = (m_j - 1)(m_i - 1)$$

In the case that a smaller number of parameters $M_j < m_j$ and $M_i < m_i$ with one constraint are estimated, then the degrees of freedom are given by

$$m_j m_i - (M_j + M_i - 1) \tag{10.26}$$

In the case where some of the possible total scores have zero frequency, the available number of independent cells and constraints need to be adjusted. Because the number of cells for a given total score depends on the total score, this adjustment can be done on a case-by-case basis. The example in section 10.6 illustrates this adjustment.

10.4.2. *The conditional test of fit based on class intervals*

In some cases, as in the example of section 10.6, the frequencies within cells conditional on the total scores will be small. For example, if two instruments assess the same trait, and the scores range from zero to 20 or so on each instrument, there will be few if any persons in the cell with pairs of scores (one, 19) given a total score of 20. In addition, if the sample size is relatively small compared to the number of cells, then the cell frequencies will be small. Therefore, in formalizing the comparison of observed and expected frequencies, it might be helpful to combine adjacent cells, conditional on the total score. Because of the potential for low expected frequencies in cells, a routine formation of class intervals involves pooling adjacent cells, conditional on a total score, to give just two class intervals for each total score. This can be formalized as a representation of the set $\{L(r), \ldots, U(R)\}$ of possible scores on instrument j as a disjoint union

$$\{L(r), \ldots, U(R)\} = A_r \cup B_r$$

yielding the test statistic

$$\chi^2 = \sum_{r=1}^{R} \frac{\left(\sum_{x \in A_r} f_x(r) - \sum_{x \in A_r} F(r)\hat{P}\{(x, r-x)|r\}\right)^2}{\sum_{x \in A_r} F(r)\hat{P}\{(x, r-x)|r\}} + \sum_{r=1}^{R} \frac{\left(\sum_{x \in B_r} f_x(r) - \sum_{x \in B_r} F(r)\hat{P}\{(x, r-x)|r\}\right)^2}{\sum_{x \in B_r} F(r)\hat{P}\{(x, r-x)|r\}} \quad [10.27]$$

10.4.2.1. *Degrees of freedom for the conditional test of fit based on class intervals*

To calculate the number of degrees of freedom for [10.27], we note that the number of possible total scores is $m_j + m_i - 1$. With two adjacent class intervals for each total score, the number of class intervals in the matrix is $2(m_j + m_i - 1)$. However, within each total score, there is a constraint. Therefore, the effective number of independent class intervals is $m_j + m_i - 1$. The maximum number of parameters that can be estimated is $m_j + m_i - 1$. Therefore, if this number is estimated, there are $m_j + m_i - 1 - (m_j + m_i - 1) = 0$ degrees of freedom available for testing the fit of the responses to the model. However, if the number of parameters estimated is $M_j + M_i - 1$ where $M_j < m_j$, $M_i < m_i$, then the number of degrees of freedom is given by

$$m_j + m_i - 1 - (M_j + M_i - 1) = (m_j + m_i) - (M_j + M_i) \quad [10.28]$$

Again, in the case where some of the possible total scores r have zero frequency, then the available number of independent cells and constraints need to be adjusted. In this case, the adjustment is simply to subtract the total number of total scores with zero observed frequencies from $(m_j + m_i) - (M_j + M_i)$. This is illustrated in the example in section 10.6.

10.4.3. *Graphical test of fit based on total scores*

Given the estimates of the parameters $(\hat{\psi}_{jx})$, $(\hat{\psi}_{i,r-x})$, we can obtain

$$\hat{E}[X_j|r] = \sum_{x=L(r)}^{U(r)} x_j \hat{P}((x, r-x)|r) \quad [10.29]$$

and $\hat{V}[X_j|r] = \sum_{x=L(r)}^{U(r)} x_j^2 \hat{P}(((x, r-x)|r) - (\hat{E}[X_j|r])^2$.

For the $F(r)$ persons with a total score of r,

$$\hat{E}[\bar{X}_j|r] = E[X_j|r], \quad V[\bar{X}_j|r] = V[X_j|r]/F(r) \quad [10.30]$$

Therefore, it is possible to compare the average scores of instrument j in scoregroup r, $\bar{X}_j|r$, with its expectation, $\hat{E}[\bar{X}_j|r]$, relative to $\sqrt{\hat{V}[\bar{X}|r]}$. With discrete distributions of the PRM, and conditional on the total score, the variance is a function of the probabilities of a response and of the total score. Thus, $\hat{V}[\bar{X}_j|r]$ is a function of both the number of persons $F(r)$ in each score group r, and of r itself. For total scores close to one and $m_j + m_i - 1$, the minimum and maximum, respectively, that can be used in the test of fit, $\hat{V}[\bar{X}_j]$ will be small. Therefore, it is reasonable to approximate confidence intervals in the usual way. A graphical plot of the observed mean $\bar{X}_j|r$ together with 95% confidence intervals given by $\hat{E}[X_j|r] \pm 1.96\sqrt{\hat{V}[\bar{X}_j|r]}$ for each score r is illustrated in the example.

10.4.4. *Graphical test of fit based on person estimates*

An estimate $\hat{\theta}_r$, the estimate of proficiency for a score of r, can be obtained directly by the ML estimation. Such an estimate can be obtained because r is a sufficient statistic for $\hat{\theta}_r$. Thus, taking the two instruments' parameter estimates as given, the ML solution equation for $\hat{\theta}_r$ for each total score r, and which must be solved iteratively for each r, is

$$\begin{aligned} r &= \sum_{j=1}^{2} \hat{E}[X_{nj}] = \sum_{j=1}^{2} \sum_{x_j=0}^{m_j} x_j \hat{P}(X_{vj} = x_j) \\ &= \sum_{j=1}^{2} \sum_{x_j=0}^{m_j} x_j \exp(\hat{\psi}_{xj} + x_j \hat{\theta}_r)/\gamma_{vj} \end{aligned} \quad [10.31]$$

Further, for any value of θ, from [10.31] it is possible to obtain the expected value $\hat{E}[X_j]$ for each instrument according to

$$\hat{E}[X_j|\theta] = \sum_{x_j=0}^{m_j} x_j \hat{P}(X_{vj} = x_j|\theta_v = \theta) \qquad [10.32]$$

Then, a plot of $\hat{E}[X_j|\theta]$ against θ provides an instrument characteristic curve for instrument j. In principle, the observed mean of responses on instrument j for each total score, $\bar{X}_j|\hat{\theta}_r$ can be compared with $\hat{E}[X_j|\hat{\theta}_r]$. If the sample size for each score r is relatively small, class intervals of adjacent total scores can be formed and the observed mean of scores in each class interval plotted against the expected value curve at the point where θ is the average of the estimates in the person estimates in a class interval. With two instruments j and i, the graphical plot of the test of fit of i is complementary to the plot of instrument j.

10.5. Equating procedures

There are two procedures for equating the scores of the two instruments, one based on the probabilities conditional on the raw scores and the other based on the estimate of the person parameters taking the estimates of the instruments' parameters as given.

10.5.1. *Equating using conditioning on total scores*

Equating raw scores follows immediately from [10.29]. Thus, because

$$\hat{E}[X_j|r] + \hat{E}[X_i|r] = r \qquad [10.33]$$

$$\hat{E}[X_i|r] = r - \hat{E}[X_j|r]; \quad \hat{E}[X_j|r] = r - \hat{E}[X_i|r] \qquad [10.34]$$

Therefore, [10.34] is the transformation for equating the scores between instruments j and i. Clearly, [10.34] is unlikely, for any integer score on one instrument, to provide an equivalent integer score on the other instrument – both scores will almost certainly be non-integers. However, that kind of relationship, where integer scores do not have direct equivalents, follows from all methods of equating. If it is required to convert an integer score of one instrument to a score on the other instrument, then various plausible rounding numerical approximations may be made. One of these approximations is shown in the example of section 10.6.

10.5.2. *Equating through person estimates*

Equating through person estimates requires estimating the person parameters given the estimated instrument parameters as fixed. These estimates are derived according to [10.31]. The use of person estimates to equate scores is also illustrated in the example in the next section.

10.6. Example

The two instruments equated involve subsets of items from two scales, the WhoQol BREF scale [SKE 04] and the SF12 scale [WAR 96]. The first scale is composed of four items and the second of seven items. The two sets of items are considered to assess the same trait, a trait concerned with the psychological quality of life. The four psychological items of the WhoQol BREF are scored in five ordered categories, with scores therefore ranging from zero to four each. In this chapter, we do not concern ourselves with the empirical ordering of these categories for each item, although in any analysis concerned with improving the scale or application at the individual level, it is recommended that the empirical evidence be investigated. Instead, the scores on the four items are summed to provide a single instruments score with a range of possible scores from zero to 16. The seven items from SF12 have three dichotomous items scored zero to one, one item with three categories scored zero to two, and three items with six categories scored zero to five. When summed to form an instrument score, the range of possible scores is 0 to 20. Data from a sample of 233 persons from the French ANRS CO-8 multicenter cohort study [PRO 07, MES 08] are considered. Details about the items are given in Table 10.6.

Instrument	Item	Item wording
WhoQoL HIV BREF	wq_1	How much do you enjoy life?
	wq_2	How satisfied are you with your ability to learn new information?
	wq_4	How much do you value yourself?
	wq_5	Do you have negative feelings, mood, despair, anxiety, depression?
SF12	sf_4	Does your health now limit you in moderate activities such as moving a table, pushing a vacuum cleaner, ...?
	sf_6	During the past four weeks, have you accomplished less than you would like?
	sf_7	During the past four weeks, were you limited in the kind of work or other regular activities you do?
	sf_9	During the past four weeks, did not you do work or other regular activities as carefully as usual?
	sf_10	How much time have you felt calm and peaceful during the past four weeks?
	sf_11	How much of the time during the past four weeks did you have a lot of energy?
	sf_12	How much time during the past four weeks have you felt down?

Table 10.6. *Item wording for the items in the two instruments that are equated*

10.6.1. *Person threshold distribution*

A four moment reduced parameterization for each instrument was applied in the first instance. Before conducting tests of fit and equating based on how well the data fit the model with four moments, it is judicious to check the alignment of the estimated locations of the person and threshold distributions. Figure 10.1 depicts this alignment of 233 persons and 36 threshold estimates.

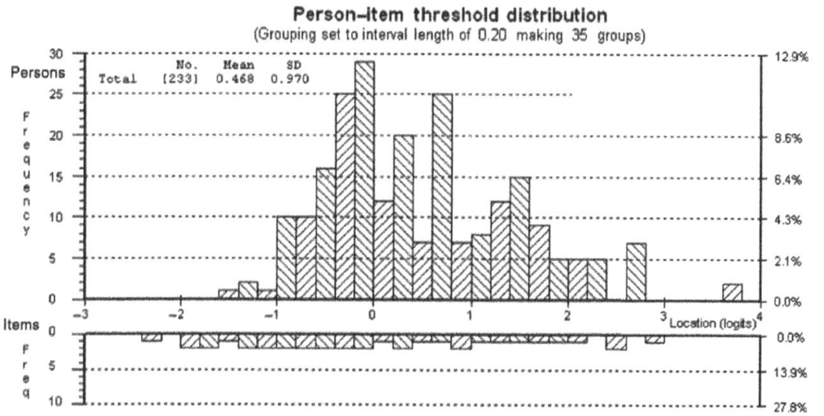

Figure 10.1. *Distribution of the persons and threshold locations with a parameterization with four moments for each instrument*

There were only two persons with a maximum score of 36, no person with a score of 35, and no persons with a score below six. It is evident that the alignment is sound and that further analysis can be interpreted without concern for the alignment.

10.6.2. *The test of fit between the data and the model*

The tests of fit, with the parameterization of the polytomous Racsh model with both four, and then two, moments of the thresholds are now presented. In the WhoQol BREF(4), scores of zero and one had a zero frequency, and in SF12(7), the score of zero had a zero frequency. These zero frequencies were no impediment to the estimation algorithm.

10.6.2.1. *Conditional χ^2 test of fit based on cells of the data matrix and four moments estimated*

We consider first the conditional fit according to [10.23] when the first four moments of the thresholds are estimated. There are $(16+1)(20+1)-2 = 355$ cells in the matrix of response pairs when the cells with total scores of $r = 0$ and $m_j + m_i = r$ are eliminated. In addition, seven different total scores, one, two, three, four, five, eight, 35, have a zero frequency. Therefore, the corresponding seven sets of cells are not involved in the test of fit. The adjusted degrees of freedom are given by subtracting this corresponding number of cells with zero frequency, which was 31, and ensuring that the number of constraints originally counted is not counted a second time. According to [10.25], and with this adjustment, the degrees of freedom from [10.26] are

$$m_j m_i - (M_j + M_j - 1) = 20 \cdot 16 - 7 - (31 - 7) = 289$$

The calculated χ^2 value from [10.23] is 262.961. Thus, the test of fit according to [10.23] gives

$$\chi^2 = 262.961, df = 289, p = 0.862$$

This indicates an excellent fit to the model.

Many cells had very low expected frequencies, many even less than one. Given the small sample size, even smaller than the degrees of freedom, any confidence in this conclusion is reduced. The example is provided only illustratively.

10.6.2.2. *Conditional χ^2 test of fit based on class intervals of the data matrix and four moments estimated*

Because many cells had small frequencies, for each total score just two class intervals of adjacent cells were formed and a χ^2 statistic according to [10.27] was calculated. If there were no total scores with zero frequency, the number of degrees of freedom given by [10.28] would be $m_j + m_i - M_j - M_i = 20 + 16 - 4 - 4 = 28$. However, with seven non-extreme scores with zero frequencies, the degrees of freedom are 21.

The calculated χ^2 value according to [10.27] is 23.806. Thus, the test of fit according to [10.27] gives

$$\chi^2 = 23.806, df = 21, p = 0.303$$

This test again shows an excellent fit of data to the model. More confidence can be placed in this χ^2 test, in which class intervals were formed, than in the one in which cells were used. However, once again we note the relatively small sample size.

10.6.2.3. *Conditional χ^2 test of fit based on cells of the data matrix and two moments estimated*

The parameterization with two moments, $M_j = M_j = 2$, is specifically that of [10.12] in which the successive thresholds for each instrument are constrained to be equidistant.

With this parameterization, there are four more degrees of freedom than when four moments, are estimated giving $df = 298 + 4 = 293$.

The χ^2 values is 292.913, giving the summary fit as

$$\chi^2 = 292.913, df = 293, p = 0.4904$$

Again, however, it is important to recognize the small sample size relative to the large degrees of freedom, and that despite evidence of fit, little confidence with such a small sample size and large degrees of freedom can be placed in the result.

10.6.2.4. *Conditional χ^2 test of fit based on class intervals of the data matrix and two moments estimated*

When class intervals are formed for each total score, the χ^2 values is 23.561, giving the summary fit as

$$\chi^2 = 23.561, df = 25, p = 0.545$$

This fit again is excellent, with the observed χ^2 value a little smaller than its expected value. In this case, more confidence can be placed on the test of fit than when cell frequencies are used.

It is stressed that only three independent parameters are estimated in this parameterization. It seems remarkable even with the caution of the smallness of the sample size that the two instruments can be equated with the PRM and just three parameters. Table 10.7 summarizes the test of fit for the two parameterizations of the real data.

Real data	Cells	Class intervals
Four moments	$\chi^2 = 262.961$ $df = 289$ $p = 0.862$	$\chi^2 = 23.806$ $df = 23$ $p = 0.303$
Two moments	$\chi^2 = 292.913$ $df = 293$ $p = 0.4904$	$\chi^2 = 23.561$ $df = 25$ $p = 0.545$

Table 10.7. *Summary of the conditional test of fit for parameterizations with four and two moments for each instrument respectively*

10.6.3. *Further analysis with the parameterization with two moments for each instrument*

Because of the successful fit of the data to the model with two moments estimated, the rest of the chapter focuses on further results from this analysis. The results from the four moment parameterization are virtually identical.

10.6.3.1. *Parameter estimates from two moments*

First, the parameter estimates, which have a clear interpretation in the case where two moments are estimated, that of location and average half distance between successive thresholds, are shown in Table 10.8. This output used the parameterization of [10.12].

Instrument	$\hat{\delta}_j$ (SE)	$\hat{\lambda}_j$ (SE)
SF12 (7)	0.230 (0.032)	0.113 (0.004)
WhoQol BREF (4)	−0.230 (0.037)	0.146 (0.006)

Table 10.8. *Estimates of the location and the half distance between successive thresholds with two moments of the instruments estimated*

10.6.3.2. *Score characteristic curves*

In this case, the score characteristic curves are simple, symmetrical and elegant. These curves are shown in Figure 10.2. They show the probability of a response in any score as a function of the location of a person on the trait. Thresholds $\hat{\delta}_3$ and $\hat{\delta}_{12}$ in each instrument are highlighted. The successive threshold estimates within each instrument are equidistant with a value of $2\hat{\lambda}_j$: in SF12(7), this distance is $2\lambda_j$ $2(0.113) = 0.226$; in WhoQol(4), it is $2(0.146) = 292$.

10.6.3.3. *Observed and expected frequencies in class intervals*

With the substantially fewer cells when two class intervals for each total score are formed for each total score, it is possible to show the observed and expected frequencies for these class intervals. Table 10.9 shows the observed and expected frequencies in the class intervals for each raw score, where the frequencies in the two class intervals are complementary. It is evident that even with some small expected frequencies, the observed and expected frequencies are very similar and consistent with the summary test of fit of $\chi^2 = 23.561, df = 25, p = 0.545$.

10.6.3.4. *Graphical test of fit based on conditioning on total scores*

Figure 10.3 shows the plot of the observed mean for each total score relative to its expected value, together with the 95% confidence intervals for each total score according to [10.30]. These two figures are complementary and both are produced for completeness. The plot is discrete, and the expected value points for each total score are interpolated for ease of interpretation. Again, the evidence is that the data fit the model exceptionally well. We note that, because there are different numbers of persons with each total score, and because the variance of the mean is a function of the total score, that the confidence intervals vary across the total scores. It is evident from the location of the observed means within their confidence intervals that the graphical test of fit is consistent with the conditional χ^2 reported in Table 10.7.

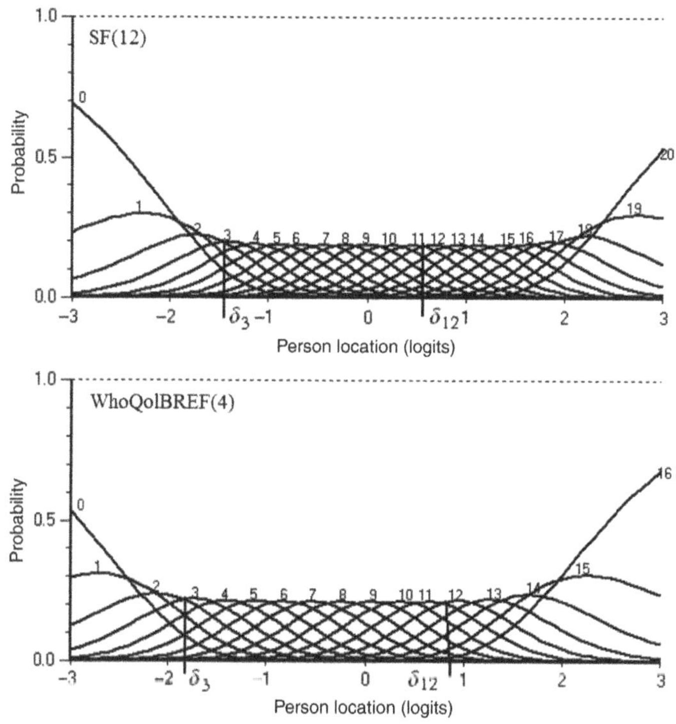

Figure 10.2. *Score characteristic curves with two moments estimated for each instrument*

10.6.3.5. *Graphical test of fit based on person estimates*

Figure 10.4 shows the results of the graphical test of fit based on person estimates: it shows the expected value curve for each of the tests with the observed mean of the responses in each six class intervals. The two plots are complementary. Clearly, the observed means are close to the expected values and confirm, given the power of the sample size, that these two instruments can be equated.

r	$F(r)$	Class Interval 1 observed	Class Interval 1 expected	Class Interval 1 residual	Class Interval 2 observed	Class Interval 2 expected	Class Interval 2 residual
6	1	0	0.201	−0.201	1	0.799	0.201
7	2	1	0.668	0.332	1	1.332	−0.332
9	1	0	0.367	−0.367	1	0.633	0.367
10	5	2	1.271	0.729	3	3.729	−0.729
11	5	3	2.013	0.987	2	2.987	−0.987
12	6	1	1.711	−0.711	5	4.289	0.711
13	4	1	1.757	−0.757	3	2.243	0.757
14	7	0	2.224	−2.224	7	4.776	2.224
15	9	5	4.286	0.714	4	4.714	−0.714
16	13	5	4.573	0.427	8	8.427	−0.427
17	12	1	2.897	−1.897	11	9.103	1.897
18	15	2	2.299	−0.299	13	12.701	0.299
19	14	1	1.254	−0.254	13	12.746	0.254
20	12	0	0.576	−0.576	12	11.424	0.576
21	6	1	0.634	0.366	5	5.366	−0.366
22	14	1	0.814	0.186	13	13.186	−0.186
23	7	1	0.866	0.134	6	6.134	−0.134
24	10	0	0.698	−0.698	10	9.302	0.698
25	15	2	2.159	−0.159	13	12.841	0.159
26	7	0	0.583	−0.583	7	6.417	0.583
27	8	0	1.333	−1.333	8	6.667	1.333
28	12	1	1.191	−0.191	11	10.809	0.191
29	15	1	2.913	−1.913	14	12.087	1.913
30	9	0	1.082	−1.082	9	7.918	1.082
31	5	0	1.170	−1.170	5	3.830	1.170
32	5	1	0.755	0.245	4	4.245	−0.245
33	5	4	1.498	2.502	1	3.502	−2.502
34	7	2	1.272	0.728	5	5.728	−0.728
Sum	231	36	43.065	−7.065	195	187.935	7.065

Table 10.9. *Observed and expected frequencies in two class intervals for each total score with two moments estimated for each instrument*

10.6.4. *Equated scores based on the parameterization with two moments of the thresholds*

We first report equating the two instruments using the expected values conditional on total scores using [10.34].

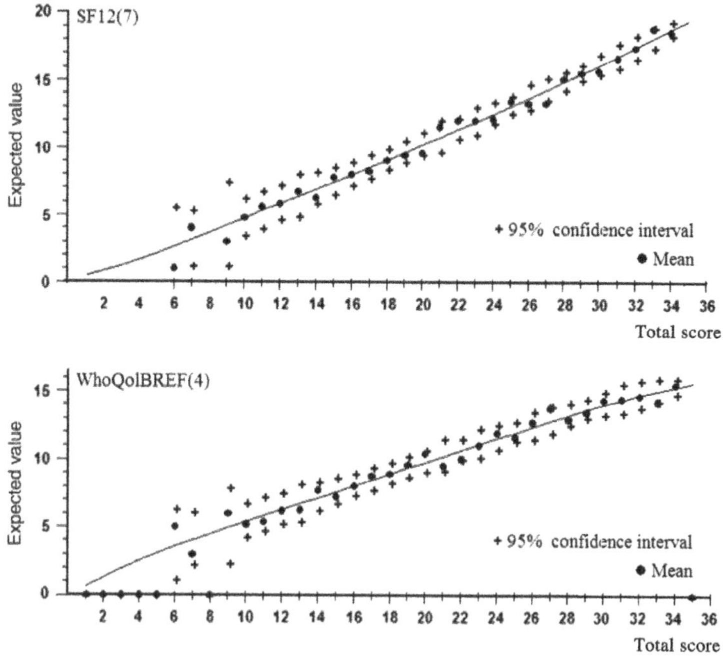

Figure 10.3. *Expected values conditional on the total score, the observed means and their 95% confidence interval, with two moments of the estimated thresholds*

10.6.4.1. *Equated scores conditional on the total score*

Table 10.10 shows the equivalent scores on the two instruments according to [10.34]. The second pair of columns for each total score shows the expected values in the first two columns, but with the scores rounded to the nearest integer. It is evident that for the same integer score on either instrument, there may be more than one corresponding rounded integer score on the other instrument. However, at most they have two different successive scores except in one case where rounded, a score of 15 on the first instrument has 17, 18 and 19 on the second instrument. This range is at the higher end of the continuum where the larger range of scores on SF12(7) is manifested. With different maximum scores, such a result for some scores is inevitable. This effect is not a function of the procedure, but of the data. Thus, the overwhelming impression is that the two sets of scores are very similar except that the different possible maximum scores on the two instruments play a role at the extremes. This effect can be seen in Figure 10.7, which shows the plot of the two sets of values, together with a linear trend line to provide a frame of reference for visualizing the curvature of the relationship in the extremes.

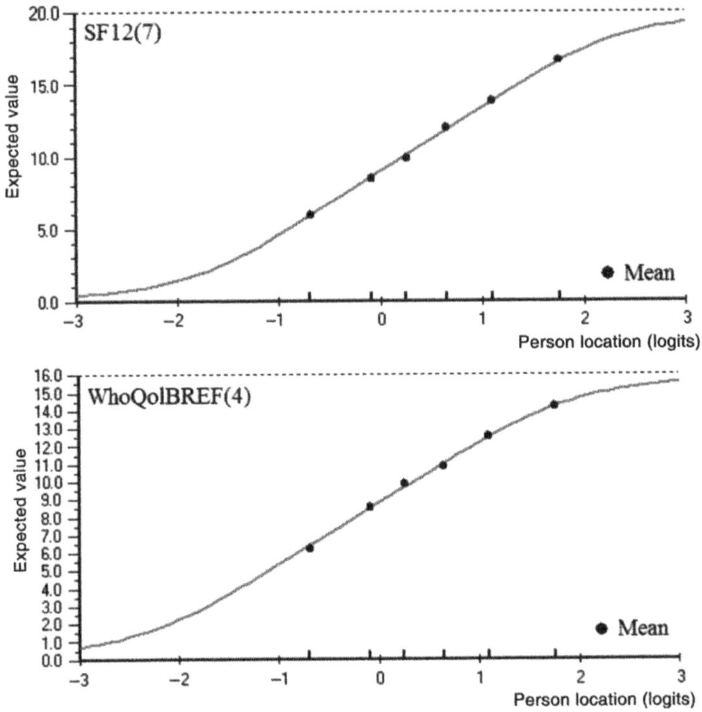

Figure 10.4. *Expected values given person estimates, and the observed means for six class intervals*

In clinical work, the approximate integer score from one instrument or the other can be used in any equating. In research, where means and standard deviations of samples from populations might be considered, non-integer values for equating can be used.

For completeness, Figure 10.6 shows the plot of the equivalence of WhoQol(4) against SF12(7). It is evident that the relationship is curvilinear.

10.6.4.2. *Equated scores given the person estimate*

To equate the two instruments using the person estimates, Table 10.11 shows the person location for each total score, and the expected values for the two instruments according to [10.32]. Again, one pair of scores is rounded to the nearest integer. It is evident that the equating based on estimates of person locations gives similar values to those based on the raw scores. There are slight differences at the extreme scores of one and 35. Figure 10.6 shows the expected value curves for each instrument. The curves are a function of the location parameter θ taken as a continuous variable, although in real data, there is only one location estimate for each total score.

Total Score	WhoQol(4)	SF12(7)	WhoQol(4)	SF12(7)
1	0.623	0.377	1	0
2	1.277	0.723	1	1
3	1.921	1.079	2	1
4	2.528	1.472	3	1
5	3.085	1.915	3	2
6	3.594	2.406	4	2
7	4.067	2.933	4	3
8	4.519	3.481	5	3
9	4.960	4.040	5	4
10	5.398	4.602	5	5
11	5.835	5.165	6	5
12	6.272	5.728	6	6
13	6.708	6.292	7	6
14	7.145	6.855	7	7
15	7.581	7.419	8	7
16	8.017	7.983	8	8
17	8.454	8.546	8	9
18	8.890	9.110	9	9
19	9.327	9.673	9	10
20	9.763	10.237	10	10
21	10.200	10.800	10	11
22	10.636	11.364	11	11
23	11.072	11.928	11	12
24	11.508	12.492	12	12
25	11.943	13.057	12	13
26	12.376	13.624	12	14
27	12.804	14.196	13	14
28	13.222	14.778	13	15
29	13.623	15.377	14	15
30	14.000	16.000	14	16
31	14.348	16.652	14	17
32	14.666	17.334	15	17
33	14.964	18.036	15	18
34	15.267	18.733	15	19
35	15.603	19.397	16	19

Table 10.10. *Equivalent expected values, and expected values rounded to the nearest integer, with two moments of the thresholds estimated conditional on total scores*

Total Score	Person Estimate	WhoQol(4)	SF12(7)	WhoQol(4)	SF12(7)
1	−2.682	0.430	−0.080	0	0
2	−2.304	1.104	0.280	1	0
3	−2.047	1.758	0.696	2	1
4	−1.844	2.377	1.163	2	1
5	−1.672	2.956	1.673	3	2
6	−1.519	3.497	2.217	3	2
7	−1.377	4.003	2.783	4	3
8	−1.243	4.485	3.366	4	3
9	−1.113	4.946	3.954	5	4
10	−0.985	5.395	4.542	5	5
11	−0.859	5.836	5.127	6	5
12	−0.732	6.274	5.706	6	6
13	−0.606	6.710	6.280	7	6
14	−0.479	7.146	6.850	7	7
15	−0.352	7.582	7.416	8	7
16	−0.225	8.018	7.981	8	8
17	−0.098	8.454	8.546	8	9
18	0.029	8.891	9.109	9	9
19	0.156	9.329	9.673	9	10
20	0.284	9.767	10.236	10	10
21	0.411	10.208	10.799	10	11
22	0.538	10.651	11.362	11	11
23	0.665	11.097	11.924	11	12
24	0.792	11.549	12.488	12	12
25	0.919	12.004	13.055	12	13
26	1.046	12.461	13.629	12	14
27	1.175	12.918	14.213	13	14
28	1.307	13.369	14.814	13	15
29	1.442	13.808	15.438	14	15
30	1.583	14.232	16.087	14	16
31	1.732	14.634	16.761	15	17
32	1.897	15.013	17.459	15	17
33	2.089	15.371	18.177	15	18
34	2.330	15.708	18.901	16	19
35	2.686	16.032	19.612	16	20

Table 10.11. *Equivalent expected values, and expected values rounded to the nearest integer, on the two instruments with two principal components estimated and based on person estimates*

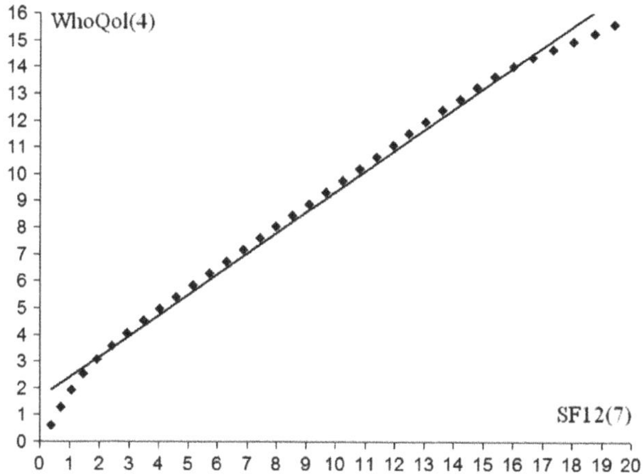

Figure 10.5. *Graphical relationship between scores on the two instruments with two moments of the thresholds conditional on total scores*

A possible advantage in using the person estimates over those based on the conditional raw score equation is that for a particular score on one instrument, the expected value on the other instrument can be obtained easily. This involves estimating the person location on one instrument given the score on that instrument, and then calculating the expected value, given the particular estimate, on the other instrument. An example is shown in Figure 10.6 where the location estimate associated with a score of 13 on the WhoQol(4) is 1.199, and the expected value on the SF12(7) for this location value is 14.321.

Figure 10.5 shows the plot of the two sets of values together with a linear trend line to provide a frame of reference for visualizing the curvature of the relationship between the scores in the extremes. The plot is similar to that obtained by conditioning on the total score shown in Figure 10.5.

10.7. Discussion

Some interpretations that arise from the equating of two instruments using the PRM in the way described above are now considered.

First arises a question of terminology regarding the different parameterizations. In some nomenclature, the reparameterization in terms of the moments of the thresholds would be considered a model different from the original parameterizations. Likewise, the parameterizations with four moments might be considered a different model from the one with just two moments for each instrument. Clearly, the parameterizations are different. However, it is suggested that it is more efficient to consider that in all cases,

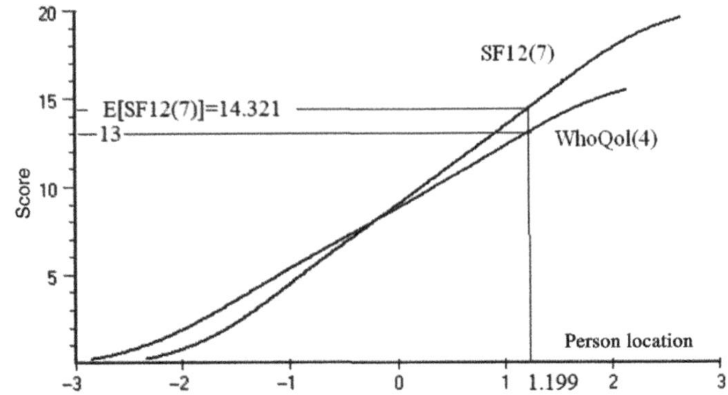

Figure 10.6. *Expected value curves for the two instruments with two moments of the thresholds as a function of the person location estimate for each total score*

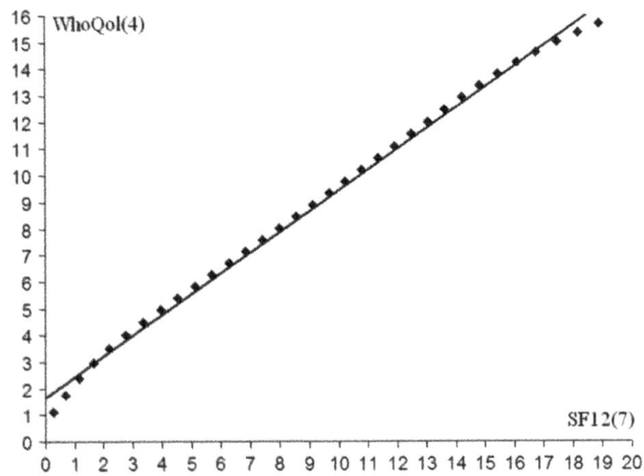

Figure 10.7. *Graphical relationship between equivalent scores on the two instruments with two moments of the thresholds based on the person estimates*

we have a single, generic model, the PRM, and to describe the cases where moments of the thresholds are estimated, and then different numbers of moments, as simply different parameterizations.

The reason for the emphasis on the generic model, in particular the Rasch model, is that this terminology is well understood to belong to the class of models with sufficient statistics. This perspective also leads to the second point of discussion. As broached earlier in the chapter, the model implies that no distributional assumptions need to be made in the equating – the persons might be somewhat more or less to the right on the continuum, and may be more or less normally distributed, or distributed in any other way, and such differences should have no impact on the equating. The equating is an intrinsic property relating the two instruments, which is independent of the distribution of persons used in the equating. This independence from this distribution seems to be a powerful property of the approach. Of course, the quality of the equating will depend on the fit of the data to the model, but other than equipercentile scaling methods, where the equality of distributions is imposed empirically, this dependence on fit is present whenever a model is used. And as shown in the chapter, rigorous tests of fit of the data to the model are available. It is left for other occasions to make comparisons between the method considered in this chapter and other methods found in the literature.

A third point of discussion when using the PRM in the way proposed, and in the example used for illustrative purposes, is whether equating should be based on the estimates of the item parameters, when they can be obtained, rather than based on the estimates of the instrument parameters. The advantage of the approach proposed based on estimates of the instrument parameters directly is that any relative degree of dependence among items within each instrument which might be greater than the degree of dependence between items from the different instruments, generally referred to as local dependence, is absorbed into the response structure of the thresholds. As a result, the equating is based on the variable that is common to the two instruments, that is, the latent variable defined by the trait common to the two instruments. If there is no local dependence within the instruments, then the two methods, directly at the instrument level and at the item level, will give similar results. If the full complement of thresholds were estimated in both approaches, and if there were no local dependence within instruments, then the two approaches would give identical results. Of course, this question does not arise if the only data available are at the level of instruments. The advantage of equating at the level of instruments, when the data fit the chosen parameterization of the model, is that the number of parameters estimated is relatively small. With a small number of parameters, their estimates should be more stable than if more parameters were estimated from the same data.

10.8. Bibliography

[AND 72] ANDERSEN E.B., "The numerical solution of a set of conditional estimation equations", *Journal of the Royal Statistical Society (Series B)*, vol. 34, pp. 42–54, 1972.

[AND 77] ANDERSEN E.B., "Sufficient statistics and latent trait models", *Psychometrika*, vol. 42, pp. 69–81, 1977.

[AND 78] ANDRICH D., "A rating formulation for ordered response categories". *Psychometrika*, vol. 43, pp. 561–573, 1978.

[AND 82] ANDRICH D., "A two parameter extension of the Rasch model for ratings". *Psychometrika*, vol. 47, pp. 105–113, 1982.

[AND 85] ANDRICH D., "A latent trait model for items with response dependencies: implications for instrument construction and analysis", in EMBRETSON S. (ed.), *Test Design: Contributions from Psychology, Education and Psychometrics*, Academic Press, New York, NY, pp. 245–273, 1985.

[AND 03] ANDRICH D., LUO G., "Conditional pairwise estimation in the Rasch model for ordered response categories using principal components", *Journal of Applied Measurement*, vol. 4, pp. 205–221, 2003.

[AND 10] ANDRICH D., SHERIDAN B., LUO G., RUMM2030, Computer software and manual, RUMM Laboratory, Perth, Australia, 2010.

[LEU 76] LEUNBACH G., *A Probabilistic Measurement Model for Assessing Whether Instruments Measure the Same Personal Factor*, Danish Institute for Educational Research, Copenhagen, 1976.

[LUO 05] LUO G., ANDRICH D., "Estimating parameters in the Rasch model in the presence of null categories", *Journal of Applied Measurement*, vol. 6, pp. 128–146, 2005.

[MES 08] MESBAH M., BOISSON V., SPIRE B., "Longitudinal Analysis of Partially Equated Health Related Quality of Life Scales", *First International Symposium on Biopharmaceutical Statistics*, Shanghai, China, 2008.

[PRO 07] PROTOPOPESCU C., MARCELLIN F., SPIRE B., PRAU M., VERDON R., PEYRAMOND D., RAFFI F., CHNE G., LEPORT C., CARRIERI M., "Health-related quality of life in HIV-1-infected patients on HAART: a five-years longitudinal analysis accounting for dropout in the APROCOCOPILOTE cohort ANRS CO-8", *Quality of Life Research*, vol. 16, pp. 557–591, 2007.

[RAS 61] RASCH G., "On general laws and the meaning of measurement in psychology", *Proceedings of the Fourth Berkeley Symposium on Mathematical Statistics and Probability, IV*, University of California Press, Berkeley, CA, pp. 321–334, 1961.

[SKE 04] SKEVINGTON S.M., LOTFY M., O'CONNELL K.A., "The world health organization's WHOQOL-BREF quality of life assessment: psychometric properties and results of the international field trial. A report from the WHOQOL group", *Quality of Life Research*, vol. 13, pp. 299–310, 2004.

[VON 04] VON DAVIER A.A., HOLLAND P.W., THAYER D.T., *The Kernel Method of Instrument Equating*, Springer, New York, NY, 2004.

[WAR 96] WARE J.E., KOSINSKI M., KELLER S.D., "A 12-Item Short-Form Health Survey: Construction of scales and preliminary tests of reliability and validity", *Medical Care*, vol. 34, pp. 220–233, 1996.

[WIL 93] WILSON M., MASTERS G.N., "The partial credit model and null categories". *Psychometrika*, vol. 58, pp. 87–99, 1993.

[WRI 82] WRIGHT B.D., MASTERS G.N., *Rating Scale Analysis: Rasch Measurement*, MESA Press, Chicago, IL, 1982.

Chapter 11

A Multidimensional Latent Class Rasch Model for the Assessment of the Health-Related Quality of Life

11.1. Introduction

The World Health Organization [WHO 95] defined the Quality of Life (QoL) as:

> "*the individuals' perceptions of their position in life in the context of their culture and the value systems in which they live, and in relation to their goals, expectations, standards and concerns. It is a broad-ranging concept affected in a complex way by the persons' physical health, psychological state, level of independence, social relationships, personal beliefs, and their relationship to the salient features of their environment.*"

In a survey about QoL, Fayers and Machin [FAY 00] defined the Health related Quality of Life (HrQoL) as:

> "*the way, which according to the health of a person it influences his/her capacity to lead on physical and social normal activities.*"

The "normality" of an activity is a variable concept, because it depends on the reference population. The use of indicators about HrQoL in clinical and epidemiological contexts is various: *in primis* these indicators give additional information to evaluate the effect of care therapies on a patient. More and more, HrQoL is considered as a secondary end point of clinical trials, because the main

---

Chapter written by Silvia BACCI and Francesco BARTOLUCCI.

focus is on survival. However, in some contexts, such as that of pain therapies for terminal cancer patients, it rises to a primary end point.

The main problem related to HrQoL concerns its measurement because this characteristic is not directly observable. Rather, suitable measurement methods based on qualitative information coming from *ad hoc* questionnaires can be translated into quantitative information (see [MES 10] for a detailed illustration about statistical aspects involved in the measurement of HrQoL). In such a way it is possible to evaluate the patient's condition in relation to the general condition of the population so as to provide clinicians with information useful for the care and therapy decisional process. In this context, the Rasch model [RAS 61] is an important tool to measure HrQoL, but some important aspects must be taken into account.

First of all, HrQoL is a latent multidimensional concept and its proper evaluation requires consideration of several dimensions corresponding to different latent traits that reflect individual health conditions and how well patients are coping with the stress due to illness. It is common to distinguish between physical and psychological macro-dimensions. These are further partitioned into subdimensions, such as bodily pain and physical functioning in the former case, and mental health or vitality in the latter case. The latent traits corresponding to the different dimensions are often highly correlated, and are also correlated with other latent traits, such as those corresponding to some psychopathological disturbances, mainly anxiety and depression. However, the classic Rasch model is based on the assumption of unidimensionality. The easiest approach that is adopted when this assumption is not realistic consists of estimating separate Rasch models for subsets of items measuring different latent traits, but this method does not allow us to measure the correlation between these latent traits. A more suitable approach is based on multidimensional extensions of Rasch models.

The second aspect is that, in many applications, it is of interest to detect homogeneous classes of individuals with very similar latent characteristics. Detecting these classes of individuals cannot be only more realistic, but also more convenient, for the decisional process because individuals in the same class will receive the same clinical treatment.

In order to analyse HrQoL data, taking these aspects into account, we propose the use of a version of the Rasch model that belongs to the class of multidimensional Item Response Theory (IRT) models proposed by Bartolucci [BAR 07]. The model is characterized by two main features: (1) more latent traits are simultaneously considered (*multidimensionality assumption*); and (2) these latent traits are represented by a random vector having a *discrete* distribution common to all subjects (*discreteness assumption*). Each support point of this distribution identifies a different class of individuals. Obviously, these are latent classes, in the sense that we do not know to which class a given individual belongs; moreover, we do not know how many latent classes exist. Bartolucci's model is related to the latent class (LC) model [LAZ 68, GOO 74] and will be referred to as the *multidimensional LC Rasch model.*

The LC model originates as a method to classify individuals on the basis of categorical responses, but, more recently, the same discrete latent structure on which this model is based has been employed to account for the unobserved heterogeneity between subjects into other models. Using this structure can be considered an alternative to the inclusion of continuous random effects, which avoids a parametric specification of the distribution of these effects. A semi-parametric model then results. In particular, this structure has been used to define a unidimensional LC Rasch model [LIN 91, FOR 95], which is a special case of the model that we adopt here. An alternative generalization of the Rasch model connected with the LC analysis is represented by the mixture Rasch model [ROS 90]. This allows for different sets of item parameters within each latent class.

Another model that is strongly related to the multidimensional LC Rasch model is the LC factor model proposed by Magidson and Vermunt [MAG 01]. However, in the first approach, each item response is affected by only one of the latent traits and these latent traits may be correlated, whereas Magidson and Vermunt assume that each item response is simultaneously affected by two or more mutually independent latent traits. We also note that alternative specifications of multidimensional Rasch models have been proposed, e.g. the multidimensional marginally sufficient Rasch model proposed by Hardouin and Mesbah [HAR 04].

The aim of this chapter is also to study the correlation between the latent dimensions of HrQoL in cancer patients and the latent dimensions behind some psychopathological disturbances. This analysis involves two tests of dimensionality. The first is a likelihood ratio (LR) test that is based on the multidimensional LC Rasch model that exploits the discrete (or LC) marginal maximum likelihood (MML) approach. The second test is based on the Martin-Löf test (ML) approach [MAR 70] and exploits the conditional maximum likelihood (CML) estimation method (see also [GLA 95a]). Alternative tests have been proposed by several authors (for a review see [VER 01]). Note also that Christensen *et al.* [CHR 02] discuss a test similar to the first test we use here. This test is based on the assumption that the latent traits follow a multivariate normal distribution.

The remainder of this chapter is structured as follows. In section 11.2 we describe the data set used for the illustrative application. In section 11.3 we present the multidimensional LC Rasch model of Bartolucci [BAR 07], with special attention to model assumptions and estimation. In section 11.4 we illustrate how to estimate the correlation between latent traits on the basis of the estimated parameters of this model. In the same section we describe our tests of dimensionality based on the MML and CML approaches. Finally, we present the results of the application to the data set described in section 11.2.

11.2. The data set

To illustrate the approach presented in this chapter, we analyze data from an Italian multicenter clinical study. These data concern 275 oncological patients recruited from three different centers (Ancona, Perugia and Messina). Patients were asked to fill in some questionnaires about different latent characteristics; here, we consider HrQoL, anxiety and depression. In particular, HrQoL is assessed by the "36-item Short-Form Health Survey" (SF-36) [WAR 02], whereas anxiety and depression are assessed by the "Hospital Anxiety and Depression Scale" (HADS) [ZIG 83]. The response rate is equal to 74% (203 patients out of 275 filled out the questionnaires). However, the sample of respondents is here assumed to be representative of the entire sample, since there is no significant difference between the distributions of age, gender, marital status, education and cancer diagnosis (see Table 11.1 for a comparison of distributions of these variables between the entire sample and the sample of respondents).

SF-36 is a multidimensional test developed in the 1990s to evaluate HrQoL during the last four weeks of illness; it has been validated in many different languages. It consists of 36 polytomous items divided into nine subsets (corresponding to different latent traits):

1) PF: physical functioning (ten items);

2) RF: role functioning (four items);

3) BP: bodily pain (two items);

4) GH: general health (five items);

5) VT: vitality (four items);

6) SF: social functioning (two items);

7) RE: role-emotional (three items);

8) MH: mental health (five items);

9) HC: health change (one item).

The items have different numbers of response categories. To simplify the illustration of the results, in the present study, all the items are dichotomized, with category one indicating the presence of a symptom or limitation (related to a low level of HrQoL), and category zero indicating its absence (related to a high level of the HrQoL). Table 11.2 shows how the items were dichotomized. For the item coding used for the questionnaire SF-36 see [WAR 02].

HADS is a questionnaire designed to assess anxiety and depression in patients with organic diseases, such as cancer. The questionnaire is composed of 14 items referred

	Entire sample	Respondents
Age (years)		
Mean	54.6	54.3
Standard deviation	13.4	11.5
Gender (%)		
Female	66.9	68.9
Male	33.1	31.1
Marital status (%)		
Single	10.1	9.8
Married	79.4	80.3
Divorced	4.2	3.3
Widowed	6.3	6.6
Education (%)		
Primary school	12.6	12.9
Middle school	29.5	30.3
High school	38.8	37.6
University	19.1	19.1
Cancer diagnosis (%)		
Colon-rectum	24.4	23.9
Mammary	45.6	46.7
Uterine	4.1	3.8
Pulmonary	8.8	8.7
Prostate	4.1	3.8
Other	13.0	13.0
Size	275	203

Table 11.1. *Entire and respondent sample distributions of age, gender, marital status, education and cancer diagnosis (column percentages)*

to two dimensions:

1) anxiety (seven items);

2) depression (seven items).

All items have four response categories that have been dichotomized for our analysis, with category one (corresponding to original categories two and three) indicating the presence of anxiety (or depression) and category zero (corresponding to original categories zero and one) indicating its absence. For the item coding used for the questionnaire HADS see [ZIG 83].

Note that, in both questionnaires, every item is assumed to measure only one latent trait, but the traits may be correlated.

Item*	Dichotomized responses	
	0	1
1	1, 2, 3	4, 5
2	1, 2, 3	4, 5
3a–3l	3	1, 2
4a–4d	2	1
5a–5c	2	1
6	1, 2, 3	4, 5
7	1, 2, 3	4, 5, 6
8	1, 2, 3	4, 5
9a, 9d, 9e, 9h	1, 2, 3, 4	5, 6
9b, 9c, 9f, 9g, 9i	5, 6	1, 2, 3, 4
10	3, 4, 5	1, 2
11a, 11c	4, 5	1, 2, 3
11b, 11d	1, 2, 3	4, 5

Table 11.2. *SF-36: original response categories and their dichotomization. Item labels refer to the Italian version of SF-36*

11.3. The multidimensional latent class Rasch model

In the following, we describe the model that we propose for the analysis of HrQoL data. This model is a version of the Rasch model that belongs to the class of IRT models proposed by Bartolucci [BAR 07]. The main differences between this model and the classic Rasch model [RAS 61] are that (1) multidimensionality is assumed; and (2) the latent traits are assumed to have a discrete distribution. To facilitate the illustration of the model, we make explicit reference to the data set described in the previous section.

11.3.1. *Model assumptions*

Let n denotes the number of subjects in the sample and suppose that they respond to k test items that measure D different latent traits or dimensions. Also let $\mathcal{I}_d$, $d = 1, \ldots, D$, be the subset of $\mathcal{I} = \{1, \ldots, k\}$ containing the indices of the items measuring the latent trait of type d and let k_d denotes the cardinality of this subset, so that $k = \sum_{d=1}^{D} k_d$. Since we assume that every item measures only one latent trait, the subsets $\mathcal{I}_d$ are disjoint. In our study, $n = 203$ and $k = 50$ (36 items from SF-36 and 14 items from HADS) and, on the basis of validation studies about these questionnaires, we know that the items measure $D = 11$ different latent traits: nine related to HrQoL and two related to psychopathological disturbances.

In this context, the classic Rasch model, based on the assumption:

$$\text{logit}[p(X_i = 1 \mid \Theta = \theta)] = \theta - \beta_i, \quad i = 1, \ldots, k, \qquad [11.1]$$

where Θ can be discrete or continuous, is extended to a multidimensional model in the following way:

$$\text{logit}[p(X_i = 1 \mid \boldsymbol{\Theta} = \boldsymbol{\theta})] = \sum_{d=1}^{D} \delta_{id}\theta_d - \beta_i, \quad i = 1, \dots, k. \qquad [11.2]$$

In the above expressions, X_i is the random variable corresponding to the response to item i; in particular, $X_i = 1$ means the presence of the symptom or disturb detected by the item and $X_i = 0$ means its absence. In the unidimensional version, Θ is the latent random variable corresponding to the trait of the interest and θ denotes one of its possible values, whereas β_i is the difficulty of item i. In the multidimensional version, $\boldsymbol{\Theta} = (\Theta_1, \dots, \Theta_D)'$ is the vector of latent variables corresponding to the different traits measured by the test items, $\boldsymbol{\theta} = (\theta_1, \dots, \theta_D)'$ denotes one of its possible realizations and δ_{id} is an indicator variable equal to one if item i belongs to $\mathcal{I}_d$ (and therefore measures the dth latent trait) and zero otherwise.

Note that the model is based on a specific formulation of multidimensionality, in which each item measures only one latent trait; in other words we assume so-called *between-item multidimensionality*. This is different from *within-item multidimensionality*, where each item measures more than one latent trait (see [ADA 97] for a detailed description).

Another important point is that the unidimensional formulation based on [11.1] is a special case of that in [11.2]. In particular, one of the situations in which formulation [11.2] specialises into [11.1] is when the possible ability vectors $\boldsymbol{\theta}$ have elements equal to each other. To clarify this point, consider a simple example involving only two latent traits, so that $\boldsymbol{\Theta} = (\Theta_1, \Theta_2)'$, which may assume the values represented in Figure 11.1.

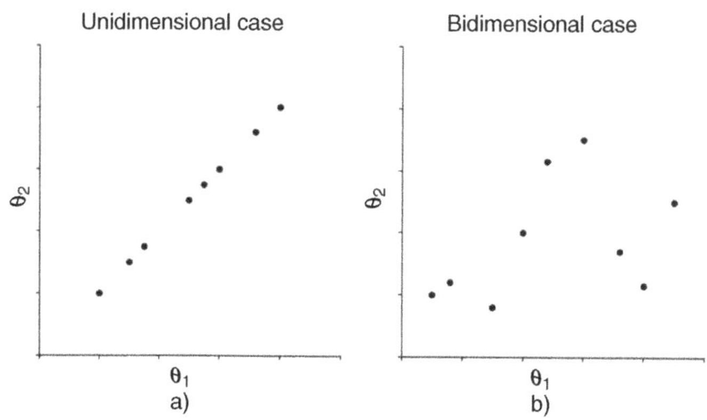

Figure 11.1. *Plots of (θ_1, θ_2) possible values*

We observe that panel a) corresponds to unidimensionality, because all points are aligned with the bisector. In other words, one latent trait coincides with the other and the actual number of dimensions is one. In panel b) the points are not on the bisector and there is no complete ordering of them; in this case, it is not possible to completely determine one latent trait from the other so that the two latent traits correspond to two distinct dimensions.

To complete the model specification, we need a distribution of the vector $\boldsymbol{\Theta}$, since we use a random-effects rather than a fixed-effects approach. In the latter, a distinct vector of parameters is estimated for each subject, but this does not allow certain analyses that are of interest in the present context.

In a standard formulation, a continuous distribution $\pi(\boldsymbol{\theta})$, such as the normal distribution, is adopted for Θ. In such a case, the *manifest distribution* of the full response vector, $\mathbf{X} = (X_1, \ldots, X_k)'$, is given by:

$$p(\mathbf{x}) = p(\mathbf{X} = \mathbf{x}) = \int_{\boldsymbol{\theta}} p(\mathbf{x}|\boldsymbol{\theta})\pi(\boldsymbol{\theta})d\boldsymbol{\theta}, \qquad [11.3]$$

where, because of the assumption of *local independence*,

$$p(\mathbf{x}|\boldsymbol{\theta}) = p(\mathbf{X} = \mathbf{x}|\boldsymbol{\Theta} = \boldsymbol{\theta}) = \prod_{i=1}^{k} p(X_i = x_i \mid \boldsymbol{\Theta} = \boldsymbol{\theta}). \qquad [11.4]$$

Note that, because of the between-item multidimensionality assumption, we assume local independence separately for each dimension and therefore:

$$\begin{aligned}\prod_{i=1}^{k} p(X_i = x_i \mid \boldsymbol{\Theta} = \boldsymbol{\theta}) &= \prod_{d=1}^{D}\prod_{h=1}^{k_d} p(X_{dh} = x_{dh} \mid \boldsymbol{\Theta} = \boldsymbol{\theta}) \\ &= \prod_{d=1}^{D}\prod_{h=1}^{k_d} p(X_{dh} = x_{dh} \mid \Theta_d = \theta_d), \qquad [11.5]\end{aligned}$$

where X_{dh} denotes the response variable for the h'th item measuring dimension d. The notation X_{dh} is equivalent to the previous notation, in the sense that each X_i coincides with a certain X_{dh} for suitable d and h. However, in this way we make explicit the dimension measured by this item.

It is worth recalling that the theory about the Rasch model does not require the latent trait of interest to have a continuous distribution. Moreover, assuming a discrete distribution may have some advantages [LIN 91, FOR 95]. Among other advantages, it can lead to more parsimonious models in certain situations: and it can be used to test the additivity assumption of the Rasch model and to construct empirical Bayes estimators of abilities [LIN 91]. We adopt this alternative approach and assume that the random vector $\boldsymbol{\Theta}$ has a discrete distribution with support set $\{\zeta_1, \ldots, \zeta_C\}$. In other words, we assume that the population is composed of C latent classes or subpopulations.

We also assume that the number of latent classes is the same for each dimension. In theory, it should also be possible to assume a more general model with a latent class structure that differs between dimensions, but in this case the interpretability of the parameters would not be straightforward. Similar to the conventional LC model [LAZ 68, GOO 74], the manifest distribution of the full response vector is given by:

$$p(\mathbf{x}) = p(\mathbf{X} = \mathbf{x}) = \sum_{c=1}^{C} p(\mathbf{x}|\boldsymbol{\zeta}_c)\pi_c, \qquad [11.6]$$

where $\pi_c = p(\boldsymbol{\Theta} = \boldsymbol{\zeta}_c)$ is the probability that a subject belongs to latent class c. According to equation [11.4], $p(\mathbf{x}|\boldsymbol{\zeta}_c)$ is defined as:

$$p(\mathbf{x}|\boldsymbol{\zeta}_c) = p(\boldsymbol{X} = \mathbf{x}|\boldsymbol{\Theta} = \boldsymbol{\zeta}_c) = \prod_{d=1}^{D}\prod_{h=1}^{k_d} p(X_{dh} = x_{dh} \mid \Theta_d = \zeta_{cd}), \quad c = 1, \ldots, C. \qquad [11.7]$$

The specification of the multidimensional LC Rasch model, based on the assumptions illustrated above, depends on the number of latent classes (C) and on how items are associated to the different dimensions (i.e. the subsets $\mathcal{I}_d$, $d = 1, \ldots, D$). Maximum likelihood estimation of this model is illustrated in the following section.

11.3.2. *Maximum likelihood estimation and model selection*

Assuming that the subjects in the sample are independent, the log-likelihood of the model is:

$$\ell(\boldsymbol{\eta}) = \sum_{\mathbf{x}} n(\mathbf{x}) \log[p(\mathbf{x})], \qquad [11.8]$$

where $\boldsymbol{\eta}$ is the vector containing all the parameters, $n(\mathbf{x})$ is the frequency of the response pattern $\mathbf{x}$ and the probability $p(\mathbf{x})$ is defined as in equation [11.6] depending on $\boldsymbol{\eta}$. Moreover, the sum $\sum_{\mathbf{x}}$ is over all the possible configurations of the response vector.

In order to maximize $\ell(\boldsymbol{\eta})$ to obtain the (discrete) MML estimate of $\boldsymbol{\eta}$, we use the EM algorithm [DEM 77], which is an iterative algorithm based on alternating two steps (E and M). The expectation (E) step consists of calculating the expected value of the complete log-likelihood evaluated at the current value of the parameters.

The maximization (M) step consists of updating these parameters by maximizing the expected log-likelihood found at the E step. These parameters are then used to determine the distribution of the latent variables at the next E step. The two steps are performed until convergence. See [BAR 07] for a detailed description of this estimation algorithm and its initialization.

At this stage we only stress that, in order to prevent the problem of the multimodality of the model likelihood, it is advisable to try different starting values chosen by both deterministic and random rules. We denote by $\hat{\eta}$ the MML estimate of η, that is the value that, at convergence of EM algorithm, corresponds to the highest log-likelihood. A similar notation is adopted for the single parameters.

Once the model is fitted, we can allocate each subject to one of the latent classes. The allocation depends on the specific item response pattern $\mathbf{x}$ provided by the subject. In particular, for each pattern $\mathbf{x}$ it is possible to estimate the *posterior probabilities* of belonging to latent class c as:

$$\hat{p}(\boldsymbol{\zeta}_c|\mathbf{x}) = \hat{p}(\boldsymbol{\Theta} = \boldsymbol{\zeta}_c|\mathbf{X} = \mathbf{x}) = \frac{\hat{p}(\mathbf{x}|\boldsymbol{\zeta}_c)\hat{\pi}_c}{\sum_{h=1}^{C} \hat{p}(\mathbf{x}|\boldsymbol{\zeta}_h)\hat{\pi}_h}, \quad c = 1, \ldots, C. \qquad [11.9]$$

An individual is assigned to the latent class with the highest posterior probability.

An important phase related to the estimation process is that of model selection, with special attention to the choice of the number of latent classes (C). A first approach [KIE 56] would suggest using the value of C corresponding to the saturation point beyond which the likelihood of the assumed model fails to increase. For the unidimensional LC Rasch model, the existence of this saturation point was established by Lindsay *et al.* [LIN 91]. However, in our context, this number of classes could be so large that the model becomes non-identifiable or almost non-identifiable. To avoid this, several authors suggest the use of information criteria. These typically penalize the log-likelihood by a factor that takes model complexity (as measured by the number of parameters) into account.

One of the most well-known information criteria is represented by the Bayesian information criterion (BIC) of Schwarz [SCH 78] given by:

$$BIC = -2\hat{\ell} + g\ln(n),$$

where $\hat{\ell}$ is the maximum value of the log-likelihood and g is the number of free parameters. For the multidimensional LC Rasch model, in particular, we have:

$$g = (C - 1) + DC + (k - D), \qquad [11.10]$$

since there are $C - 1$ mass probabilities for the classes, DC ability parameters and $k - D$ difficulty parameters (we have to consider that the D of them are constrained to 0 in order to ensure model identifiability). Among different models, the model with the smallest value of the BIC index is to be preferred. For an illustration in the context of mixture models, which is strongly related to the present model, see [MCL 00, Chapter 6].

11.3.3. *Software details*

In our application, we used the software accompanying the paper [BAR 07] to estimate the model and choose the number of classes. This software can be downloaded from the Web page:

`http://www.stat.unipg.it/bartolucci`

and is quite simple to use. The program is based on a Matlab® function, named `lcest.m`, which requires the following inputs:

– a matrix with each row corresponding to a different configuration of item responses and each column corresponding to an item (responses are coded by 0 or 1 and are suitably separated);

– a vector with the frequencies of the observed response configurations;

– the number of latent classes;

– the type of starting values (deterministic or random);

– the type of model (LC model, multidimensional LC Rasch model or multidimensional LC two-parameter logistic model);

– a matrix indicating the multidimensional structure of the set of items (any row contains the set of items referred to the same dimension).

The following output is obtained from `lcest.m` for the estimated model:

– maximum log-likelihood;

– estimated probabilities of the latent classes;

– BIC index;

– estimated difficulty parameters (and discriminating indices for the LC two-parameter logistic model);

– estimated support points for each latent class and each latent dimension;

– estimated probability of responding 1 to every item for each latent class;

– estimated posterior probabilities of belonging to the latent class for each response configuration.

Function `lcest.m` also allows us to select the optimal number of latent classes. We have to estimate a multidimensional LC Rasch model with an increasing number of latent classes and the best model is chosen on the basis of a given selection criterion, such as BIC. In a similar way, we can estimate the multidimensional LC Rasch model with different multidimensional structures in order to choose the optimal number of dimensions and to evaluate the possibility of collapsing two dimensions into a single dimension (see later sections for theoretical details an illustration using the data set).

Other outputs, such as the correlations between latent dimensions or between every item and the corresponding dimension, cannot be obtained directly by `lcest.m`, but a little extra programming is sufficient.

The analyses proposed here can also be performed by means of the R function `est_multi_poly` [BAR 12]. Input and output are analogous to those of `lcest.m`.

11.3.4. *Concluding remarks about the model*

It is a crucial assumption of the multidimensional LC Rasch model described above that the latent trait distribution is discrete. Alternatively, we could assume that the vector $\boldsymbol{\Theta}$ follows a multivariate normal distribution of dimension D. However, if the variance–covariance matrix of this distribution is unconstrained, calculating the manifest distribution of $\boldsymbol{X}$ would require complex numerical tools when D is greater than two, as in our application, because a high-dimensional integral is involved (see equation [11.3]). This has obvious implications on the parameter estimation and on the possibility of making a comparison with our model, which is based on a discrete latent trait distribution.

On the other hand, the model based on a multivariate normal distribution for the latent traits would be easily estimable under the constraint that the variance–covariance matrix is diagonal, so that the latent traits are independent. In fact, estimating this model is equivalent to estimating a separate unidimensional normal Rasch model for each dimension. This is also true for the model with a discrete latent trait distribution. It is worth noting that, with the same number of latent classes (C), the latter model involves more free parameters than the multidimensional LC Rasch model that we propose to use. In fact, this model has $D(C-1)+DC+(k-D)$ parameters that is larger than the number of parameters given in [11.10].

Though estimating separate unidimensional Rasch models does not allow us to study the correlation between the latent traits, this may be useful for assessing whether the assumption of discreteness of the latent trait distribution is suitable or not for the data at hand. This amounts to comparison of the global fit of these models under this assumption with the global fit statstics under the assumption of normality. The comparison may be based on standard criteria, such as BIC.

Finally, we remark that the multidimensional LC Rasch model may be easily extended to deal with polytomous items and incomplete data. Concerning the first issue, the extension would be based on adopting a suitable parameterization of the conditional response distribution given the latent traits, which extends that in [11.2]. For this aim, we can use one of the parameterizations illustrated by Samejima [SAM 96] in her review of IRT models for polytomous data. For incomplete data, we have to clarify that the model and the estimation algorithm can be easily extended to treat the case of incomplete responses by design, because it is sufficient to drop, for each subject, the items to which the subject does not respond. The extension to the case of informative missing responses is not so obvious.

11.4. Correlation between latent traits

In our context, the main interest is on the study of the correlation between the latent traits corresponding to the different dimensions. First of all, for two dimensions d_1 and d_2 (e.g. BP and SF), the correlation may be measured through the index:

$$\hat{\rho}_{d_1 d_2} = \sum_{c=1}^{C} \hat{\zeta}^*_{cd_1} \hat{\zeta}^*_{cd_2} \hat{\pi}_c, \qquad [11.11]$$

where $\hat{\pi}_c$ is the estimate of the weight of the cth latent class and $\hat{\zeta}^*_{cd}$, $c = 1, \ldots, C$, $d = 1, \ldots, D$, is the standardized estimate of the latent trait level referred to dimension d for the subjects in latent class c. In practice, this is the dth element of $\hat{\boldsymbol{\zeta}}_c$, once the average latent trait level has been subtracted from each element and this difference has been divided by the standard deviation.

A crucial point is how to test the hypothesis that two dimensions d_1 and d_2 are perfectly correlated. This hypothesis is strongly related to the hypothesis that the items in $\mathcal{I}_{d_1}$ and $\mathcal{I}_{d_2}$ measure the same latent trait. Given the parameterization in [11.2], the latter may be expressed as $H_0 : \zeta_{cd_2} = \zeta_{cd_1} + a$, with $c = 1, \ldots, C$, where a is an arbitrary constant. In the following, we deal with two different approaches to test H_0.

The first approach is directly based on the LR statistic between the multidimensional latent class Rasch model, in which a separate latent variable is used to represent each dimension, and a restricted version of this model in which dimensions d_1 and d_2 are collapsed into a single dimension. Both models are estimated by the discrete MML method, and the EM algorithm illustrated at the end of section 11.3. From this estimation we obtain the maximum log-likelihood of the general model ($\hat{\ell}_1$) and that of the restricted model ($\hat{\ell}_0$). Recall that both models are based on the same number of latent classes; they only differ in the number of latent variables and in how items are allocated to these variables. On the basis of these likelihoods, we obtain the following LR test statistic for the null hypothesis H_0:

$$LR_1 = -2(\hat{\ell}_0 - \hat{\ell}_1). \qquad [11.12]$$

Under H_0, LR_1 has an asymptotic chi-square distribution with $C - 1$ degrees of freedom, where C is the selected number of latent classes. We reject H_0 for high values of LR_1, that is values larger than a suitable percentile of the asymptotic distribution; otherwise, we do not reject this hypothesis, implying that the two dimensions are indeed collapsible. In order to measure the evidence provided by the data in favor of H_0, we can also calculate a p-value, as the value of the survival function of the asymptotic distribution at LR_1.

One of the main advantages of the above LR test is that, if properly extended, it can be also used when items discriminate differently among subjects (i.e. when the Rasch paradigm does not hold); however, this aspect is beyond the purposes of the current chapter. A disadvantage is, this approach requires the choice of the number of latent classes and the results may depend on this choice. For this reason we also consider a second approach for testing if two sets of items measure the same dimension, which does not require us to formulate any assumption on the distribution of the latent variables. This approach is based on the ML test [GLA 95a]. See [MAR 70] for the original version of the test for dichotomous items split into two dimensions and [CHR 02] for a generalization to polytomous items and to situations with more than two dimensions. It is worth mentioning that, in the psychometric literature, alternative tests are available that may be more powerful in certain situations. We refer, in particular, to the class of one degree of freedom tests proposed by Verhelst [VER 01].

The ML test is also an LR test between two models. The main difference with respect to the test based on statistic LR_1 is that the maximum log-likelihoods of the two models under comparison are obtained from CML estimates [RAS 61, AND 70, AND 72]. The maximum log-likelihood of the general model obtained in this way is denoted by $\tilde{\ell}_1$, whereas that of the restricted model is denoted by $\tilde{\ell}_0$. The resulting LR test statistic is then:

$$LR_2 = -2(\tilde{\ell}_0 - \tilde{\ell}_1). \qquad [11.13]$$

In particular, the first log-likelihood is obtained as:

$$\tilde{\ell}_1 = \tilde{\ell}_{1c}^{(1)} + \tilde{\ell}_{1c}^{(2)} + \tilde{\ell}_{1m}, \qquad [11.14]$$

where $\tilde{\ell}_{1c}^{(1)}$ is the maximum conditional log-likelihood for the items in $\mathcal{I}_{d_1}$ (e.g. PF), $\tilde{\ell}_{1c}^{(2)}$ is the maximum conditional log-likelihood for the items in $\mathcal{I}_{d_2}$ (e.g. RF), both obtained through the CML method, and $\tilde{\ell}_{1m}$ is the maximum marginal log-likelihood of the multinomial model for the distribution of the scores. The latter may be expressed as:

$$\tilde{\ell}_{1m} = \sum_{r_1=0}^{k_{d_1}} \sum_{r_2=0}^{k_{d_2}} n_{r_1 r_2} \log(n_{r_1 r_2}/n), \qquad [11.15]$$

where r_1 is the test score for the items in the subset $\mathcal{I}_{d_1}$, r_2 is the test score for the items in the subset $\mathcal{I}_{d_2}$, and $n_{r_1 r_2}$ is the frequency of subjects with scores r_1 and r_2 at the two subsets (see [VER 01] for details). We recall that the test score is the number of items that are responded by category one and that k_{d_1} and k_{d_2} are the number of items in the first dimension (e.g. PF) and in the second dimension (e.g. RF), respectively.

A decomposition similar to that in [11.14] holds for $\tilde{\ell}_0$. We have:

$$\tilde{\ell}_0 = \tilde{\ell}_{0c} + \tilde{\ell}_{0m}, \qquad [11.16]$$

where $\tilde{\ell}_{0c}$ is the maximum conditional log-likelihood for the items in $\mathcal{I}_{d_1} \cup \mathcal{I}_{d_2}$, and

$$\tilde{\ell}_{0m} = \sum_{r=0}^{k_{d_1}+k_{d_2}} n_r \log(n_r/n). \qquad [11.17]$$

In the above expression, r is the test score achieved at the items in both subsets, the frequency of which is denoted by n_r. Under H_0, the test-statistic LR_2 has an asymptotic chi-square distribution with $k_{d_1} k_{d_2} - 1$ degrees of freedom.

Though the ML test has the advantage of not requiring the choice of the number of latent classes neither the formulation of distribution assumptions on the latent variables, Verhelst [VER 01] and Christensen *et al.* [CHR 02] found that its power is significantly affected by the number of items and that it may be disappointingly low with strongly correlated latent dimensions. More precisely, it can be verified that the null distribution may deviate from the asymptotic chi-square distribution when the number of items is large and the sample size is small. In the psychometric literature there are several proposals to solve this problem. For example, Christensen and Kreiner [CHR 07] proposed a Monte Carlo test procedure for computing p-values. Another problem connected with the ML test concerns the fact that this test can be used only when the Rasch model holds, since otherwise the CML method cannot be applied.

In order to take into account advantages and disadvantages of the two tests described in this section, in our empirical study we apply both. The ML test is performed by means of STATA as concerning the computation of the maximum conditional log-likelihoods ($\tilde{\ell}_{0c}$, $\tilde{\ell}_{1c}^{(1)}$, $\tilde{\ell}_{1c}^{(2)}$), and through a suitable Matlab® function as concerning the marginal counterparts ($\tilde{\ell}_{0m}$, $\tilde{\ell}_{1m}$). The same methods could be applied by alternative statistical softwares, such as MULTIRA of Carstensen and Rost [CAR 01], the %pml SAS macro of Christensen and Bjorner [CHR 03] or DIGRAM of Kreiner [KRE 03].

Finally, we stress that the above methodology gives valid results provided that the Rasch paradigm holds for each dimension.

11.5. Application results

First we verified that the Rasch model holds for only five dimensions for the data set described earlier. Three of these dimensions (BP, SF and VT) are HrQoL dimensions, whereas the other two (anxiety and depression) measure psychopathological disturbances. Therefore, we based our analysis on the responses to the items referred to these five dimensions, whereas the items referred to the other dimensions were discarded. Overall, the data analyzed contains 22 items.

The first step of the analysis was focused on verifying if a discrete latent structure, on which the LC Rasch model is based, is indeed more suitable for the data at hand than a continuous latent structure based on the normal distribution. As explained in section 11.3.4, we cannot directly compare the multidimensional LC Rasch model with its normal counterpart because of the difficulties in estimating the latter. However, we can indirectly perform this comparison by estimating separate undimensional (LC and normal) Rasch models for each dimension. The results of this comparison are reported in Table 11.3 in terms of maximum log-likelihood and BIC index for each model.

The assumption that the distribution of the latent traits is discrete is preferable to the assumption that the distribution is normal. In fact, for each dimension, a unidimensional LC Rasch model always attains a higher maximum log-likelihood than its normal counterpart, while the minimum BIC index is always smaller. The same happens at global level (see the last two rows of Table 11.3). Then, we fitted the multidimensional LC Rasch model with an increasing number of latent classes. In this regard, in Table 11.4 we report the values of the maximum log-likelihood and of the BIC index obtained with a number of latent classes (C) from one to seven.

According to the adopted selection criterion, we chose $C = 6$ latent classes corresponding to $BIC = 4,175.0$. We observe that this model has a better fit than the model that is equivalent to separate independent unidimensional LC Rasch models. For the latter we have 4,277.1 as minimum value of the BIC index; this value is reached with two latent classes (see Table 11.3). For the multidimensional LC Rasch model with $C = 6$ latent classes, we obtained the parameter estimates (support points and class weights) displayed in Table 11.5. In particular, we estimated five support points (corresponding to the number of dimensions) for each of the six latent classes. Owing to the parameterization, given by equation [11.2], very low values of these support points correspond to a negligible probability of response 1, whereas very high values correspond to a negligible probability of response 0. To facilitate the interpretation of the results, the latent classes are ordered on the basis of the conditional probability of response 1 for the first dimension (BP).

Dimension		normal RM	LC Rasch model – number of latent classes (C)						
			1	2	3	4	5	6	7
BP	$\hat{\ell}$	−193.4	−206.9	**−190.5**	−190.5	−190.5	−190.5	−190.5	−190.5
	BIC	402.7	424.4	**402.2**	412.8	423.5	434.1	444.8	455.4
SF	$\hat{\ell}$	−157.8	−163.1	**−147.2**	−147.2	−147.2	−147.2	−147.2	−147.2
	BIC	331.5	336.9	**315.7**	326.4	337.0	347.6	358.3	368.9
VT	$\hat{\ell}$	−495.1	−511.0	−454.6	**−446.8**	−446.8	−446.8	−446.8	−446.8
	BIC	1016.7	1043.2	941.2	**936.2**	946.8	957.5	968.1	978.8
Anx.	$\hat{\ell}$	−671.6	−753.5	−653.4	**−642.7**	−641.0	−641.0	−641.0	−641.0
	BIC	1385.8	1544.3	1354.8	**1343.9**	1351.1	1361.8	1372.4	1383.0
Depr.	$\hat{\ell}$	−636.5	−701.6	−607.7	**−602.0**	−602.0	−602.0	−602.0	−602.0
	BIC	1315.5	1440.4	1263.2	**1262.4**	1273.0	1283.6	1294.2	1304.9
Overall	$\hat{\ell}$	−2154.4	−2336.1	**−2053.5**	−2029.2	−2027.5	−2027.5	−2027.5	−2027.5
	BIC	4452.2	4789.2	**4277.1**	4281.7	4331.4	4384.7	4437.7	4491.0

Table 11.3. *Maximum log-likelihood and BIC index for the unidimensional Rasch model fitted for each dimension by the MML method under the assumption that the latent trait has a normal distribution and under the assumption that it has a discrete distribution with a number of support points (latent classes) between one and seven; for each dimension, the data in bold refer to the model with the smallest BIC*

	Number of latent classes (C)						
	1	2	3	4	5	6	7
$\hat{\ell}$	−2321.8	−2066.7	−2016.3	−1989.8	−1966.9	**−1949.3**	−1937.7
BIC	4760.6	4282.1	4213.2	4192.1	4178.3	**4175.0**	4183.7

Table 11.4. *Maximum log-likelihood and BIC index for the multidimensional latent class Rasch model with a number of latent classes between one and seven; the data in bold refer to the model with the smallest BIC*

A crucial point of the present study is the interpretation of the latent classes, which defines homogeneous groups in the population. This interpretation is not always easy, but some useful suggestions come from the estimates of the support points and class probabilities. In particular, the smallest classes are the first (4.2% of subjects) and the last (8.6% of subjects). These classes contain patients with the highest tendency to psychopathological disturbances and with the highest impairment regarding BP and SF, respectively. The second class contains more subjects (22.3%); these subjects are in the best conditions with respect to all dimensions, with the exception of BP. The third class is the largest (38.3% subjects) and includes subjects with an intermediate tendency to be ill with respect to each dimension. Finally, the fourth and fifth latent classes have a very similar size (13.4% and 13.1% of subjects) and include subjects with the worst conditions with respect to VT and the best conditions with respect to SF, respectively.

	Latent class					
Dimension	1	2	3	4	5	6
BP	$-\infty$	−2.17	−0.92	−0.91	−0.20	**1.48**
SF	−2.56	$-\infty$	−1.71	−2.92	$-\infty$	**0.79**
VT	−2.36	*−3.28*	−0.46	**1.09**	−2.23	0.93
Anxiety	**0.00**	*−4.87*	−3.40	−1.85	−1.55	−0.05
Depression	**1.30**	*−4.10*	−1.99	0.12	−1.50	0.76
Probability	0.042	0.223	0.383	0.134	0.131	0.086

Table 11.5. *Estimated support points and probabilities of the latent classes (for each dimension, the highest support points are in bold; the smallest support points are in italic)*

Note that individuals belonging to the second and the fifth latent classes show a very good level with respect to SF.

As already mentioned, it is important to analyze the correlation between the different dimensions of HrQoL and the correlation with anxiety and depression. Table 11.6 reports the correlation coefficients estimated on the basis of equation [11.11] for every pair of dimensions.

	SF	VT	Anxiety	Depression
BP	0.679	0.794	0.932	0.989
SF		0.934	0.388	0.596
VT			0.530	0.707
Anxiety				0.971

Table 11.6. *Estimated correlation matrix between latent traits*

As regards the dimensions of HrQoL, we observe that all three dimensions (BP, SF and VT) are strongly correlated, especially VT with the other psychological dimension SF ($\hat{\rho} = 0.934$). As regards the association between the dimensions of HrQoL measured by the SF-36 questionnaire and the psychopathological disorders measured by the HADS questionnaire, both anxiety and depression show a very high correlation with BP ($\hat{\rho} = 0.932$ and $\hat{\rho} = 0.989$, respectively). On the other hand, the association of anxiety with SF and VT is much weaker ($\hat{\rho} = 0.388$ and $\hat{\rho} = 0.530$, respectively), and the association of depression with SF and VT assumes intermediate values ($\hat{\rho} = 0.596$ and $\hat{\rho} = 0.707$, respectively). Finally, as we may expect, the correlation between anxiety and depression is very high ($\hat{\rho} = 0.971$).

When the correlation between two latent traits is high, it is interesting to verify if the corresponding items actually measure the same dimension. For this aim, we performed both tests described in the previous section, that is the LR tests based on the discrete MML and the CML methods, for every pair of dimensions. LR statistics and the corresponding p-values are shown in Table 11.7 for the first test and in Table 11.8 for the second.

	SF	VT	Anxiety	Depression
BP	27.1 (0.000)	14.0 (0.007)	22.2 (0.000)	27.5 (0.000)
SF		12.5 (0.014)	32.1 (0.000)	26.3 (0.000)
VT			51.2 (0.000)	70.3 (0.000)
Anxiety				9.1 (0.059)

Table 11.7. *Results from the test of dimensionality based on the discrete MML parameter estimates; in brackets the p-values*

	SF	VT	Anxiety	Depression
BP	23.0 (0.000)	38.6 (0.000)	53.7 (0.000)	57.0 (0.000)
SF		30.7 (0.000)	42.9 (0.000)	36.3 (0.001)
VT			126.7 (0.000)	112.7 (0.000)
Anxiety				83.3 (0.001)

Table 11.8. *Results from the test of dimensionality based on the CML parameter estimates (ML test); in brackets the p-values*

We observe that the values of the test statistic based on the discrete MML method are almost always smaller than the corresponding values calculated on the basis of the CML method, but the main conclusions are similar. In fact, both test statistics have a null asymptotic chi-square distribution, but the second is based on a larger number of degrees of freedom. Nevertheless, both kinds of test do not show any evidence of unidimensionality. A weak evidence of unidimensionality appears under the test based on the discrete MML estimates for anxiety and depression (p-value equal to 0.059) and for VT and SF (p-value equal to 0.014). Then, the present study confirms that the dimensions defined by the SF-36 and HADS questionnaires are indeed separate, and that collapsing some of them would imply an inappropriate simplification of the phenomena investigated by the test items.

11.6. Acknowledgments

The authors are grateful to A. Bonacchi of the University of Florence (Italy) for making available the data. F. Bartolucci acknowledges the financial support from PRIN07 (grant 2007XECZ7L003) and from the Einaudi Institute for Economics and Finance, Rome, Italy.

11.7. Bibliography

[AND 70] ANDERSEN E.B., "Asymptotic properties of conditional maximum likelihood estimators", *Journal of the Royal Statistical Society, Series B*, vol. 32, pp. 283–301, 1970.

[AND 72] ANDERSEN E.B., "The numerical solution of a set of conditional estimation equations", *Journal of the Royal Statistical Society, Series B*, vol. 34, pp. 42–54, 1972.

[ADA 97] ADAMS R.J., WILSON M., WANG W.C., "The multidimensional random coefficients multinomial logit model", *Applied Psychological Measurement*, vol. 21, pp. 1–23, 1997.

[BAR 07] BARTOLUCCI F., "A class of multidimensional IRT models for testing unidimensionality and clustering items", *Psychometrika*, vol. 72, pp. 141–157, 2007.

[BAR 12] BARTOLUCCI F., BACCI S., GNALDI M., "Multidimensional latent class Item Response Theory models", R package version 1.0, available at http://CRAN.R-project.org/package=MULTILCIRT, 2012.

[CAR 01] CARSTENSEN C.H., ROST J., MULTIRA (Version 1.65), Computer software and manual, available at http://www.multira.de.

[CHR 02] CHRISTENSEN K.B., BJORNER J.B., KREINER S., PETERSEN J.H., "Testing unidimensionality in polytomous Rasch models", *Psychometrika*, vol. 67, pp. 563–574, 2002.

[CHR 03] CHRISTENSEN K.B., BJORNER J.B., SAS macros for Rasch based latent variable modelling, Res. Rep. No. 03/13, Department of Biostatistics, University of Copenhagen, 2003.

[CHR 07] CHRISTENSEN K.B., KREINER S., "A Monte Carlo approach to unidimensionality testing in polytomous Rasch models", *Applied Psychological Measurement*, vol. 31, pp. 20–30, 2007.

[DEM 77] DEMPSTER A.P., LAIRD N.M., RUBIN D.B., "Maximum likelihood from incomplete data via the EM algorithm (with discussion)", *Journal of the Royal Statistical Society, Series B*, vol. 39, pp. 1–38, 1977.

[FAY 00] FAYERS P.M., MACHIN D., *Quality of Life: Assessment, Analysis and Interpretation*, Wiley, 2000.

[FOR 95] FORMANN A.K., "Linear logistic latent class analysis and the Rasch model", in FISCHER G.H., MOLENAAR I.W. (eds), *Rasch Models: Foundations, Recent Developments, and Applications*, Springer-Verlag, New York, pp. 239–255, 1995.

[GLA 95a] GLAS C.A.W., VERHELST N.D., "Testing the Rasch model", in FISCHER G.H., MOLENAAR I.W. (eds), *Rasch Models: Foundations, Recent Developments, and Applications*, Springer-Verlag, New York, pp. 69–95, 1995.

[GLA 95b] GLAS C.A.W., VERHELST N.D., "Tests of fit for polytomous Rasch models", in FISCHER G.H., MOLENAAR I.W. (eds), *Rasch Models: Foundations, Recent Developments, and Applications*, Springer-Verlag, New York, pp. 325–352, 1995.

[GOO 74] GOODMAN L.A., "Exploratory latent structure analysis using both identifiable and unidentifiable models", *Biometrika*, vol. 61, pp. 215–231, 1974.

[HAR 04] HARDOUIN J.B., MESBAH M., "Clustering binary variables in subscales using an extended Rasch model and Akaike information criterion", *Communication in Statistics – Theory and Methods*, vol. 33, pp. 1277–1294, 2004.

[KIE 56] KIEFER J., WOLFOWITZ J., "Consistency of the maximum likelihood estimator in the presence of infinitely many incidental parameters", *The Annals of Mathematical Statistics*, vol. 27, pp. 887–906, 1956.

[KRE 03] KREINER S., Introduction to DIGRAM, Res.Rep.No. 03/10, Department of Biostatistics, University of Copenhagen, 2003.

[LAZ 68] LAZARSFELD P.F., HENRY N.W., *Latent Structure Analysis*, Houghton Mifflin, Boston, 1968.

[LIN 91] LINDSAY B., CLOGG C., GREGO J., "Semiparametric estimation in the Rasch model and related exponential response models, including a simple latent class model for item analysis", *Journal of the American Statistical Association*, vol. 86, pp. 96–107, 1991.

[MAG 01] MAGIDSON J., VERMUNT J.K., "Latent class factor and cluster models, bi-plots, and related graphical displays", *Sociological Methodology*, vol. 31, pp. 223–264, 2001.

[MCL 00] MCLACHLAN G.J., PEEL D., *Finite Mixture Models*, Wiley, 2000.

[MAR 70] MARTIN-LÖF P., *Statistika Modeller: Anteckningar Från Seminarier Lasåret 1969–1970* [Statistical Models: Notes from Seminars in the Academic Year 1969–1970], with the Assistance of Rolf Sundberg, Stockholm, Institütet för Försäkringsmatemetik och Matematiks Statistik vid Stockholms Universitet, 1970.

[MES 10] MESBAH M., "Statistical quality of life", in BALAKRISHNAN N. (ed.), *Methods and Applications of Statistics in the Life and Health Sciences*, Wiley, New York, pp. 839–864, 2010.

[RAS 61] RASCH G., "On general laws and the meaning of measurement in psychology", *Proceedings of the IV Berkeley Symposium on Mathematical Statistics and Probability*, vol. 4, pp. 321–333, 1961.

[ROS 90] ROST J., "Rasch models in latent classes: an integration of two approaches to item analysis", *Applied Psychological Measurement*, vol. 14, pp. 271–282, 1990.

[SAM 96] SAMEJIMA F., "Evaluation of mathematical models for ordered polychotomous responses", *Behaviormetrika*, vol. 23, pp. 17–35, 1996.

[SCH 78] SCHWARZ G., "Estimating the dimension of a model", *Annals of Statistics*, vol. 6, pp. 461–464, 1978.

[VER 01] VERHELST, N.D., "Testing the unidimensionality assumption of the Rasch model", *Methods of Psychological Research Online*, vol. 6, pp. 231–271, 2001.

[WAR 02] WARE J.E., KOSINSKI M., DEWEY J.E., *How to Score Version 2 of the SF-36 Health Survey (Standard & acute forms)*, Quality Metric Incorporated, Lincoln RI, 2002.

[WHO 95] WHOQOL GROUP, "The World Health Organization Quality of Life Assessment (WHOQOL): position paper from the World Health Organization", *Social Science and Medicine*, Special issue on Health-Related Quality of Life: What is It and How Should We Measure It?, vol. 41, no. 10, pp. 1403–1409, 1995.

[ZIG 83] ZIGMOND A.S., SNAITH R.P., "The hospital anxiety and depression scale", *Acta Psychiatrika Scandinavica*, vol. 67, pp. 361–370, 1983.

Chapter 12

Analysis of Rater Agreement by Rasch and IRT Models

12.1. Introduction

Comparing different evaluations of the same medical situation is an important part of medical diagnostics. Establishing treatment standards may involve having an expert panel rate the appropriateness of certain medical procedures. Quality control to evaluate staff training, comparisons of laboratory measurement to ensure inter-lab comparability or replacing one measuring device (or one medical doctor rater) with another perhaps less expensive one are other examples of comparisons that are frequent in medicine. Therefore the quantification of the agreement between raters is important.

The most basic design to compare the performances of different raters involves having all raters evaluate the same cases – a fixed-panel design. With several raters and continuous (Gaussian) responses, the standard analysis is a two-way analysis of variance. This chapter explores the use of the item response theory (IRT) model in the case of binary ratings. For the ease of description, it is assumed that the design is a fixed-panel design in which each of a number of raters returns a positive or negative evaluation of other raters in a sample from a population. It is assumed that no "gold standard" is available. The rater responses are modeled using IRT models allowing for rater-specific as well as individual-specific parameters.

Chapter written by Jørgen Holm PETERSEN.

12.2. An IRT model for modeling inter-rater agreement

The IRT model to describe inter-rater agreement for a binary response taking on values 0 and 1 corresponding to positive and negative evaluations is a two-parameter model defined as

$$P(X_{vi} = 1|\theta_v) = \frac{\exp(\alpha_i\theta_v - \beta_i)}{1 + \exp(\alpha_i\theta_v - \beta_i)} \qquad [12.1]$$

where $\theta = (\theta_1, \ldots, \theta_n)^t \in R^n$ characterizes the individuals, and $\beta = (\beta_1, \ldots, \beta_k)^t \in R^k$ and $\alpha = (\alpha_1, \ldots, \alpha_k)^t \in R^k$ similarly characterize the raters. It is assumed that all X_{vi} are independent (conditional on α, β and θ), also called local independence.

The parameter θ_v takes values from minus infinity to plus infinity and characterizes the cases in terms of how easy or difficult they are to evaluate. Easy cases are in the two ends of the θ spectrum where the probability of positive response will be either near zero or near one, regardless of which rater performs the evaluation. Difficult cases will have θ values around zero where the probability of positive response, although dependent on the rater parameter, will be around one half.

It should be noted that not all α_i and β_i are identifiable, and we arbitrarily set $\alpha_k = 1$ and $\beta_k = 0$ making the kth rater a "reference" rater. In the chosen parameterization, the parameter β_i is the difference between rater i and rater k for an average individual, that is an individual with $\theta = 0$. $\beta_i > 0$ means that the ith rater has a higher propensity than rater k to score an average individual or group of individuals positively. This constitutes rater bias – a relative bias – since we are not able to pinpoint whether one, or for that matter any, of the raters achieve the true level.

The discrimination (slope) parameters $\alpha = (\alpha_1, \ldots, \alpha_k)^t \in R^k$ account for the possibility of the different raters having different "responsiveness" to differences in the individuals' levels and may be interpreted as representing different degrees of expertise among the raters. In assessments by an expert rather than a novice, the rate at which the probability of positive response increases with increasing θ is higher. The expert rater thus has a smaller span of θ values where there is doubt about the evaluation being positive or negative. Responses from raters with steeper slopes will be more associated than from those with less steep slopes. The components of the model are shown in Figure 12.1.

An alternative interpretation of the slope parameters may be obtained by approximating the logistic ogive with the Gaussian cumulative distribution function with an appropriately chosen mean and standard deviation (σ), and we may find $\sigma = 1.7/\alpha$. The interpretation of the corresponding Gaussian-based process is therefore that each individual has an apparent trait level ($\tilde{\theta_v}$), which is assumed normally distributed with the true value (θ_v) as its mean and a measurement error (σ). The response Y_{ij} becomes 1 if $\tilde{\theta_v}$ exceeds the rater threshold level β_i, and is otherwise 0. This strength of association factor has been termed as a measurement error by Uebersax and Grove [UEB 93], because of the close relationship between the logistic model described here and a Gaussian cumulative distribution function.

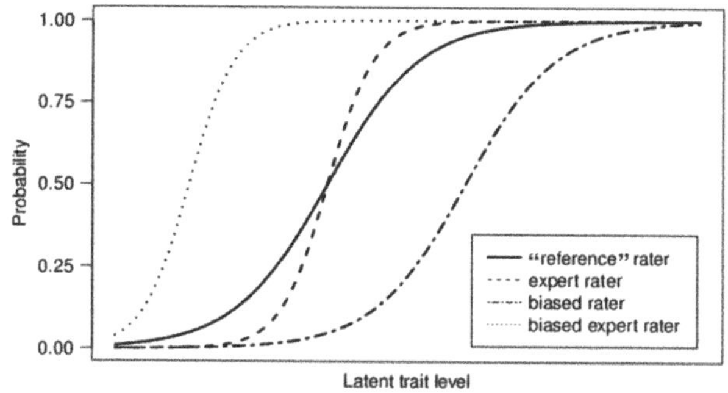

Figure 12.1. *Item characteristic curves of the rater agreement IRT model* $logit(p_{vi}) = \alpha_i\theta_v + \beta_i$ *with four different types of raters. Compared with a reference rater (*$\alpha = 1$ *and* $\beta = 0$*), a biased rater has* $\alpha = 1$ *and* $\beta \neq 0$*. An expert rater (*$\alpha > 1$ *and* $\beta = 0$*) has a better ability to distinguish between individuals than the reference rater. A biased expert would have* $\alpha > 1$ *and* $\beta \neq 0$*. Similarly, we might have a novice rater (biased or unbiased) with* $\alpha < 1$*, represented by a flatter item characteristic curve (not shown), than the "reference" rater*

12.3. Umbilical artery Doppler velocimetry and perinatal mortality

Umbilical artery Doppler velocimetry is a technique used by obstetricians to assess the status of a fetus. It is an ultrasound technique that measures the blood flow through the umbilical cord, and is used as a general indicator of how well the fetus is growing. Doppler velocimetry measurement is an important factor in deciding whether to deliver a poorly developing child prematurely by Cesarian section in order to avoid pre- or perinatal death. Doppler velocimetry is perhaps the most intensively used technique in modern obstetrics, and it is part of the standard diagnostic kit in many obstetrics departments. In Denmark, it is estimated that 20,000 examinations are performed yearly. Several studies, including a number of randomized clinical trials, have investigated the benefit of the technique. Meta analyses of the randomized clinical trials have shown a 49% reduction in perinatal mortality on using the technique on high-risk pregnancies. Later meta analyses have shown smaller reductions: 38% in 1995, 29% in 1996 and 19% (95% CI: 28–48%) after exclusion of small studies. In the most recent and comprehensive assessment of the many studies [WES 01], it is concluded that the technique is beneficial in pregnancies with inter-uterine growth retardation or hypertensive disease. The results of the original studies as well as the results of the meta analyses vary somewhat: something that, apart from the possible genetic as well as purely random variation, has been attributed to different inclusion criteria involving the various definitions of what constitutes a high-risk pregnancy. No comprehensive studies of a possibly important factor, the rater, have previously been carried out. To describe the influence of the medical doctor on the decision to make a Doppler velocimetry measurement, a study was set up [WES 01]. Data collected from 13 different randomized clinical trials on 139 perinatal deaths were sent to 32 Doppler velocimetry experts. The data included information on gestational age (GA), the estimated body weight, whether the fetus was small for its GA, and other relevant information about the child and its mother, for example whether if the placenta had loosened, hypertension, possible malformations and other relevant clinical information. No information was given about the origin of the cases, nor whether a Doppler velocimetry measurement was originally taken. The experts were asked whether each of the 139 death might have been avoided (only yes/no answers) had a Doppler velocimetry measurement been taken.

12.4. Quantifying the rater agreement in the Rasch model

Quantifying the rater variation in the Rasch model is fairly straightforward. Recall the model:

$$P(X_{vi} = 1|\theta_v) = \frac{\exp(\theta_v - \beta_i)}{1 + \exp(\theta_v - \beta_i)} \quad [12.2]$$

Two approaches to the quantification of the rater variation are considered. One in which the rater levels are described by means of fixed-effect parameters and one in which the rater levels are accounted for by introducing random effects.

12.4.1. *Fixed-effects approach*

The fixed-effect approach is particularly relevant when evaluating specific raters in a context where it is desirable for the raters to be exchangeable. Such modeling of the rater effects is seen in, for example, quality control studies where the aim of the study is to confirm that data obtained from different raters can be analyzed without taking into account that the data are collected by different raters. Alternatively, if rater differences are present, we may have to adjust for the rater differences in a final data analysis of some endpoint.

An initial analysis in which all raters are compared with all other raters gives an idea of the variation between raters and, possibly, an indication of distinct subgroups of rater, for example expert raters and ordinary raters. The result of these two-by-two comparisons are shown in Figure 12.2.

The upper part of the figure shows all two-by-two rater comparisons. Here, rater responses are compared using an exact McNemar test, which is also a (conditional) score test in the Rasch model of the hypothesis that $\beta_{i_1} = \beta_{i_2}$ (see Petersen *et al.* [PET 11]). The larger bullets indicate that rater parameters could be identical (at a 5% level). Raters two and three are seen to rate in a fairly consistent manner, whereas raters one and two tend not to agree sufficiently on many cases.

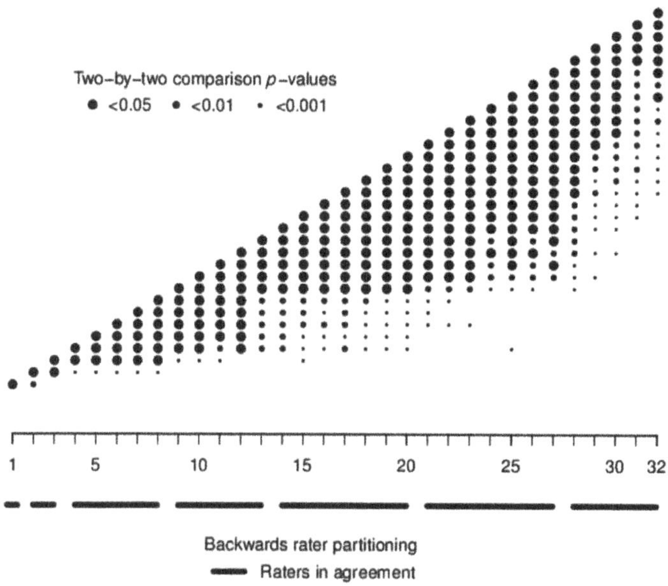

Figure 12.2. *Fixed-effects parameter comparisons. Results are based on Rasch model analyses in which rater effects are estimated as fixed parameters. Each dot in the plot represents a p-value from a comparison of two-rater parameters (McNemar's test). The lower part of the plot shows a partitioning of the raters into groups that have similar rater parameters*

A more elaborate partitioning of the raters into distinct groups of raters that are similar within groups and not similar between groups can be done in a number of ways. The only requirement is that the partitioning is consistent with the results of the two-by-two comparisons (possibly corrected for multiple testing). The lower part of Figure 12.2 shows one such partitioning. While following the observed ordering of the raters, the partitioning is based on a backward procedure where in each step of the procedure a rater is joined to a group if the rater parameter is not significantly different from the common group parameter. Groups are compared in the same way. Each step of the procedure thus reduces the number of raters (or possibly groups) by one. A joint description of these specific raters is obtained by a conditional maximum likelihood estimation in the Rasch model [12.2]. The estimates are shown in Figure 12.3.

Note that the estimates are monotone, but not linear, transformations of the rater scores. The case distribution in Figure 12.5 is markedly skewed and includes a ceiling effect for a score of 32 corresponding to all raters responding that death was unavoidable. These 39 cases (39 with score 32 and 0 with score 0) are not used in the Rasch analysis which may at first seem counter-intuitive. Although high rater agreement is reflected in either a low and a high score, these cases with maximum or minimum score do not contribute to the information about the possible rater variation. The most probable reason for the agreement is that they are very easy cases (large positive or negative θ). Because of the existence of a sufficient statistics – the individuals' scores – for the case parameter, no assumptions are necessary about the distribution among the cases of the difficulty of these cases. As a consequence, individuals are excluded from the conditional analysis if they have a maximum or minimum score. With more general IRT models, such as the two-parameter model described in section 12.6, no sufficient statistics for the case parameters exist, so a distributional assumption is necessary and all cases, also those achieving the minimum or maximum score, are included in the analysis.

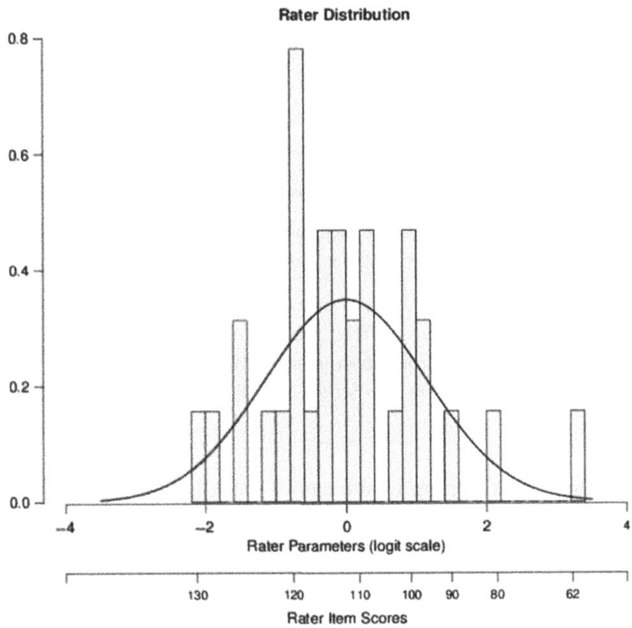

Figure 12.3. *Rater distribution. Empirical distribution of conditional maximum likelihood estimates of rater parameters in the Rasch model: logit*$P(X_{vi} = 1|\theta_v) = \theta_v - \beta_i$*. The higher values (on the logit scale) are from raters with a lower propensity to score 1 (death unavoidable) for a given subject*

The Rasch model was checked in a number of ways. This included a conditional likelihood ratio (CLR) goodness-of-fit test of Andersen [AND 73]. This test assesses whether the case difficulty changes the rater's relative tendencies to respond that death was unavoidable. The assumption of conditional independence of rater responses given the individual levels was tested using Tjur's and Rosenbaum's tests (see [TJU 82, ROS 89]). In Rosenbaum's test, the conditional distribution of two rater's responses given any third raters' response is assessed. If the Rasch model is correct, the positive correlation is required. Tjur's test assesses the conditional distribution of two raters' responses given the sum of one of the rater's responses and any third rater's response. In this conditional distribution, the association vanishes if the model is correct. Rosenbaum's and Tjur's tests are powerful tools for identifying aberrant raters and for assessing the important conditional independence assumption (between rater responses given the individuals' levels (θ_i)).

An exact score test of the hypothesis of rater homogeneity, that is the hypothesis

$$H_0 : \beta_1 = \ldots = \beta_k = 0,$$

is described in Petersen *et al.* [PET 11], and yields $p < 0.0001$. A corresponding CLR test results in a test statistic CLR $= 462.1$, which is asymptotically chi-square distributed with degrees of freedom equal to 31, so $p < 0.0001$.

12.4.2. *Random Effects approach and the median odds ratio*

A random effects approach becomes relevant when the raters are considered a random and representative sample from a population of possible raters. The aim of the analysis in this setting is to describe, and possibly draw inferences about, the variation between raters in the general rater population. The estimation of the rater variation in [12.2]:

$$P(X_{vi} = 1|\theta_v) = \frac{\exp(\theta_v - \beta_i)}{1 + \exp(\theta_v - \beta_i)} \qquad [12.3]$$

may be done by maximum likelihood estimation based on the marginal distribution of X, that is where [12.2] is integrated with respect to the distribution of θ_v and β_i. Although straightforward, in principle, matters are complicated by the presence of the individual-specific parameters (θ_v) – the number of which increases with the number of individuals in the sample. Instead, different alternative approaches are implemented.

On the basis of a model in which a fixed-effect parameter is alloted to each individual (using "lmer" in the *lme4* package in R) an estimate of the standard deviation can be obtained in the rater distribution on the logit scale of 1.132. Instead, the rater parameters could be estimated as fixed-effect parameters using conditional maximum likelihood. The standard deviation of these rater parameter estimates also provides a reasonable approach to the estimation of the rater variability. This can be carried out using "RM" in the *eRm* package in *R*, or similarly by using conditional logistic regression with "clogit" in the *survival* package in *R*. This results in an estimate of 1.144. It is noted, that a model assuming both normally distributed raters and individuals (using "lmer" in the *lme4* package in *R*) results in an estimate of 1.075.

To quantify the rater variability, a measure, called median odds ratio (MOR), suggested by Petersen *et al.* [PET 11], is used.

For two randomly chosen raters, indexed by i and j, rating a given individual, rater i's odds of rating positively is given by $\exp(-\beta_i)$. Similarly, rater j's odds of rating positively is given by $\exp(-\beta_j)$. The ratio of the rater with the highest odds, or equivalently probability, of rating positively relative to the rater with the lowest odds of rating positively is then given by $\exp(|\beta_i - \beta_j|)$. The odds ratio is a random variable characterized by the cumulative distribution function

$$F(x) = P(\exp(|\beta_i - \beta_j|) \leq x) = P(|\beta_i - \beta_j|) \leq \log x), x > 0 \qquad [12.4]$$

Because $\beta_i - \beta_j \sim N(0, 2\sigma^2)$ then $|\beta_i - \beta_j| \leq \log x$ occurs when $-\log x \leq N(0, 2\sigma^2) \leq \log x$ which in turn implies $-\frac{\log x}{\sqrt{2}\sigma} \leq N(0,1) \leq \frac{\log x}{\sqrt{2}\sigma}$. This means that

$$F(x) = P(\exp(|\beta_i - \beta_j|) \leq x) = 2\Phi\left(\frac{\log x}{\sqrt{2}\sigma}\right) - 1 \qquad [12.5]$$

where $\Phi(\cdot)$ is the cumulative distribution function of the standardized normal distribution.

The density function of the odds ratio then becomes

$$f(x) = \frac{\partial}{\partial x}F(x) = \frac{\sqrt{2}}{x\sigma}\phi\left(\frac{\log x}{\sqrt{2}\sigma}\right) \qquad [12.6]$$

where $\phi(\cdot)$ is the density function of the standardized normal distribution.

The rater variability is thus characterized by the above distribution function. Two properties of the distribution are particularly relevant, the MOR and the interval odds ratio (IOR).

The MOR is the median in the distribution and is readily found by solving $F(x) = 0.5$ resulting in an explicit formula for MOR:

$$MOR = \exp(\sqrt{2}\sigma\Phi^{-1}(0.75)) \approx 2.596^{\sigma} \qquad [12.7]$$

Another way of characterizing the rater variability is by means of a $(1 - \alpha)$ prediction interval for the above odds ratio distribution. Distributing a probability mass of $\alpha/2$ outside both endpoints of the interval results in an interval given by:

$$\left(\exp(\sqrt{2}\sigma\Phi^{-1}(0.5 + \alpha/4))\,;\,\exp(\sqrt{2}\sigma\Phi^{-1}(1 - \alpha/4))\right)$$

Another way of characterizing the rater variability distribution of the odds ratio is by means of a $(1 - \alpha)$ prediction interval for the odds ratio distribution (IOR). The lower and upper endpoints of the interval is given by solving $F(x) = \alpha/2$ and $F(x) = 1 - \alpha/2$, respectively. A 95% prediction interval (IOR_{95}) is calculated using:

$$\text{IOR} = \left(\exp(\sqrt{2}\sigma\Phi^{-1}(0.025));\ \exp(\sqrt{2}\sigma\Phi^{-1}(0.975))\right)$$

This approach may be useful in the presence of rater-specific covariates, for example gender, number of years of training or others.

12.5. Doppler velocimetry and perinatal mortality

The data are shown in Figure 12.4. The presence of bands – white or black – for some raters and not others is an indication of inter-rater variation.

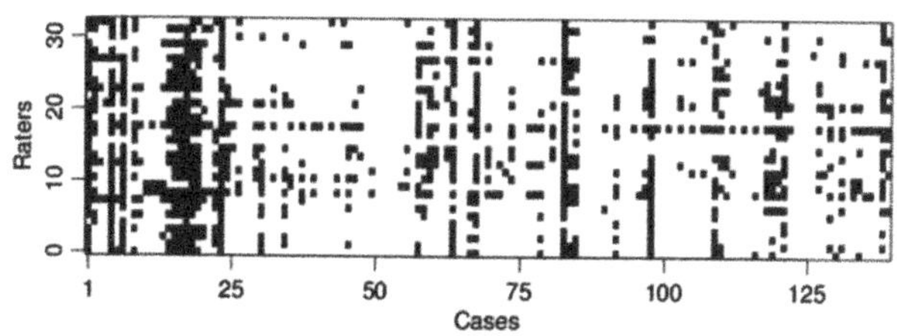

Figure 12.4. *Data on 139 cases evaluated by 32 raters. A white square signifies that death was inevitable and a black square that death could possibly have been avoided using the information in the Doppler velocimetry measurement. Vertical bands – white or black – for some cases signify that many raters agree. Horizontal bands indicate rater variation*

The bands – white or black – for some cases signify that many raters agree, that is the cases are easy. Other cases are difficult and the raters are more in disagreement as indicated by the presence of many black and white squares.

It is somewhat surprising that with such a well-established technique there is still considerable variation between raters. More information about the variability is obtained from the case and rater scores in Figure 12.5.

The rater score is much less skewed, but indicates some degree of variability. Both histograms are affected by all the sources of variability considered here. So, the case score distribution is affected by not only the true case variability but also the inter-rater variability and the randomness induced by the probabilistic part of the model – what could be called the measurement noise. It is through the statistical modeling of the data that we can separate the different sources of variation.

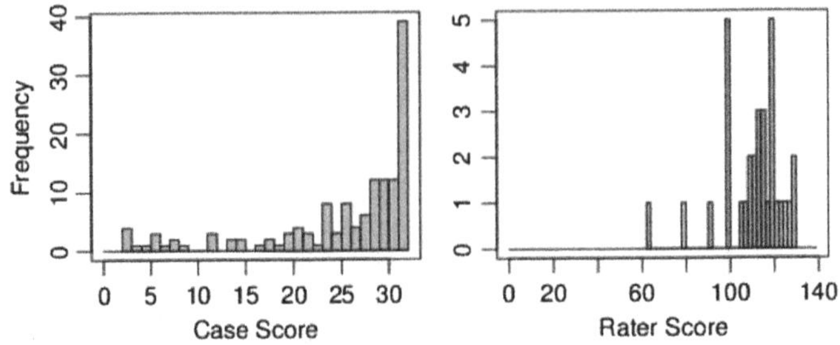

Figure 12.5. *Case and rater scores. The left-hand histogram shows the distribution of the sum of the 32 raters for each case. A high score signifies that many raters agree that death was unavoidable. The right-hand histogram shows the distribution of the sum of the 139 cases for each of the 32 raters. Raters with relatively high scores relative to other raters therefore have a higher tendency to believe that death was unavoidable*

Also, testing the Rasch model against a larger model: $\text{logit}(\text{P}(Y_{ij} = 1|\theta_i, \alpha_j)) = \beta_j\theta_i + \alpha_j$ (see [MOL 83]). Finally, when quantifying the rater agreement, testing the Gaussian assumption is carried out as described in [CHR 04].

Corresponding to the estimated standard deviation on the logit scale of 1.144, an estimate of the rater variability of MOR = 2.98 (95% CI: 2.77–3.52) is obtained. The odds ratio distribution and the rater variability measures MOR and IOR_{95} are shown in Figure 12.6.

The interpretation of MOR is straightforward. For two randomly selected raters who are asked to give their opinion in a particular case, the generally more optimistic of the two has a 2.98 times higher propensity (as measured by the odds) than the less optimistic of the two to say that death was avoidable. If two raters are different, one rater finds that 50% of some group of women would benefit from the use of the Doppler technique and the other rater would find it beneficial in 75% of the women. From this it is obvious that great care should be taken while designing studies to assess the benefits of this technique – especially in defining the inclusion criteria. It is also clear that the knowledge of the medical indications for the use of the technique is either not defined precisely enough or are not known in sufficient detail by the medical doctors who are using the technique.

It is clear from these considerations that the variations in previously reported effects of using the ultrasound technique may in part be attributed to the considerable rater variation. Being on the same scale, the magnitude of the effect is directly comparable with the effects of potential individual risk factors, for example hypertension or inter-uterine growth retardation.

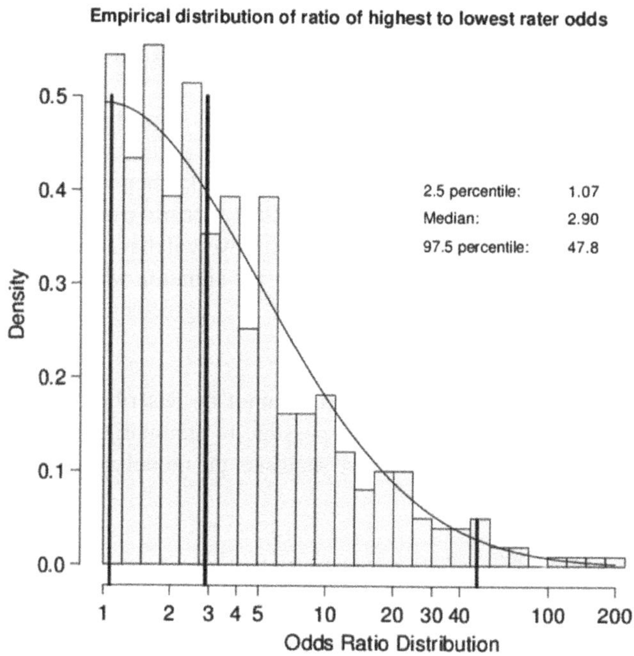

Figure 12.6. *Empirical distribution of ratio of highest to lowest rater odds. The 2.5, 50 and 97.5 percentiles are indicated with vertical black lines. The corresponding estimates are also shown in the figure. Based on the normal distribution assumption, the same percentiles are estimated to be 1.05, 2.98 and 37.6, respectively*

If an effort to reduce the variability between raters were to be considered, the three raters with the lowest scores, see Figure 12.5, would be obvious candidates for an audit.

12.6. Quantifying the rater agreement in the IRT model

Quantifying the rater variation in the IRT model

$$P(Y_{vi} = 1|\theta_v) = \frac{\exp(\alpha_i\theta_v - \beta_i)}{1 + \exp(\alpha_i\theta_v - \beta_i)}, \quad [12.8]$$

is not straightforward.

In the case $\exists j : \alpha_j \neq 1$, the odds ratio of one rater relative to another (for a given individual) is in the form:

$$\text{OR}_{2 \text{ vs } 1} = \exp((\alpha_2 - \alpha_1)\theta_v - (\beta_2 - \beta_1)). \quad [12.9]$$

The rater differences thus depend on the rated individual's level. It is seen that $\text{OR}_{2 \text{ vs } 1}$ is monotonously increasing ($\alpha_2 - \alpha_1 > 0$) or decreasing ($\alpha_2 - \alpha_1 > 0$). Also, $\text{OR}_{2 \text{ vs } 1} = 1$ for $\theta_{\text{OR}=1} = (\beta_2 - \beta_1)/(\alpha_2 - \alpha_1)$. The monotonicity and the fact that the raters have the same probability of positive response for $\theta_{\text{OR}=1}$ have consequences that make it difficult to summarize the rater agreement. Assuming that $\alpha_2 - \alpha_1 > 0$, then for individuals with $\theta > \theta_{\text{OR}=1}$, rater two will have a higher probability of positive response than rater one. Conversely, for individuals with $\theta < \theta_{\text{OR}=1}$, rater two will have a lower probability of positive response than rater one. So, except for the situation where $\alpha_1 = \alpha_2$ (i.e. the Rasch model), it is not possible to quantify the rater agreement along the same lines as with the Rasch model.

As the relationship between two raters cannot be described without taking the individual's level into account, it is not possible to summarize the rater variability in a measure similar to MOR. Still, as we shall see, the model can provide insight into the rater differences.

Fitting the IRT model

$$\mathrm{P}(Y_{vi} = 1|\alpha_i, \beta_i, \theta_v) = \frac{\exp(\alpha_i\theta_v - \beta_i)}{1 + \exp(\alpha_i\theta_v - \beta_i)}, \qquad [12.10]$$

where

$$\begin{pmatrix} \alpha_i \\ \beta_i \end{pmatrix} \sim N\left(\begin{pmatrix} 1 \\ 0 \end{pmatrix}, \begin{pmatrix} \sigma_\alpha^2 & \rho\sigma_\alpha\sigma_\beta \\ \rho\sigma_\alpha\sigma_\beta & \sigma_\beta^2 \end{pmatrix}\right) \text{ and } \theta \sim N(\mu, \sigma_\theta^2)$$

is, not possible in any standard software packages. Here the estimation has been carried out by first estimating in the model assuming α_i and β_i were fixed-effects (θ_v Gaussian), and, second, by calculating the empirical variance–covariance matrix of the (α_i, β_i) estimates. The fixed-effects estimates are shown in Figure 12.7.

Five expert raters have been excluded from this analysis. A likelihood ratio test comparing the two-parameter model ($\log \text{L} = -1203.21$) with the Rasch model where all discrimination parameters are one ($\log \text{L} = -1229.01$), yields $\chi^2 = 51.6$, $\text{df} = 26$, $p = 0.002$. The following estimates were obtained $\sigma_\alpha = 0.33$, $\sigma_\beta = 1.48$, $\rho = -0.64$.

Assuming two raters have the same discrimination parameter (α), the interpretation of the location parameter (β_i) is straightforward. For a rater with a high location parameter relative to another rater, the probability that the rater of death being unavoidable is lower – the rater is less optimistic of the two about the usage of the Doppler technique. A high discrimination parameter (α_i) results in the item characteristic curve being steeper – these raters are experts relative to the others.

Notice the tendency for raters with high location parameters to have low discrimination parameters. This means that raters that tend to think that perinatal death was avoidable, also have the less steep item characteristic curves. Conversely, raters with low location parameters have high discrimination parameters, that is they are experts. This means that experts more often than "ordinary" raters tend to think that perinatal death was unavoidable. Taken at face value this is an indication that the Doppler technique is used more often than is strictly necessary. The dotted lines in Figure 12.7 connect the estimates in the two-parameter model with the location parameter estimates obtained in the Rasch model: logit $p(Y_{vi} = 1|\theta_v) = \theta_v - \beta_i$, that is where all α_is are 1. The estimates are not exactly those presented in section 12.5, because five "expert" raters have been excluded *a priori* from the analysis, and because the estimation here is marginal maximum likelihood, that is assuming θ_v is Gaussian, as opposed to the conditional maximum likelihood estimates reported previously where no distributional assumption about θ_v is necessary.

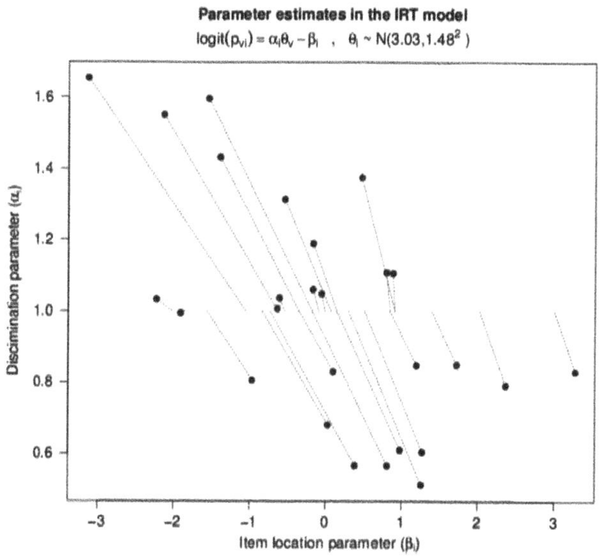

Figure 12.7. *Parameter estimates in the two-parameter model. A high item location parameter (β_i) results in lower probability of death being unavoidable – the rater is more optimistic about the usage of the Doppler technique. A high discrimination parameter (α_i) results in the item characteristic curve being steeper – these raters are experts. The dotted lines connect the estimates in the two-parameter model with the location parameter estimates obtained in the Rasch model where ($\forall i : \alpha_i = 1$)*

12.7. Discussion

This chapter discusses the use of IRT models for the analysis of agreement between raters in a situation where all raters have supplied dichotomous ratings of the same cases in a sample. The models allow raters to have different propensities to score a given set of individuals positively or negatively. This has been termed rater bias and, in the model, it is captured by the rater-specific parameters β_i. Also, some raters might be more sensitive than other raters to small differences in the latent traits (differences in θ) among the rated individuals. Such different sensitivities of the raters is captured in the model by the rater-specific parameters α_i.

For practical reasons, it may not be possible to have all raters evaluate all cases, resulting in missing data. The IRT model approach still works, provided the design matrix has full rank and that data are missing at random. A full rank design matrix basically means that the raters are connected through the cases: two raters are connected if they evaluate the same case, or if a third rater shares cases with one rater and is connected with the other.

The attractive properties of the IRT models hold true provided the model is correct. The basic assumptions are the conditional independence assumption, the logistic form which is closely related to the partitioning of the rater/individual-effect into additive terms and finally, the distributional assumption for the rater (and possibly individual) effects. These assumptions have been studied extensively in the IRT literature, see [GLA 95] for an overview. Deviations from the assumption of additive effects of the raters and individuals is particularly interesting because of its interpretation in terms of the substance matter. Although the described approached could be carried out with any distributional assumptions (for raters and individuals), the chosen distribution should also be critically assessed.

The basic premise of this exposition is that there is not a single way of performing inter-rater agreement analysis, not even in the case of binary responses. The IRT models are explicit about the assumptions being made. If the model fits the data well, which can be checked using existing methods, the data can be summarized through the model parameters in a way that allows discussion with subject matter researchers or other users of the results.

12.8. Bibliography

[AND 73] ANDERSEN E.B., "A goodness of fit test for the Rasch model", *Psychometrika*, vol. 38, pp. 123–140, 1973.

[CHR 04] CHRISTENSEN K.B., KREINER S., "Testing the fit of latent regression models", *Commun Stat A*, vol. 33, pp. 1341–1356, 2004.

[GLA 95] GLAS C.A.W., VERHELST N.D., "Testing the Rasch Model", in FISCHER G.H., MOLENAAR I.W. (eds), *Rasch Models – Foundations, Recent Developments, and Applications*, Springer-Verlag, Berlin, pp. 69–95, 1995.

[MOL 83] MOLENAAR, I.W., "Some improved diagnostics for failure of the Rasch model", *Psychometrika*, vol. 48, pp. 49–72, 1983.

[PET 11] PETERSEN J.H., LARSEN K., KREINER S., "Assessing and quantifying inter-rater variation for dichotomous ratings using a Rasch model", *Statistical Methods in Medical Research*, first published on December 22, 2010.

[ROS 89] ROSENBAUM P.R., "Criterion-related construct validity", *Psychometrika*, vol. 54, pp. 625–633, 1989.

[TJU 82] TJUR T., "A connection between Rasch's item analysis model and a multiplicative Poisson model", *Scandinavian Journal of Statistics*, vol. 9, pp. 23–30, 1982.

[UEB 93] UEBERSAX J.S., GROVE W.M., "A latent trait finite mixture model for the analysis of rating agreement", *Biometrics*, vol. 49, pp. 823–835, 1993.

[WES 01] WESTERGAARD H.B., LANGHOFF-ROSS J., LINGMAN G., MARSAL K., KREINER S., "A critical appraisal of the use of umbilical artery doppler ultrasound in high-risk pregnancies: use of meta-analysis in evidence-based obstetrics", *Ultrasound Obstet Gynecol*, vol. 17, pp. 466–476, 2001.

Chapter 13

From Measurement to Analysis

13.1. Introduction

In previous chapters, the Rasch model, its underlying properties, the statistical estimation of its parameters and the statistical evaluation of goodness of fit (GOF) were presented. The Rasch model is primarily a measurement model. Is it no more than a stochastic measurement model? Answering this question needs some caution. Can we use it to only estimate (i.e. to *measure*) the latent value for each person, and then, in a second, separate, step, forget the item responses, and analyze change of these estimates (*measurements*) between groups or between occasions (longitudinal). This is known as a two-step method of analysis.

Another approach is to use latent regression to analyze change between groups and between occasions. A latent regression model is a complex statistical model where the response variable is an unobserved latent variable. Observations are the item responses. In most cases, the analysis model linking the latent variable to covariates is a classical linear regression model, while the measurement model linking the items to the latent variable is, *marginally*, a Rasch model. The aim of a latent regression model is neither the estimation of the values of the latent variable or estimation of the item parameters, nor the inference about any underlying property of the measurement model.

The aim of the latent regression model is to allow us direct inference about associations between the latent unobserved variable and any other observed covariate. Should two-step methods or latent regression analysis be used for this? Two-step methods are easier to implement, whereas inference under a latent regression model

---

Chapter written by Mounir MESBAH

is not trivial. Both methods need preliminary validation of the questionnaire by examining the fit to the Rasch model. The two-step method requires a preliminary scoring step before the analysis step.

Latent variable models involve a set of observable variables $A = \{\mathbf{X}_1, \mathbf{X}_2, \ldots, \mathbf{X}_k\}$ and a latent (unobserved) variable θ, which may be either unidimensional (i.e. scalar) or vector valued of dimension $d \leq k$. Analysis (regression) models involve a set of observed covariates $B = \{\mathbf{Z}_1, \mathbf{Z}_2, \ldots, \mathbf{Z}_p\}$. In such models, the dimensionality of A is defined by the number d of components of θ. When $d = 1$, the set A is unidimensional.

The two-step method uses an estimate S_v of θ_v and the structure is illustrated by the graphical representation in Figure 13.1 for which $k = 5$, $d = 1$ and $p = 4$.

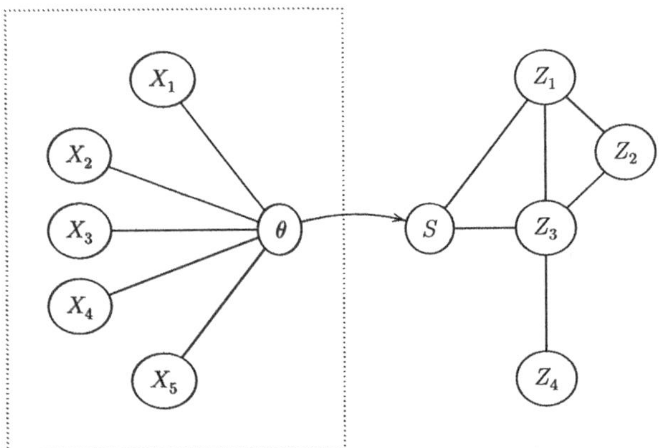

Figure 13.1. *Illustration of a two-step model: $X_1, \ldots, X_5$ are the observed item responses, θ is the unobserved latent variable, S is the estimate of the latent variable and $Z_1, \ldots, Z_4$ are the observed covariates*

The (Rasch) measurement model in the box in Figure 13.1 is used to estimate the value of the latent variable θ_v for each individual. Then, in a second step, the distribution of the estimates S_v is analyzed using the analysis model. We have discussed in previous chapters the issue of estimation of the person parameter. We will get back to that issue in the following section, which is crucial for medical evaluation of the person. It is also crucial for the evaluation of health policies with a view to two-step analysis. In the analysis step, the individual scores S_v are used as observed surrogates of the unobserved true latent values θ_v.

Latent regression models, as illustrated in Figure 13.2, include the latent variable θ, the measurement model and the analysis model, but do not explicitly include the surrogate variable S. Latent regression models are one-step models where the surrogate values S_v are exactly the true latent values θ_v. For this reason there is no loss of information and inference about associations between observed covariates and the latent variable will be more powerful. In section 13.2, we present the general form of the likelihood for both kinds of models, then we come back to the measurement model (section 13.3) and their validation (section 13.4). In section 13.5, we focus on scoring methods and present some real examples analysed with a two-step method. Finally, in section 13.6, we present some real examples of latent regression models.

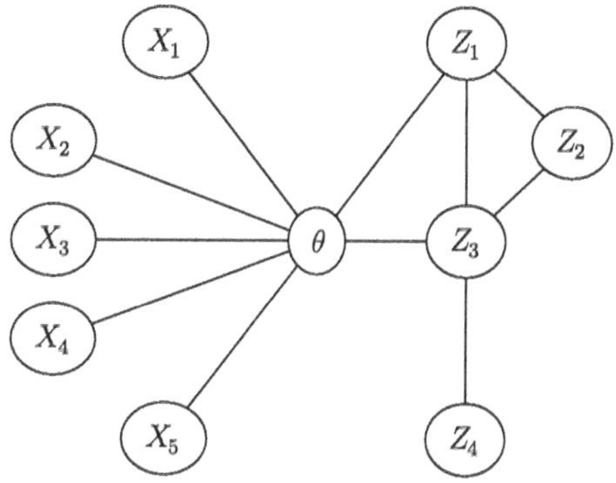

Figure 13.2. *Independence graph of latent regression model: $X_1, \ldots, X_5$ are the observed item responses, θ is the unobserved latent variable and $Z_1, \ldots, Z_4$ are the observed covariates*

13.2. Likelihood

Figures 13.3 and 13.4 show the simplest two-step and latent regression models, respectively. To simplify the explanation, there is only one observed variable $\mathbf{X}$ and only one covariate $\mathbf{Z}$. The variable $\mathbf{X}$ represents the set of items $\mathbf{X}_i$, where $i = 1, \ldots, k$, and $\mathbf{Z}$ represents the set of covariates $\mathbf{Z}_i$, where $i = 1, \ldots, p$.

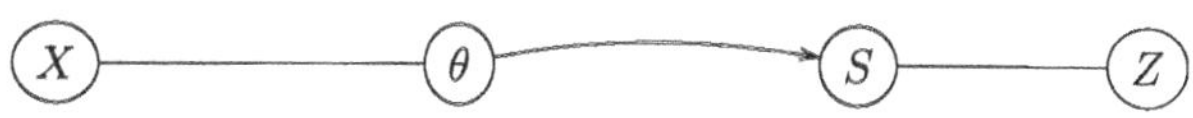

Figure 13.3. *Illustration of a two-step method: X is the vector of observed item responses, θ is the unobserved latent variable, S is a surrogate of the latent variable and Z are the observed covariates*

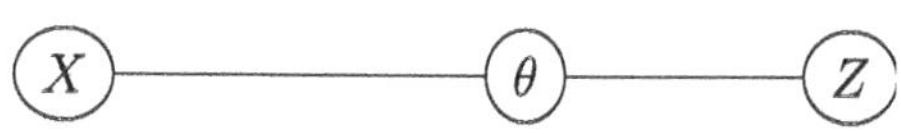

Figure 13.4. *Independence graph of simplest latent regression model: X is the vector of observed item responses, θ is the unobserved latent variable and Z are the observed covariates*

13.2.1. *Two-step model*

The probabilistic measurement model is a specification of the distribution of $\mathbf{X}$ conditional to θ as a function of the item parameter: $f(\mathbf{X}/\theta; \beta)$. Likelihood methods as presented in previous chapters allow us to estimate each individual value θ_v. We refer to this as $\mathbf{S}_v$. The regression analysis model is a specification of the distribution of the surrogate $\mathbf{S}$ of the latent variable, conditional on $\mathbf{Z}$, or the distribution of $\mathbf{Z}$, conditional to $\mathbf{S}$, depending on which variable is the response in the regression model. The likelihood is easily deduced as a function of all individuals observed scores $\mathbf{S}_v$, and all individual observed values of the variable $\mathbf{Z}_v$ and the specific parameters of the distribution (typically regression or correlation parameters).

13.2.2. *Latent regression model*

There is only one distribution to specify and to analyze and no need to introduce a surrogate $\mathbf{S}$. Note that a direct consequence of the independence graph in Figure 13.4 is that $\mathbf{X}$ and $\mathbf{Z}$ are conditionally independent given θ. This is an important assumption of latent regression models and this assumption must be validated in the validation step of the measurement model (the assumption of no differential item functioning, DIF). The only associations that we will test are the associations between $\mathbf{Z}$ and θ. Once more, depending on which is the response in the regression model, the joint distribution of the observed outcomes $f(\mathbf{X}, \mathbf{Z})$ and the latent θ will be specified:

– The latent θ is the response of the regression model:

$$f(X, Z, \theta) = f(X/\theta) \times f(\theta/Z) \times f(Z).$$

– Z is the response of the regression model:

$$f(X, Z, \theta) = f(X/\theta) \times f(Z/\theta) \times f(\theta).$$

Marginal likelihood estimation methods can be used to estimate the parameters of the regression model. The statistical properties need to be carefully investigated for each practical example. The use of conditional likelihood estimation methods is, here, an issue.

13.3. First step: measurement models

We begin by recalling an older model used in a classical test theory that can be considered the precursor of the Rasch model: the parallel model. The random response of a subject v to an item i is denoted $\mathbf{X}_{vi}$. The random variable generating responses to an item i is denoted $\mathbf{X}_i$.

The parallel model is a *classical* latent variable model describing the unidimensionality of a set $A = \{\mathbf{X}_1, \mathbf{X}_2, \ldots, \mathbf{X}_k\}$ of quantitative observable variables.

Define $\mathbf{X}_{vi}$ as the measurement of a subject v, $v = 1, \ldots, n$, given by a variable $\mathbf{X}_i$, where $i = 1, \ldots, k$, then:

$$\mathbf{X}_{vi} = \tau_{vi} + \varepsilon_{vi}, \qquad [13.1]$$

where τ_{vi} is the true measurement corresponding to the observed measurement $\mathbf{X}_{vi}$ and ε_{vi} is the measurement error. Specification of τ_{vi} as:

$$\tau_{vi} = \beta_i + \theta_v,$$

defines the parallel model. In this setting, β_i is an unknown fixed (non-random) parameter describing the effect of variable i and θ_v is an unknown random parameter describing the effect of subject v. It is generally assumed to have zero mean and unknown standard error σ_θ. The first of these assumptions is an arbitrary identifiability constraint with consequences for the interpretation of the parameter: its value must be interpreted comparatively to the mean population value. *For instance, θ_v is the true Health-Related Quality of Life score that the doctor would like to know, to monitor the health status of the patient.* It is a zero mean individual random part of all observed subject responses X_{vi}, the same whatever is the item X_i in a health questionnaire. The ε_{vi}s are the independent random effects with mean zero and standard error σ corresponding to the additional measurement error. Moreover, the true measure and the error are assumed uncorrelated: $cov(\theta_v, \varepsilon_{vi}) = 0$. This model is known as the parallel model, because the regression lines relating the observed items $(X_i)_{i=1,\ldots,k}$ to the true unique latent measure θ_v are parallel.

Another way to specify the same model is through conditional moments of the observed responses. So, the conditional mean of a subject response is specified as:

$$E[X_{vi}/\theta_v; \beta_i] = \beta_i + \theta_v. \qquad [13.2]$$

Again, β_i, $i = 1, \ldots, k$, are fixed effects and θ_v, $v = 1, \ldots, n$, are independent random effects with zero mean and standard error σ_θ. The conditional variance of a subject response is specified as:

$$V[X_{vi}/\theta_v; \beta_i] = V(\varepsilon_{vi}) = \sigma^2. \qquad [13.3]$$

These assumptions are classical in experimental design. This model defines relationships between different kinds of variables: the observed score X_{vi}, the true score τ_{vi} and the error ε_{vi}. It is interesting to make some remarks about assumptions underlying this model. The random part of the true measure given by the response of individual v to a question i is the same whatever might be variable i. θ_v does not depend on i. The model is unidimensional. We can assume that in their random part all observed variables (items X_i) are generated by a common unobserved θ_i. More precisely, let $X^*_{vi} = X_{vi} - \beta_i$ denote the calibrated version of the response to item i of person v. The model given by [13.2] and [13.3] can be rewritten as:

$$E[X^*_{vi}/\theta_v; \beta_i] = \theta_v; \ \forall i, \qquad [13.4]$$

with same assumptions on β and θ and with the same conditional variance model. An important consequence of the previous assumptions, when item responses are assumed normally distributed, is a conditional independence property: whatever i and i', two observed items X_i and $X_{i'}$ are independent conditional to the latent θ_v. So, even when normality cannot be assumed, it is essential to add this property to the model.

It is important to note that the choice of the identifiability constraints is essential. Without adding identifiability constraints, the model parameters are not identifiable. There are two kinds of identifiability constraints: (1) the sum of item parameters equal to zero and (2) one specific item parameter is set to zero. So, in the first case, the interpretation of any item parameters must be performed relative to the mean difficulty of all items involved in the questionnaire. In the second case, the interpretation must be done relative to the difficulty of the reference item whose difficulty level was arbitrarily fixed to be zero.

Modern ideas about measurement models start from this simple model, but instead of arbitrarily defining the relationship between observed and the true latent by an additive function, let us focus on the joint distribution $f(X, \theta)$ of the observed item responses and the latent variable.

This leads us naturally to think about the conditional independence graphical modeling when we build models. The interpretation of an independence graph is easy. Each multivariate distribution is represented by graph, composed of nodes and edges between nodes. Nodes represent one-dimensional random variables (observed or latent) and a missing edge between two variables means that those two variables are conditionally independent given the remaining variables. Since the pioneering work of Lauritzen and Wermuth [LAU 89] many monographs on graphical modeling are now available [LAU 96, WHI 90, EDW 00]. Graphical models and Rasch models have been combined [KRE 02].

One way to define *latent unidimensionality* in the context of graphical models is straightforward: a set of variables X is unidimensional, if there exists one and only one *scalar* latent variable θ such that each variable X is related to θ and only to θ. The unidimensionality is a consequence of the dimension of θ. The word *latent* means more than the fact that θ is not observed (or hidden). The observed items X_i are caused by the true unobserved θ and not any other variable. This causal property is induced by the conditional independence property. If X_i is independent of $X_{i'}$ conditionally to θ, then knowledge of θ is enough. Such directed graphical models are also known as causal graphs or Bayesian networks.

The graphical model framework is helpful to explain relationships between variables, when some of them are observed and others are not. Historically, the Rasch model was established earlier, mainly as a measurement model more appropriate to binary responses. Nevertheless, its connection with graphical models through conditional independence properties included in it is recent. In the latent variable modeling context, conditional independence is known as local independence, which is a more general definition: the value of the latent variable can be assumed as a fixed parameter in $P(X|\theta)$.

The parallel model presented here is a linear mixed model. When item responses are binary, ordinal and categorical, the parallel model is inappropriate. For instance, when the item response is a Bernoulli variable X_{vi} taking values x_{vi} (coded, for instance, 0 (failure or false or no) or 1 (success or correct or yes)), theories of exponential family and of generalized linear models [MCC 89] suggest an adapted *generalized* linear *mixed* model alternative to the model [13.2]. Instead of the linear *mixed* model,

$$E[X_{vi}/\theta_v; \beta_i] = \beta_i + \theta_v, \qquad [13.5]$$

define the *generalized* linear *mixed* model, using the canonical link associated with the Bernoulli distribution,

$$\text{logit}(E[X_{vi}/\theta_v; \beta_i]) = \beta_i + \theta_v, \qquad [13.6]$$

as previously β_i is a fixed effect and θ_v is independent random effects with zero mean and standard error σ_θ. This model is a Rasch model with random effects. This is the version of the Rasch model used for marginal maximum likelihood (MML) estimation (see Chapter 3). It should be noted that *mixed Rasch model* is an inappropriate term for this model, because mixed Rasch models already exist in the psychometric literature and are completely different models.

The partial credit model (PCM) [MAS 82] is an another member of the family Rasch models for ordinal categorical responses. When, for $i = 1, \ldots, k$, the item X_i takes values $\{0, 1, \ldots, m_i\}$ let $P_{vix} = P(X_{vi} = x)$, then:

$$P_{vix} = \frac{\exp\left(x\theta_v - \sum_{l=1}^{x} \beta_{il}\right)}{\sum_{h=0}^{m_j} \exp\left(h\theta_v - \sum_{l=1}^{h} \beta_{il}\right)}. \qquad [13.7]$$

The models [13.5, 13.6 and 13.7] are the models for measuring a latent trait when the measurement instrument is a questionnaire consisting of a set of unidimensional items with responses quantitative [13.5], binary [13.6] and ordinal [13.7], respectively. All these models constitute the family of Rasch models. The models [13.6] and [13.7] came historically later. They all have interesting measurement properties. The models [13.6] and [13.7] are the focus of the current volume that is devoted to Rasch models and their use in health sciences.

13.4. Statistical validation of measurement instrument

Before using measurements of the latent variable in the regression analysis step, we need to carefully check that the underlying properties of the measurement model are confirmed with our data. This is the statistical validation of the measurement *instrument*, i.e. the *questionnaire*. Note, we must validate the measurement instrument, not the measurement model, which is assumed to be the perfect model. This is generally done by the way of GOF tests. The null hypothesis of such GOF test is: the responses (**X**) (observed data) produced by the instrument follows the measurement model (Rasch model). If we reject the null hypothesis, we conclude that there is a significant departure of the distribution of the observed data from the data predicted by the measurement model. In practice, we can interpret such a result in two different ways:

– There is a problem with the measurement model. We must improve the model. Do not change the instrument!

– There is a problem with the measuring instrument. We must improve the instrument. Do not change the model!

These two opposite strategies following the same result of a preliminary statistical test of fit are very common. Adapting the measurement model to the data, to get a better fit, and then interpreting the results are often termed the "model fitting" philosophy. Adapting the measurement instrument, without changing the model (Rasch model), is referred to as the "measurement" or the "Rasch" paradigm. The most important underlying properties of Rasch family models are:

1) *Unidimensionality*,

2) *Monotonicity*,

3) *Local Sufficiency*,

4) *Local Independence*,

5) *No DIF*.

(see Chapter 1 and Chapter 2). The first property is an essential property for latent variable models. It is included in all Rasch models through the fact that the latent parameter is a scalar, related to k different items. The monotonicity property concern the "positive correlation" between the item and the latent variable. This property is equivalent to the mean function, $E(X_i/\theta)$ is a non-decreasing function of θ. When item responses are dichotomous the mean function is the probability function, $E(X_i/\theta) = P(X_i = 1/\theta)$. This property is obviously included in the quantitative parallel model or in the Rasch dichotomous model through the linear or logistic link, and it can easily be proven that it is also included in the PCM model.

Mokken models [MOL 88] do not assume the logistic link, but replace it with a non-parametric monotone link function: this can be interesting for practical application, but relaxing the assumption of a logistic link, we loose the sufficiency property of the total score, which is the most interesting characteristic property of Rasch models. This property justifies the use of simple scores as a surrogate for the latent score.

Local independence and *no DIF* are conditional independence properties that can be expressed in a graphical model: there are no direct edges between nodes corresponding to two different items or between any item and an external variable. Items are only connected to the latent variable.

We will not discuss practical tests that we can use to check these properties since this was done in previous chapters. In the following, we will show, how validation of unidimensionality can be elegantly performed with a simple graphic.

A measurement instrument gives us values that we call observed measure. The reliability ρ of an instrument is defined as the ratio of the true over the observed measure. Under the parallel model, we can show that the reliability of any variable X_j (as an instrument to measure the true value) is given by:

$$\rho = \frac{\sigma_\theta^2}{\sigma_\theta^2 + \sigma^2}, \qquad [13.8]$$

which is also the constant correlation between any two items; the intra-class coefficient. The reliability coefficient ρ can be interpreted as a correlation coefficient between repeated locally independent measurements. When the parallel model is assumed, the reliability of the sum of k variables equals:

$$\tilde{\rho}_k = \frac{k\rho}{k\rho + (1-\rho)}. \qquad [13.9]$$

This formula is known as the Spearman–Brown formula. The maximum likelihood estimator of $\tilde{\rho}_k$, under parallel model and normal distribution assumption, is known as Cronbach's coefficient α (CAC) [CRO 51, KRI 63]. Its expression is given by:

$$\alpha = \frac{k}{k-1}\left(1 - \frac{\sum_{j=1}^{k} S_j^2}{S_{tot}^2}\right), \qquad [13.10]$$

where

$$S_j^2 = \frac{1}{n-1}\sum_{i=1}^{n}(X_{ij} - \overline{X_j})^2$$

and

$$S_{tot}^2 = \frac{1}{nk-1}\sum_{i=1}^{n}\sum_{j=1}^{k}(X_{ij} - \overline{X})^2.$$

The Spearman–Brown formula [13.9] indicates a simple relationship between $\tilde{\rho}_k$ and the number of items k. It is easy to show that $\tilde{\rho}_k$ is an increasing function of k. Figure 13.5 shows, drawn on the same graph, the theoretical reliability curves corresponding to $\rho = 0.1, 0.2, \ldots, 0.9$.

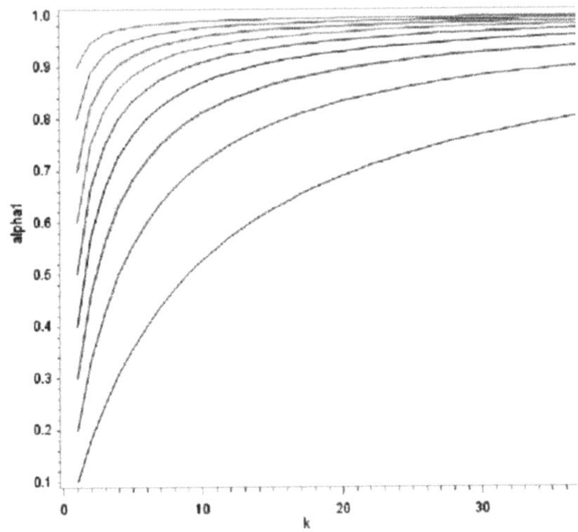

Figure 13.5. *Theoretical relationship between α and the number of items*

So, *if the parallel model is true*, increasing the number of items will increase the reliability of a questionnaire. Moreover, this coefficient lies between 0 and 1. A zero value indicates a totally unreliable scale, while a unit value means that the scale is perfectly reliable. Of course, in practice, these two scenarios never occur.

The α-coefficient is an estimate of the reliability of the raw score (sum of item responses) of a person *if the model generating those responses is a parallel model*. It could be a valid criterion of the unidimensionality of such responses, if, again, those item responses are *generated by a parallel model*. Let us now present a graphical tool, which is helpful in the step of checking the unidimensionality of a set of variables. It consist of a curve to be drawn in a stepwise manner, using estimates of reliability of subscores.

The first step uses all variables and compute's CAC. Then, at each successive step, one item is removed from the score. The removed variable is the variable that leaves the score on the remaining set of variables with a maximum CAC value. This procedure is repeated until only two items remain. If the parallel model is true, increasing the number of items increases the reliability of the total score that is consistently estimated by Cronbach's coefficient α. Thus, a decrease of such a curve after adding a variable would lead us to strongly suspect that the added variable did not constitute a unidimensional set together with variables already included. This algorithm was successfully used in various previous medical applications [MOR 93, CUR 97, NOR 05].

Drawing the Backward Reliability Curve (BRC) of a set of *unidimensional* items is an essential tool in the validation process of a health questionnaire. When use develops a health questionnaire, generally, the main goal is to measure some unidimensional latent subjective traits (such as sociability and mobility). The use of the BRC in empirical data is very helpful to detect non-unidimensional subsets of items. When the BRC is not an increasing curve, we can remove one or more items to get an increasing curve. So, if the reduced set gives an increasing curve, it is, in some sense, *more valid in terms of unidimensionality* than the previous curve.

13.5. Construction of scores

Measuring individual traits is frequently done by calculating scores. This approach assumes that the set of items represent a single dimension (one score) or multiple dimension (multiple scores). These scores can be considered statistics, and a function of individual measurements (for instance, item responses). They must have good statistical properties.

Cronbach α-coefficient, as an indicator of reliability of an instrument, is probably one of the most used in health fields or in applied psychology. The main problem with Cronbach α as a reliability coefficient is the lack of a clear scientific rule to decide whether or not a score is reliable. We need to know a threshold to decide that the score is reliable or not. Following Nunnaly [NUN 78], a scale is satisfactory when it has a Cronbach's α above 0.7. The "Nunnally rule" is an empirical rule without any clear scientific justification. *So reliability is not a direct operational indicator*. The Spearman–Brown formula [13.9] is a direct consequence of the parallel model assumptions. It implies that, when adding an item, or more generally increasing the number of items, the reliability of the sum of item responses must increase. This property is of course a *population property* characterizing the parallel model. Its sampling version is probably less regular. A Cronbach α coefficient is the sampling estimate of theoretical reliability of the sum of item responses. So, the use of the BRC as an empirical rule to validate the parallel model (and thus the *unidimensionality* of the item set) graphically, is straight forward.

Measurement models considered here are very simple models based on unidimensionality principle. They can be defined as Rasch-type models: a parallel model for quantitative items and Rasch model or PCM for ordinal items. Each "*unidimensional*" set of items is related to one and only one latent variable. There is no *confusion between "concepts"*, so an item cannot be related directly to two latent variables. An item can be related to another latent variable only through its own latent variable. It is of course a strong property, hard to get in practice. Health questionnaires are built using questions drawn with words and often health concepts (psychological, sociological or even physical concepts) are not clearly separated. Anyway, measurement is generally considered as the beginning of science, and science is hard to achieve.

So, correlations between each item and all unidimensional scores must be computed. This can be considered as part of the internal validation in a multidimensional setting. To ensure the *separability* of the subsets, we must check that for any item:

1) *Specificity:* there is a strong correlation between the item and a surrogate of the underlying latent variable, and

2) *Separability:* this correlation must be higher than the correlation between the item and surrogates of other latent variables.

Under the parallel model, correlation is the same for all items, and is also known as the intra-class coefficient. The Cronbach α is a monotone function of that value. It must be evaluated for each subscale. Item correlations between each item and all subsores must be tabulated.

1) *Sum of item responses:* this score is sufficient statistics for the latent parameter under Rasch model. Under the parallel model, its reliability is estimated by Cronbach's coefficient α. It is the simplest and easiest score to derive.

2) *Weighted sum of item responses:* this score is more complicated than the previous score. The weights are generally fixed and obtained with PCA previously performed in a "large representative population".

3) *Percentage of item responses:* this score is similar to the first, with different range of its values. This range is between 0% and 100%. When a dimension includes k ordinal items with responses coded $0, 1, \ldots, m$, (all items with the same maximum level m), then this score is obtained by dividing the first score by km.

13.6. Two-step method to analyze change between groups

13.6.1. *Health-related quality of life and housing in europe*

This example is based on a data set from WHO's "Housing and Health" large analysis and review of European housing and health status (LARES) survey [BON 04, BON 03, FRE 09, MES 09], a large survey done in eight big European cities. A total of 8,519 questionnaires from all the people in the selected dwellings were collected, but only people older than 18 years are considered here. In total, 6,920 valid questionnaires were retained. A Health-related Quality of Life (HrQoL) score was derived after a preliminary exploratory phase based mainly on principle component analysis (PCA) with varimax rotation, followed by a confirmatory phase using BRC method (see Figure 13.6, the curve for the *Quality of Life* (QoL) scale finally built) and other GOF tests of Rasch models.

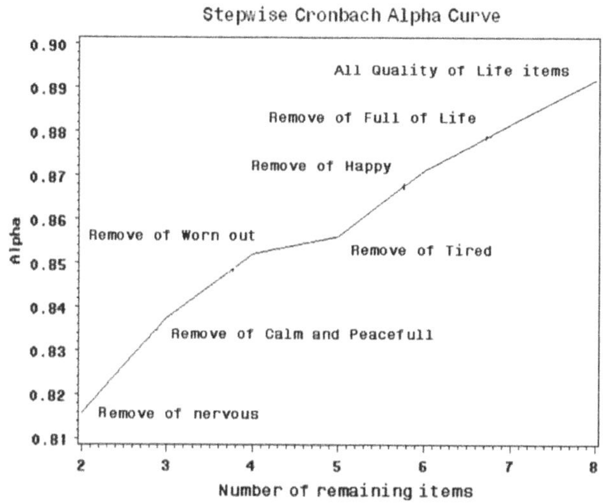

Figure 13.6. *The empirical backward reliability curve for the quality of life scale*

This score can be interpreted as the estimated probability of good HrQoL or as a proportion of the best HrQoL possible. This proportion is actually the ratio of two numbers: the numerator is the number of responses positively associated with good QoL, the denominator is the maximum possible value of the numerator. So, we can analyze this score by multiple logistic regression and present odds-ratio as a measure of association. All computations were done using statistical analysis software (SAS). The obtained odds-ratios were estimated under multiple logistic regression models. The final model was chosen after a parsimonious stepwise selection of models. Table 13.1 shows the odds-ratio between this validated QoL score and some selected significant housing condition factors. Odds-ratios greater than one means that the factor is positively associated with QoL. On the other side, when the odds-ratio is smaller than one, this means that the factor is negatively associated with the QoL. The 95% confidence interval of this odds-ratio is indicated in parentheses.

Nevertheless, we must be aware of the fact that the LARES survey [BON 04, BON 03, FRE 09, MES 09] was transversal (instead of longitudinal) and observational (instead of interventional) slightly limits the causal interpretation of housing factors revealed. Setting the evidence of a causal relationship is a more complex work.

	OR (95% CI)
Panel block	0.962 (0.932; 0.993)
Semi-detached housing unit	1.134 (1.077; 1.194)
Multifamily apartment block, up to six residential units	1.122 (1.084; 1.162)
In the urban center close to a busy street	1.095 (1.057; 1.135)
Window can be opened in flat	1.080 (1.037; 1.124)
Window cannot be closed in flat	0.929 (0.910; 0.947)
Single-glazed windows	1.047 (1.020; 1.075)
Condensation signs at windows	0.937 (0.900; 0.975)
Wallpaper, paint, etc., gets off wall	0.950 (0.924; 0.977)
Shared spaces are well maintained/taken care of	1.055 (1.027; 1.083)
One or two Graffitis	0.891 (0.861; 0.923)
Vegetation/greenery visible on facades/windows/balconies	1.029 (1.006; 1.053)

Table 13.1. *HrQoL and housing information*

13.6.2. *Use of surrogate in an clinical oncology trial*

The motivation of the following models is an HrQoL clinical trial involving analysis of a longitudinal HrQoL variable and an event time. In such clinical trial, the longitudinal HrQoL variable is often unobserved at dropout time. The model proposed by Dupuy and Mesbah (DM model) [DUP 02] works when the longitudinal HrQoL is directly observed at each time visit except, of course, at dropout time. We propose to extend the DM model to the latent context case, i.e. when the HrQoL variable is obtained through a questionnaire. In this example, QoL was assessed among subjects involved in a cancer clinical trial [AWA 02]. Quantitative "surrogate" scores were obtained via an HrQoL instrument by auto-evaluation. There were two treatment groups and a non-ignorable dropout analysis was performed.

Let T be a random time to some event of interest, and θ be the HrQoL longitudinally measured. Let C be a random right-censoring time. Let $X = T \wedge C$ and $\Delta = 1_{\{T \leq C\}}$. Suppose that T and C are independent conditionally on S the assessment of HrQoL, i.e. a surrogate of the true unobserved HrQoL. Following, the Cox proportional hazards model [COX 72], the hazard function of T has the form:

$$\lambda(t|S) = \lambda(t) \exp(\beta^T S(t)). \qquad [13.11]$$

The observations are $[X_i, \Delta_i, \theta_i(u), 0 \leq u \leq X_i]_{1 \leq i \leq n}$. The unknown parameters are β and $\Lambda(t) = \int_0^t \lambda(u)\, du$. Let us assume that C is non-informative for β and λ. Dupuy and Mesbah [DUP 02] suggest a method that supposes a non-ignorable missing process, taken into account the unobserved value of the longitudinal HrQoL variable at dropout time and use a joint modeling approach of event time and longitudinal variable. In this setting, HrQoL assessments: $t_0 = 0 < \ldots < t_{j-1} < t_j < \ldots < \infty$.

θ: takes value $S(t)$ at time t and constant value S_j in the intervals $(t_{j-1}, t_j]$. Z_j is unobserved until t_j. Dupuy and Mesbah's [DUP 02] model assumes that:

$$\lambda(t|S) = \lambda(t) \exp(W(t)\beta_0 S_{a_d} + \beta_1 S_d) \qquad [13.12]$$

with

– S has a density satisfying a Markov property: $f_S(s_j|s_{j-1}, \ldots, s_0; \alpha) = f_S(s_j|s_{j-1}; \alpha)$, $\alpha \in \mathbb{R}^p$,

– C is non-informative for α and does not depend on $S(t)$.

Let $W(t) = (S_{a_d}, S_d)^T$ and $\beta^T = (\beta_0, \beta_1)$. The observations are $Y_i = (X_i, \Delta_i, S_{i,0}, \ldots, S_{i,a_d})_{1 \leq i \leq n}$. The unknown parameters of the model are $\tau = (\alpha, \beta, \Lambda)$. There are hidden variables in the model, the missing values of S at dropout time, S_{i,a_d}. The objective is to estimate τ from n independent vectors of observations Y_i.

The likelihood for one observation y_i $(1 \leq i \leq n)$ is obtained as:

$$\begin{aligned} L^{(i)}(\tau) &= \int \lambda(x_i)^{\delta_i} \exp\left[\delta_i \beta^T w_i(x_i) - \int_0^{x_i} \lambda(u)\, e^{\beta^T w_i(u)}\, du\right] \\ &\quad \times f\left(s_{i_0}, \ldots, s_{i_{a_d}}, s_d; \alpha\right) ds_d \\ &= \int l(y_i, s_d, \tau)\, ds_d. \end{aligned}$$

The parameter τ is identifiable. First, suppose that the functional parameter τ is a step function $\Lambda_n(t)$ with jumps at event times X_i and taking unknown values $\Lambda_n(X_i) = \Lambda_{n,i}$, then rewrite the likelihood and estimate α, β and $\Lambda_{n,i}$. The contribution of y_i to the likelihood obtained is now taken to be:

$$\begin{aligned} L^{(i)}(\tau) &= \int \Delta\Lambda_{n,i}^{\delta_i} \exp\left[\delta_i \beta^T w_i(x_i) - \sum_{k=1}^{p(n)} \Delta\Lambda_{n,k} e^{\beta^T w_i(x_k)} 1_{\{x_k \leq x_i\}}\right] \\ &\quad \times f(s_{i_0}, \ldots, s_{i_{a_d}}, s_d; \alpha)\, ds_d, \end{aligned}$$

where $\Delta\Lambda_{n,k} = \Delta\Lambda_n(X_k) = \Lambda_{n,k} - \Lambda_{n,k-1}$, $\Delta\Lambda_{n,1} = \Lambda_{n,1}$ and $X_1 < \ldots < X_{p(n)}$ $(p(n) \leq n)$ are increasingly ordered event times. The maximizer $\hat{\tau}_n$ of $\sum_{i=1}^n \log L^{(i)}(\tau)$ over $\tau \in \Theta_n$ satisfies:

$$\sum_{i=1}^n \frac{\partial}{\partial \tau}\left[L_{\hat{\tau}_n}^{(i)}(\tau)\right]_{|\tau = \hat{\tau}_n} = 0,$$

where $L_{\hat{\tau}_n}^{(i)}(\tau) = E_{\hat{\tau}_n}[\log l(Y, S; \tau)|y_i]$. Let us refer $\sum_{i=1}^n L_{\hat{\tau}_n}^{(i)}(\tau)$ to as the EM log likelihood. An expectation-maximization (EM) algorithm that is used to solve the maximization problem is described by [DUP 06]. A maximizer $\hat{\tau}_n$=$(\hat{\alpha}_n, \hat{\beta}_n, \hat{\Lambda}_n)$ of $\sum_{i=1}^{n} \log L^{(i)}(\tau)$ over $\tau \in \Theta_n$ exists and under some additional conditions,

$$(\sqrt{n}(\hat{\alpha}_n - \alpha_t), \sqrt{n}(\hat{\beta}_n - \beta_t), \sqrt{n}(\hat{\Lambda}_n - \Lambda_t)) \sim G,$$

where G is a tight Gaussian process in $l^{\infty}(H)$ with zero mean and a covariance process $\text{cov}[G(g), G(g^*)]$ [DUP 06]. From this we deduce, for instance:

1) $\sqrt{n}(\hat{\beta}_n - \beta_t)$ converges in distribution to a bivariate normal distribution with mean 0 and variance–covariance matrix $\Sigma_{\tau_t}^{-1}$,

2) consistent estimate of Σ_{τ_t} is obtained,

and similar results for $\hat{\alpha}_n$ and $\hat{\Lambda}_n$ are obtained. The results are shown in Table 13.2. [MES 04]

	Arm	A	Arm	B	Test	Statistics
	Random	NI	Random	NI	Random	NI
$\hat{\beta}_0$	−0.16	0.13	−0.17	0.09	0.033	0.35
SE($\hat{\beta}_0$)	0.08	0.08	0.08	0.08	–	–
$\hat{\beta}_1$		−0.36		−0.32	–	−0.37
SE($\hat{\beta}_1$)		0.09		0.09	–	–
$\hat{\alpha}$	0.96	0.95	0.96	0.95	0.35	0.32
SE($\hat{\alpha}$)	0.01	0.01	0.01	0.01	–	–
$\hat{\sigma}_e^2$	0.70	0.71	0.571	0.576	2.19565	2.18126
SE($\hat{\sigma}_e^2$)	0.046	0.047	0.04	0.04	–	–
Loglikelihood	−963.9	−896.4	−927.2	-857.2	–	–

Table 13.2. *HrQoL analysis in a cancer clinical trial*

In this example, HrQoL, excepted for its value at dropout time, was just considered an observed continuous score S. But in fact, HrQoL is not directly observed. It is an unobserved latent variable. In practice, HrQoL data always consists of a multidimensional binary or a categorical observed variable (QoLS) used to measure the true unobserved latent variable HrQol. From the QoLS, we can derive HrQoL scores, i.e. statistics. These scores are surrogate of the true unobserved latent variable HrQol. In the following section, we will show, how to use a latent regression model, to derive a likelihood not based on a surrogate S, but on item responses effectively observed.

13.7. Latent regression to analyze change between groups

In the same example presented in the previous section, the true HrQoL variable θ was considered as observed (excepted for the last unobserved dropout value θ_d), and its value replaced by its surrogate, the score S. The true likelihood for one individual y_i, $(1 \leq i \leq n)$, *if θ was directly observed*, is:

$$\begin{aligned} L^{(i)}(\tau) &= \int \lambda(x_i)^{\delta_i} \exp\left[\delta_i \beta^T w_i(x_i) - \int_0^{x_i} \lambda(u) e^{\beta^T w_i(u)}\, du\right] \\ &\quad \times f\left(\theta_{i_0}, \ldots, \theta_{i_{a_d}}, \theta_d; \alpha\right) d\theta_d \\ &= \int l(y_i, \theta_{i_d}, \tau)\, d\theta_{i_d}, \end{aligned}$$

where $y_i = (x_i, \delta_i, \theta_{i_0}, \ldots, \theta_{i_{a_d}}) = (x_i, \delta_i, \theta_{i_obs})$, and all the previous statistical inference, based on the likelihood,

$$L^{(i)}(\tau) = \int l(x_i, \delta_i, \theta_{i_{obs}}), \theta_d, \tau)\, d\theta_d, \qquad [13.13]$$

is highly validated by theoretical asymptotic results and well working computer algorithms. In the latent variable context, $\theta_{i_{obs}}$ is in fact not directly observed. The k item responses Q_{ij} of a subject i (response or raw vector Q_i) are observed and must be used to recover the latent HrQoL values θ_i through a measurement model. The obvious choice in our context is the Rasch model, which is for binary responses:

$$P\left(Q_{ij} = q_{ij} \mid \theta_i, \zeta_j\right) = f\left(q_{ij}, \theta_i, \zeta_j\right) = \frac{e^{(\theta_i - \zeta_j) q_{ij}}}{1 + e^{\theta_i - \zeta_j}}. \qquad [13.14]$$

So, currently, observations are $Y_i = (X_i, \Delta_i, Q_{i_0}, \ldots, Q_{i_{a_D}})_{1 \leq i \leq n}$; with $Q_i = (Q_{i1}, \ldots, Q_{ip})$ for a unidimensional scale of p items. Unknown parameters of the model are $\tau = (\alpha, \beta, \Lambda)$ and nuisance parameters ζ. The objective is now to estimate τ from n independent vectors of observations Y_i. Let us suppose the following two assumptions hold:

1) The DM analysis model holds for the true unobserved QoL θ and dropout D or survival T.

2) The Rasch measurement model relates the observed response items Q to QoL θ.

First, we have two main issues:

– Specification of a model for the data and the true latent QoL.

– Choice of a method of estimation.

Similar to Rasch model, for categorical ordinal responses (with number of levels m_j different per item), the PCM is given by:

$$p_c = P(Q_{ij} = c \mid \theta_i, \zeta_j) = \frac{e^{(c\theta_i - \sum_{l=1}^{c} \zeta_{jl})}}{\sum_{c=0}^{m_j} e^{(c\theta_i - \sum_{l=1}^{c} \zeta_{jl})}}. \qquad [13.15]$$

The joint distribution of Q (items), θ (latent), D (time to death or dropout) and T (treatment) can be derived, using only the conditional independence property:

$$f(Q,\theta,D,T/\theta) = \frac{f(Q,\theta,D,T)}{f(\theta)} = \frac{f(Q,\theta)}{f(\theta)} \times \frac{f(\theta,D,T)}{f(\theta)}, \qquad [13.16]$$

so, we have:

$$f(Q,\theta,D,T|\theta) = f(Q|\theta) \times f(D,T|\theta), \qquad [13.17]$$

Then, without any other assumption, we can specify two models:

– First model:

$$f(Q,\theta,D,T) = f(Q/\theta) \times f(D/\theta,T) \times f(\theta/T) \times f(T). \qquad [13.18]$$

– Second model:

$$f(Q,\theta,D,T) = f(Q/\theta) \times f(\theta/D,T) \times f(D/T) \times f(T). \qquad [13.19]$$

The right likelihood must be based on the probability function of the observations, i.e., currently, $Y_i = (X_i, \Delta_i, Q_{i_0}, \ldots, Q_{i_{a_D}})_{1\le i\le n}$. The parameters of the model are $\tau = (\alpha, \beta, \Lambda)$ and the nuisance difficulty parameter of the HrQoL questionnaire is ζ. There are non-observed (hidden) variables in the model (latent θ, missing Q): $(\theta_{i_0}, \ldots, \theta_{i_{a_D}}, \theta_{i_d}, Q_d)_{1\le i\le n}$.

Following directly from the conditional independence assumptions of the DMq model, factorization rules of the joint distribution function of the observations (Y_i), the latent HrQoL (θ) and the missing questionnaire Q_d can now be specified, and then integrating through the hidden variables, we get the likelihood:

$$L^{(i)}(\tau) = \int \prod_{j=1}^{p} \left[\frac{e^{\left(c\theta_{i_0} - \sum_{l=1}^{c} \zeta_{jl}\right)}}{\sum_{h=0}^{m_j} e^{\left(c\theta_{i_0} - \sum_{l=1}^{c} \zeta_{jl}\right)}} \times \cdots \times \frac{e^{\left(c\theta_{i_{a_d}} - \sum_{l=1}^{c} \zeta_{jl}\right)}}{\sum_{h=0}^{m_j} e^{\left(c\theta_{i_{a_d}} - \sum_{l=1}^{c} \zeta_{jl}\right)}} \right.$$
$$\left. \times \sum_{c=1}^{p} \frac{e^{\left(c\theta_{i_d} - \sum_{l=1}^{c} \zeta_{jl}\right)}}{\sum_{h=0}^{m_j} e^{\left(c\theta_{i_d} - \sum_{l=1}^{c} \zeta_{jl}\right)}} \right]$$
$$\times \Delta\Lambda_{n,i}^{\delta_i} \exp\left[\delta_i \beta^T w_i(x_i) - \sum_{k=1}^{p(n)} \Delta\Lambda_{n,k} e^{\beta^T w_i(x_k)} 1_{\{x_k \le x_i\}}\right]$$
$$\times f(\theta_{i_0}, \ldots, \theta_{i_{a_d}}, \theta_d; \alpha) d\theta_{i_0}, \ldots, \theta_{i_{a_d}}, \theta_{i_d}.$$

The marginalization over the latent variables is similar to the marginalization over the dropout missing value. Computer programs are easily extended. Nevertheless, when the number of latent components is large, computing time can be very long. So, generally, in health applications, a two-step approach is reasonably preferred.

13.8. Conclusion

The definition (or construction) of variables and indicators, and the analysis of the evolution of their joint distribution between various populations, times and areas are generally two different, well-separated steps of the work for a statistician in the field of health measurement.

The first step generally deals with calibration and metrology of questionnaires. Keywords are measurement or scoring, depending on the area of application.

The second step is certainly more known by most statisticians. Linear, generalized linear, time series and survival models are very useful models in this step, where the variables constructed in the first step are incorporated and their joint distribution with the other analysis variables (treatment group, time, duration of life, etc.) is investigated. HrQoL scores, validated during the first step, are then analyzed, with a complete omission of the real observations, i.e. item responses. The latent nature of the HrQoL concept is generally neglected.

Mesbah [MES 09] compared the simple strategy of separating the two steps with the global strategy of defining and analyzing a global model, including both the measurement and the analysis steps. If, with a real data set, we find a significant association between a built (from items) score and an external covariate, then the true association, i.e. the association between the external covariate and the true latent, is probably larger. So, if the scientific goal is to show an association between the true and the covariate, we do not need to use a global model: just use the model with the surrogate built score instead of the true latent. Conclusions with the built score also stand for the true.

But, if we get no significant association between built score and the covariate, then the true association could be anything, perhaps even larger. So, we have to consider a global model, even if we do not need to build new scores or to validate the measurement model.

Building a global model taking into account the latent trait parameter in a one-step way, i.e. without separation between measurement and analysis, is a promising latent regression approach [CHR 04, SEB 05] permitted by the increasing performance of computers. In HrQoL field, most papers are devoted to a two-step approach, where the HrQoL scores are used instead of the original item responses data. Moreover, scientific results are published in different kinds of scientific journals: those devoted to validation of measurements and instruments and numerous others, specializing on analysis of previously validated measurements.

13.9. Bibliography

[AWA 02] AWAD L., ZUBER E., MESBAH M., "Applying survival data methodology to analyze longitudinal Quality of Life Data", in MESBAH M., COLE B.F., LEE M.L.T. (eds), *Statistical Methods for Quality of Life Studies: Design, Measurement and Analysis*, Kluwer Academic, Boston, MA, pp. 231–243, 2002.

[BON 03] BONNEFOY X.R., BRAUBACH M., MOISSONNIER B., MONOLBAEV K., RÖBBEL N., "Housing and health in Europe: preliminary results of a pan-European study", *American Journal of Public Health* vol. 93, pp. 1559–1563, 2003.

[BON 04] BONNEFOY X.R., LARES GROUP, "Habitat et Santé: état des connaissances", *Les échos du logement*, vol. 4, pp. 145–153, 2004.

[CHR 04] CHRISTENSEN K.B., BJORNER J.B., KREINER S., PETERSEN J.H., "Latent regression in loglinear Rasch models", *Communication in Statistics—Theory and Methods*, vol. 33, pp. 1295–1313, 2004.

[COX 72] COX D.R., "Regression models and life tables" (with discussion), *Journal of the Royal Statistical Society, Series B*, vol. 34, pp. 187–220, 1972.

[CRO 51] CRONBACH L.J., "Coefficient alpha and the internal structure of tests", *Psychometrika*, vol. 16, pp. 297–334, 1951.

[CUR 97] CURT F., MESBAH M., LELLOUCH J., DELLATOLAS G., "Handedness scale: how many and which items?", *Laterality*, vol. 2, pp. 137–154, 1997.

[DUP 02] DUPUY J.-F., MESBAH M., "Joint modeling of event time and nonignorable missing longitudinal data", *Lifetime Data Analysis*, vol. 8, pp. 99–115, 2002.

[DUP 06] DUPUY J.-F., GRAMA I., MESBAH M., "Asymptotic theory for the Cox model with missing time dependent covariate", *Annals of Statistics*, vol. 34, pp. 903–924, 2006.

[EDW 00] EDWARDS D., *Introduction to Graphical Modelling*, 2nd ed., Springer-Verlag, New York, NY, 2000.

[FRE 09] FREDOUILLE J., LAPORTE E., MESBAH M., "Housing and mental health", in ORMANDY D. (ed.), *Housing and Health in Europe: The Who Lares Project*, Taylor and Francis, Boston, MA, 2009.

[KRE 02] KREINER S., CRISTENSEN K.B., "Graphical Rasch models", in MESBAH M., COLE B.F., LEE M.L.T. (eds), *Statistical Methods for Quality of Life Studies: Design, Measurement and Analysis*, Kluwer Academic, Boston, MA, 2002.

[KRI 63] KRISTOF W., "The statistical theory of stepped-up reliability coefficients when a test has been divided into several equivalent parts", *Psychometrika*, vol. 28, pp. 221–238, 1963.

[LAU 89] LAURITZEN S.L., WERMUTH N., "Graphical models for association between variables, some of which are qualitative and some quantitative", *Annals of Statistics*, vol. 17, pp. 31–57, 1989.

[LAU 96] LAURITZEN S.L., *Graphical Models*, Oxford University Press, Oxford, 1996.

[MAS 82] MASTERS G.N., "A Rasch model for partial credit scoring", *Psychometrika*, vol. 47, pp. 149–174, 1982.

[MCC 89] McCULLAGH P., NELDER J., *Generalized Linear Models*, Chapman and Hall, London, 1989.

[MES 04] MESBAH M., DUPUY J.F., HEUTTE N., AWAD L., "Joint analysis of longitudinal quality of life and survival processes", *Handbook of Statistics*, vol. 23, pp. 689–728, 2004.

[MES 09] MESBAH M., "Building quality of life related housing scores using LARES study: a methodical approach to avoid pitfalls and bias", in ORMANDY D. (ed.), *Housing and Health in Europe: The Who Lares Project*, Taylor and Francis, Boston, MA, 2009.

[MOL 88] MOLENAAR I.W., SIJSTMA K., "Mokken's approach to reliability estimation extended to multicategory items", *Psychometrika*, vol. 49, pp. 359–381, 1988.

[MOR 93] MORET L., MESBAH M., CHWALOW J., LELLOUCH J., "Validation interne d'une échelle de mesure: relation entre analyse en composantes principales, coefficient alpha de Cronbach et coefficient de corrélation intra-classe", *La Revue d'Epidémiologie et de Santé Publique*, vol. 41, pp. 179–186, 1993.

[NOR 05] NORDMAN J.F., MESBAH M., BERDEAUX G., "Scoring of visual field measured through Humphrey perimetry: principal component, varimax rotation followed by validated cluster analysis", *Investigative Ophtalmology and Visual Science*, vol. 48, pp. 3168–3176, 2005.

[NUN 78] NUNNALY J., *Psychometric Theory*, 2nd ed., McGraw-Hill, New York, 1978.

[SEB 05] SÉBILLE V., MESBAH M., "Sequential analysis of quality of life Rasch measurements", in NIKOULINE M., COMMENGES D., HUBER C. (eds), *Probability Statistics and Modeling in Public Health: in Honor of Marvin Zelen*, Kluwer Academic Publisher, New York, NY, 2005.

[WHI 90] WHITTAKER J., *Graphical Models In Applied Multivariate Statistics*, 1st ed., Wiley, New York, NY, 1990.

Chapter 14

Analysis with Repeatedly Measured Binary Item Response Data by *Ad Hoc* Rasch Scales

14.1. Introduction

We often encounter sets of items that tentatively measure some underlying construct, but which were never designed to measure this construct and a scale based on the set was never validated. Moreover, these items may be measured at various times in the course of a process and we may be tempted to use the information in the items as some measures of the course of the underlying construct. The present study aims at exploring the conditions under which we may use such an *ad hoc* scale based on binary items in analyses involving repeated measurements.

A typical example of the above situation is provided by data from the Diabetes Care in General Practice (DCGP) study [OLI 01]. In this study, newly diagnosed type 2 diabetes patients are followed, and regularly reviewed. At three times during the follow-up period all patients undergo an elaborate examination and respond to a questionnaire: at inclusion in the study (just after diagnosis), approximately six years after inclusion, and 14 years after inclusion. Part of these questionnaires is an inquiry into specific symptoms generally considered to be related to diabetes. Six symptoms are evaluated at all three time points: abnormal thirst, frequent urination, unintended weight loss, fatigue, visual disturbances and genital itching, as well as an inquiry into the patient's self-rated health (SRH). SRH is defined as the response to the question "How would you rate your health at present?", dichotomized into *good* (combines answer categories good and excellent) and *poor* (combines fair, poor and very poor). An overview of the symptom prevalence is shown in Table 14.1.

Chapter written by Volkert SIERSMA and Paolo EUSEBI.

Baseline (T = 1)	SRH		Total	p-value[1]
	Good	Poor		
Total	560 (45.3)	675 (54.7)	1235 (100)	
Number of symptoms				
0	114 (20.4)	51 (7.6)	165 (13.4)	0.0000
1	96 (17.1)	96 (14.2)	192 (15.6)	
2	102 (18.2)	119 (17.6)	221 (17.9)	
3	96 (17.1)	142 (21.0)	238 (19.3)	
4	97 (17.3)	146 (21.6)	243 (19.7)	
5	43 (7.7)	96 (14.2)	139 (11.3)	
6	12 (2.1)	25 (3.7)	37 (3.0)	
Mean (SD)	2.26(1.68)	2.93(1.59)	2.61(1.67)	0.0000[2]
Presence of symptoms				
1: Abnormal thirst	298 (53.2)	464 (68.7)	762 (61.7)	0.0000
2: Frequent urination	275 (49.1)	371 (55.0)	646 (52.3)	0.0403
3: Unintended weight loss	182 (32.5)	239 (35.4)	421 (34.1)	0.2832
4: Fatigue	256 (45.7)	500 (74.1)	756 (61.2)	0.0000
5: Visual disturbances	114 (20.4)	211 (31.3)	325 (26.3)	0.0000
6: Genital itching	138 (24.6)	189 (28.0)	327 (26.5)	0.1831
1st follow-up (T = 2)	SRH			
	Good	Poor	Total	p-value[1]
Total	479 (58.3)	342 (41.7)	821 (100)	
Number of symptoms				
0	332 (69.3)	105 (31.0)	437 (53.4)	0.0000
1	85 (17.8)	87 (25.7)	172 (21.0)	
2	42 (8.8)	73 (21.5)	115 (14.1)	
3	15 (3.1)	42 (12.4)	57 (7.0)	
4	4 (0.8)	26 (7.7)	30 (3.7)	
5	1 (0.2)	4 (1.2)	5 (0.6)	
6	0 (0.0)	2 (0.6)	2 (0.2)	
Mean (SD)	0.49 (0.87)	1.46(1.36)	0.89(1.20)	0.0000[2]
Presence of symptoms				
1: Abnormal thirst	32 (6.7)	55 (16.2)	87 (10.6)	0.0000
2: Frequent urination	67 (14.0)	107 (31.6)	174 (21.3)	0.0000
3: Unintended weight loss	22 (4.6)	29 (8.6)	51 (6.2)	0.0210
4: Fatigue	60 (12.5)	179 (52.8)	239 (29.2)	0.0000
5: Visual disturbances	25 (5.2)	69 (20.4)	94 (11.5)	0.0000
6: Genital itching	29 (6.1)	56 (16.5)	85 (10.4)	0.0000

Table 14.1. *Prevalence of the six selected diabetic symptoms at baseline and the two follow-up time points and their association with self-rated health (SRH)*

2nd follow-up (T = 3)	SRH		Total	p-value[1]
	Good	Poor		
Total	265 (6.8)	164 (38.2)	429 (100)	
Number of symptoms				
0	161 (61.9)	36 (22.2)	197 (46.7)	0.0000
1	65 (25.0)	52 (32.1)	117 (27.7)	
2	23 (8.9)	38 (23.1)	61 (14.5)	
3	7 (2.7)	21 (13.0)	28 (6.6)	
4	2 (0.8)	10 (6.2)	12 (2.8)	
5	1 (0.4)	4 (2.5)	5 (1.2)	
6	1 (0.4)	1 (0.6)	2 (0.5)	
Mean (SD)	0.58 (0.93)	1.59 (1.32)	0.97 (1.20)	0.0000[2]
Presence of symptoms				
1: Abnormal thirst	11 (4.2)	32 (19.8)	43 (10.2)	0.0000
2: Frequent urination	41 (15.8)	58 (35.8)	99 (23.5)	0.0000
3: Unintended weight loss	6 (2.3)	19 (11.7)	25 (5.9)	0.0000
4: Fatigue	51 (19.6)	95 (58.6)	146 (34.6)	0.0000
5: Visual disturbances	18 (6.9)	34 (21.0)	52 (12.3)	0.0000
6: Genital itching	24 (9.2)	19 (11.7)	43 (10.2)	0.4095

[1]: p-value of a Chi-squared test except where otherwise indicated.
[2]: p-value of a t-test.

Table 14.1. *(Continued.) Prevalence of the six selected diabetic symptoms at baseline and the two follow-up time points and their association with self-rated health (SRH)*

The symptoms are objective observations of the disease experience and SRH, the interpretation of these symptoms – and other health signs – by the patient. When the relationship between SRH and the symptoms is strong, the diabetic symptoms are an important part in the patient's perception of general health, and the symptoms may then form a motivational factor in the treatment. The relationship between symptoms and SRH may change in the natural development of the disease. In analyses of this relationship, the symptom burden is viewed as a single construct. This enables us to look at associations between this construct and other measures of health such as SRH.

In order for items to objectively measure an underlying construct, they must fulfill the assumptions of a Rasch model [RAS 60]. A disease burden score can be created by simply summing up the number of symptoms that is indicated. A Rasch model measures the symptom burden construct with the sum score of the symptoms, but implies strong assumptions that are obviously violated, because item responses have properties that are unwanted in that, for example, abnormal thirst and frequent urination are obviously correlated. Furthermore, various factors have previously been shown to correlate differently with specific symptoms [NIE 11].

Violations of the assumptions of the Rasch model are usually dealt with by the removal of the items that do not fit the assumptions of the model after performing a careful item analysis. This approach views the Rasch model as a prescriptive model in which we investigate *how the data fit the model* instead of the more classical statistical problem of *how the model fit the data* [BON 01]. The item deletion process can be quite expensive in terms of loss of information; the more so when not many items are available, as is the case in the diabetes data. Furthermore, in a longitudinal setting, the assumptions of the Rasch model must hold jointly in all the time points that exaggerate the problem. Also, the Rasch model is not trivially extended to longitudinal data. To avoid item deletion, we can on some occasions extend the Rasch model into a model framework that combines the measurement approach with an explanatory perspective [DEB 04], i.e. a reversion to the classical problem of model fit. In the present study, we use a *generalized multilevel Rasch model* to jointly accommodate for violations of the conventional Rasch model and account for the repeated longitudinal observations. For binary items this model is identified as a multilevel logistic regression model.

In the following we first, in section 14.2, describe the generalized multilevel Rasch model framework, the ways how violations of the Rasch model are incorporated and elaborate on the relevant research questions it stands to answer for the above introduced DCGP data. Thereafter, in section 14.3, we describe ways of identifying the violations of the Rasch model in order to perform analyses in parsimonious models; these methods are illustrated with the DCGP data. In section 14.4, we perform a simulation analysis to illustrate some general principles for longitudinal analysis of *ad hoc* scales. Finally, in section 14.5, we discuss our results.

14.2. The generalized multilevel Rasch model

14.2.1. *The multilevel form of the conventional Rasch model for binary items*

Disregarding the time aspect for the moment, the data we have to fit a Rasch model consists of binary item responses X_{vi} to k items $i = 1, \ldots, k$ for n persons $v = 1, \ldots, n$. The Rasch model then writes the probability of a positive ($X_{vi} = 1$) response by a person v to item i, i.e. π_{vi}, as the simple logit function:

$$P(X_{vi} = 1) = \pi_{vi} = \text{logit}(\eta_{vi}) = \frac{\exp(\eta_{vi})}{1 + \exp(\eta_{vi})} \qquad [14.1]$$

where

$$\eta_{vi} = \theta_v + \beta_i \qquad [14.2]$$

so that the probability π_{vi} depends on the level of the underlying construct θ_v that may be different for each person, and on the easiness of the item β_i that is the same for all persons. In the following, we use the Rasch model and its variants as tools for providing objective measurements of the latent construct, and therefore our main purpose is to estimate the person parameter θ_v and associations of other variables with this estimate; we are interested in the estimation of the item parameters β_i only to the extend it helps in the inference concerning θ_v.

In the Rasch literature there are three well-know approaches to the maximization of the likelihood [FIS 95]: the joint maximum likelihood (JML), the conditional maximum likelihood (CML) and the marginal maximum likelihood (MML). In JML person and item parameters are estimated jointly but the obtained estimates are inconsistent. In CML one of the sets of parameters is conditioned out using the item sum score and estimates are consistent. These methods assume the Rasch assumptions to hold and such procedures do not easily accommodate (specific) violations of the Rasch model. In MML one set of parameters is assumed independent random that draws from a normal distribution to obtain consistent estimates of the other set together with estimates for the two moments of the assumed Normal; estimates of the parameter set that was assumed normal can be obtained through an empirical posterior Bayes procedure. If we want to estimate person parameters in JML they will be estimated jointly with item parameters; in CML item parameters will be conditioned out; and in MML they will be integrated out. Summarizing, in MML either the person or the item parameters forms a random effect, this is in contrast to JML and CML where both are fixed effects. We expand this idea in the following.

In this chapter, we are not necessarily interested in the measurement of each of the persons on the underlying construct, but primarily in extending the framework of the Rasch model to investigate differences in the underlying construct between subgroups in the data. This leads us to adopt a perspective in which both θ_v and β_i are random instead of fixed effects. This defines the multilevel form of the Rasch model which in its basic formulation rewrites [14.2] as:

$$\eta_{vi} = \zeta_v + \varepsilon_v + \beta_i \qquad [14.3]$$

where $\varepsilon_v \sim N(0, \sigma_\varepsilon^2)$ $\beta_i \sim N(0, \sigma_\beta^2)$ and $\zeta_v = \sum_{j=1}^{J} \vartheta_j \zeta_{vj}$. The model differs from the traditional perspective in that not only the person parameter but also the item parameters are random. Furthermore, θ_v is replaced by a linear regression equation $\zeta_v + \varepsilon_v$ in which ζ_v includes the J person characteristics ζ_{vj} and ε_v is the remaining random person effect. The model is also know in literature as the latent regression Rasch model [ADA 97]. Note that once the model has been fitted, we can obtain the item and person parameters from the estimates of the conditional modes of the random effects. The estimation of the parameters of the model is done in a generalized logistic regression model procedure such as PROC GLIMMIX in SAS [DEB 04] and the lme4 package in R [DOR 07].

14.2.2. *Group comparison and repeated measurement*

The multilevel form of the Rasch model becomes useful when we want to make comparisons between subgroups in the data. In the spirit of the DCGP data, we may want to know whether there is a difference in symptom burden (at a specific time point) between those that rate their health well and those that rate their health poor. In a conventional setting where we would have observed the symptom burden, we would have compared the averages between the two groups. Now, in the multilevel form of the Rasch model, we write [14.3] as:

$$\eta_{vi} = \zeta^s \mathrm{SRH}_{vi} + \varepsilon_v + \beta_i \qquad [14.4]$$

where $\mathrm{SRH}_{vi} = \mathrm{SRH}_v$ is the indicator for poor SRH so that ζ^s denotes the average *difference* in probability (on logit scale) of a positive indication for a symptom for poor SRH compared to good SRH; the statistical significance of ζ^s assesses the evidence of this difference.

In a longitudinal setting such as the DCGP data, we are interested in modeling the effect of time on the item responses. This is naturally implemented in the multilevel form of the Rasch model since the multilevel framework that is used in the model naturally extends to the modeling of longitudinal, time-dependent relationships found in repeated measurement data. For T time points $= 1, \ldots, T$, for example the three time points in the DCGP study, the linear predictor [14.3] is written as:

$$\eta_{vit} = \zeta_t T_{vit} + \varepsilon_v + \beta_i \qquad [14.5]$$

where T_{vit} is the indicator of the time point t and ζ_t denotes the probability of a positive indication on an item (on logit scale) averaged over the items and the persons at the corresponding time point. Hence, the sequence of ζ_t characterizes the development of the latent construct over time. In the DCGP data, this model investigates the natural development of the symptom burden in diabetes patients.

One of our main interests is the relationship between symptom burden and SRH, and its development over time. An analysis into this relationship combines [14.4] and [14.5] into:

$$\eta_{vit} = \zeta_t T_{vit} + \zeta_t^s \mathrm{SRH}_{vit} T_{vit} + \varepsilon_v + \beta_i \qquad [14.6]$$

where T_{vit} is the indicator of time point t, $\mathrm{SRH}_{vit} = \mathrm{SRH}_{vt}$ is the indicator for poor SRH at time point t and $\mathrm{SRH}_{vit} T_{vit}$ is the direct product of the two. The parameter ζ_t then denotes the average probability (on logit scale) of a positive indication for a symptom at time point t for people with good SRH, and together characterize the symptom burden for those that have good SRH throughout the full follow-up period. More interesting is the parameter ζ_t^s that denotes the average *difference* (on logit scale) of the probabilities of a positive indication on a symptom between those with good SRH and those with poor SRH at time point t. Hence, it measures the strength of the relationship between symptom burden and SRH at time point t.

14.2.3. *Differential item functioning and local dependence*

The multilevel form of the Rasch model extends to the generalized multilevel Rasch model in that we can easily explicitly incorporate certain violations of the assumptions of the conventional Rasch model, most prominently differential item functioning (DIF) and local dependence (LD).

DIF occurs when patients from different subgroups in the data show differing answering probabilities to certain items beyond what can be expected from differing values of the underlying construct [HOL 93]. Typically such subgroups are defined by demographic (e.g. gender and age) and socioeconomic variables. Let Z be an indicator variable that divides the data into two groups. Uniform DIF, then, increases the probability of certain item responses in one group compared to the other. This can be easily modeled for binary items within the framework of the generalized multilevel Rasch model. The dummy variables is defined W_{vit} as:

$$W_{vit} = \begin{cases} 1 & \text{for person } v \text{ and item } i \text{ if } T = t \text{ and } Z = 1 \\ 0 & \text{otherwise} \end{cases} \qquad [14.7]$$

indicators to change the probability of a positive indication of item i if person v has group characteristic Z at time point t. These variables can be added to [14.3], [14.4], [14.5] or [14.6] as a fixed effect in the linear term:

$$\eta_{vit} = \zeta_t T_{vit} + \zeta_t^s \text{SRH}_{vit} T_{vit} + \varepsilon_v + \beta_i + \zeta_{it}^{\text{DIF}} W_{vit}, \qquad [14.8]$$

here shown added to [14.6]. Note that in this way we are able to specify DIF differently at specific time points. This is of some interest because in a longitudinal setting it may well be that a DIF effect changes with the natural development. The parameter ζ_{it}^{DIF} is interpreted as the excess probability (on logit scale) of answering positively to item i at time point t when $Z = 1$. The parameters ζ_t loose their intuitive interpretation of the development of the latent construct and, for what it is worth, are interpreted as the average probability of answering positively to an item at time point t when the excess probability due to DIF is controlled for; or, alternatively, when $Z = 0$. However, the parameters ζ_t^s retain their interpretation, since for a specific person v item i at time point t and any value z of Z, and thereby any value w for W_{vit} we find that:

$$\begin{aligned} &\eta_{vit}|_{\text{SRH}=1} - \eta_{vit}|_{\text{SRH}=0} \\ &\quad = \left(\zeta_t + \zeta_t^s + \varepsilon_v + \beta_i + \zeta_{it}^{\text{DIF}} w\right) - \left(\zeta_t + \varepsilon_v + \beta_i + \zeta_{it}^{\text{DIF}} w\right) = \zeta_t^s \end{aligned} \qquad [14.9]$$

Thus, while the actual probabilities are affected by DIF, the parameters ζ_t^s are still the average *difference* (on logit scale) of the probabilities of a positive indication on a symptom between those with good SRH and those with poor SRH at time point t.

LD is the situation where answers to two specific items are correlated beyond the dependence that is expected from them measuring the same underlying construct.

Typically this happens when two items are dependent by construction, such as in the DCGP data we know that increased thirst will be associated with frequent urination. LD changes the probability for a positive response on one item when the response to another item is positive. Similarly to DIF, LD also can typically be easily incorporated into the generalized multilevel Rasch model. The dummy variables is defined W_{vijt} as:

$$W_{vijt} = \begin{cases} 1 & \text{for person } v \text{ and } T = t \text{ and item } i \text{ or } j \\ 0 & \text{otherwise} \end{cases} \qquad [14.10]$$

that, similar to [14.7], are indicators to change the probability of a joint positive indication of items i and j for person v at time point t. To allow for LD, these variables can be added to [14.3], [14.4], [14.5] or [14.6] as a fixed effect in the linear term:

$$\eta_{vit} = \zeta_t T_{vit} + \zeta_t^s \text{SRH}_{vit} T_{vit} + \varepsilon_v + \beta_i + \zeta_{ijt}^{\text{LD}} W_{vijt}, \qquad [14.11]$$

here shown added to [14.6]. Also we are able to specify LD differently at specific time points. The parameter ζ_{ijt}^{LD} is interpreted as the excess probability (on logit scale) of answering positively to item i at time point t when item j is answered positively (and *vice versa*). Again, the parameters ζ_t lose their intuitive interpretation of the development of the latent construct and are interpreted as the average probability (on logit scale) of answering positively to an item at time point t when the excess probability due to LD is subtracted, i.e. when both item i and j are not answered positively. But as with DIF, the parameters ζ_t^s retain their interpretation in the presence of LD since for a specific person v, item i, time point t and any answer to item j, and thereby any value w for W_{vijt} we find that:

$$\eta_{vit}|_{\text{SRH}=1} - \eta_{vit}|_{\text{SRH}=0} = \left(\zeta_t + \zeta_t^s + \varepsilon_v + \beta_i + \zeta_{ijt}^{\text{LD}} w\right) - \left(\zeta_t + \varepsilon_v + \beta_i + \zeta_{ijt}^{\text{LD}} w\right) = \zeta_t^s \qquad [14.12]$$

In summary, by using dummy variables W_{vit} and W_{vijt} we are able to allow for DIF and LD in the generalized multilevel Rasch model and retain the interpretation of the parameters that are of greatest interest with respect to our research aims. In addition, we can use inference on the parameters ζ_{it}^{DIF} and ζ_{ijt}^{LD} to investigate whether the data give evidence of specific DIF or LD effects; this is exploited in the following section.

14.3. The analysis of an *ad hoc* scale

In the previous section we have identified the ways in which we can adjust for certain violations of the Rasch model in the analysis, we now have to identify which model elements are to be included in the generalized multilevel Rasch model to do this adequately. This is a model search procedure. Notably, we are not so interested in the resulting model, but more pertinently in the inference between the construct and the covariates. Therefore, we present a couple of ways to perform the model search – some more elaborate than others – and focus on the impact of these different methods on the resulting inference. The DCGP data that has six items (symptoms) are used and we investigate DIF with respect to three covariates: gender, age at diagnosis and household status (whether a person is living alone or not); for the three time points this allows for $15 \times 3 = 45$ LD instances and $3 \times 6 \times 3 = 56$ DIF instances. The following five model search heuristics (resulting in five *Model*s and inferences) are used:

– *Model 0* (empty model): This trivial method estimates model [14.6], thereby avoids model search altogether by ignoring DIF and LD. It serves as a benchmark for the other model search methods.

– *Model 1* (separate time points): There exist various computer programs dedicated to scale validation that, among other things, can be used to detect the presence of DIF and LD for single scales. These programs often use powerful inference, but do not account for repeated measurement. These programs can be used on the data for each time point separately to identify DIF and LD. We used the program DIGRAM [KRE 03] to identify DIF and LD for each of the time points. Specifically, we used a screening procedure [KRE 11] to identify a start configuration of DIF and LD, and thereafter we used a manual backward elimination (eliminating DIF or LD with highest p-value until all included DIF and LD have $p < 0.05$) and a manual forward selection (including DIF or LD with lowest p-value if $p < 0.05$) to come to a final configuration of DIF and LD. The identified DIF and LD are then included in the generalized multilevel Rasch model as dummy variables [14.7] and [14.10] in the manner of [14.8] and [14.11].

– *Model 2* (forward inclusion): Instead of relying on dedicated scale validation software we can use the inference on the generalized multilevel Rasch model itself included in the procedures that estimate the generalized logistic regression model; we use the lme4 package in R [DOR 07] for this. Now we can use a model search on the complete data including all time points since we can account for repeated measurement. Two straightforward model search heuristics are well-known: (1) backward elimination: starting from a model with all DIF and LD terms, we sequentially eliminate DIF and LD terms with the highest p-value until all DIF and LD terms that are left have $p < 0.05$, and (2) forward inclusion: starting from a model without DIF and LD terms, we sequentially include DIF and LD terms with the lowest p-value until all DIF and LD terms that are not included have $p > 0.05$ if they were to be included. The problem with backward elimination is that the complete model with all DIF and LD terms included does not compute; generally, generalized multilevel Rasch models with many DIF and LD terms take time to compute. Hence, backward elimination is not a feasible strategy and we use forward inclusion to identify DIF and LD for Model 2.

– *Model 3* (simulated annealing): A model search defines in general a discrete optimization problem where some model fit criterion is to be optimized relative to which DIF and LD terms are to be included in the model. Natural candidates for model fit criterions are the information criterions, for example Akaike Information Criterion (AIC) and Bayesian information criterion (BIC), as these balance fit with model parsimony [BUR 98]; we use BIC in the following. In theory, we could calculate the BIC of the generalized multilevel Rasch model for all possible configurations of DIF and LD and then pick the configuration that gives the lowest value for BIC. Such exhaustive search is often computationally too demanding. Therefore, it is necessary to use some other strategy to approach the optimum in not too long time. An optimization heuristic that is easily implemented and often gives surprisingly good results is simulated annealing [KIR 83]. Simulated annealing as implemented for the present model search is an iterative procedure where in each iteration a current model is changed by adding or omitting a DIF or LD term, the BIC is evaluated and the change is kept not only if the BIC of the new model is lower than that of the current model, but also – however with a probability that diminishes with the number of iterations; we used $1/(i+1)$ – if the BIC of the new model is higher than that of the current model. This last element of the algorithm protects the optimization that get stuck in a local optimum. In our implementation the simulated annealing is started with a model that includes all DIF and LD terms that were significant univariately after a Bonferroni correction ($p < 0.05/101 = 0.0005$), see Figure 14.1 (the dark gray shaded cells), and continued for a maximum of 200 iterations.

– *Model 4* (restricted simulated annealing): Reducing the search space, the number of DIF and LD terms that can be included in the model, can potentially speed up the simulated annealing as evaluation of unimportant changes may be avoided. However, we may restrict ourselves too much and we may not be able to reach the same low BIC values as in the unrestricted simulated annealing (Model 3). We implemented a restricted simulating annealing algorithm that works in much the same way as the unrestricted algorithm, only the random DIF and LD terms that are added or omitted are chosen exclusively from the terms that were significant ($p < 0.05$) univariately, see Figure 14.1 (the light gray shaded cells).

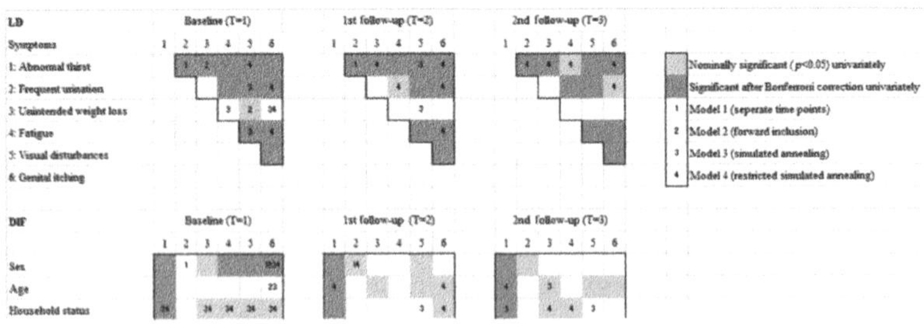

Figure 14.1. *The configurations of LD and DIF that result from the model search heuristics*

The models that result for the various model search strategies are summarized in Figure 14.1. We see that, while each of the model search methods tries to achieve a similar aim, they result in very different models. There does not seem to be consensus about a single model. Even though, the models – especially Models 2, 3 and 4 – do not differ much in quality as measured by the BIC. This is shown in Figure 14.2 that illustrates the convergence of the two iterative simulated annealing model search methods.

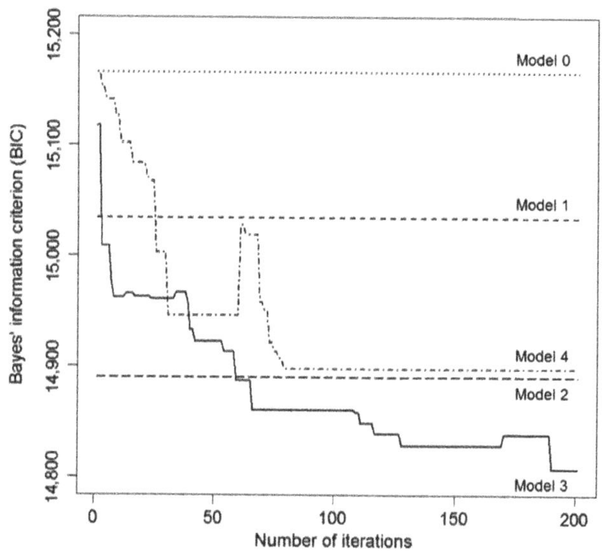

Figure 14.2. *The quality as measured by the BIC and convergence of the model search heuristics*

The present results may serve as a warning that model search is a difficult business and that we may never be sure that what we have found is some true configuration of DIF and LD. However, the aim of the model search was not to find some true model, but to adequately adjust inference on the parameters of interest for DIF and LD. Note then that to this aim we rather want too many DIF and LD terms in the model than too few; this is not reflected in the above model search methods.

The estimates and inference for the parameters of interest for the DCGP data are shown in Table 14.2. We note that the estimates for parameters ζ_t of the time variable are rather different from model to model. This coincides with the above observation that these parameters change interpretation when DIF and LD terms are added to the model. However, the estimates for the parameters ζ_t^s of the relationship between symptom burden and SRH, and the ensuing inference, are surprisingly similar between the models. While we have argued that these parameters retain their interpretation when DIF and LD terms are added to the model, it is not directly clear that omitting

DIF and LD terms from the model in a situation where there is evidence for these violations of the Rasch model does not affect estimation and inference on these parameters. Since Model 0 seems to perform just as well as the others in Table 14.2, this is apparently so for the relation between symptom burden and SRH in the DCGP data, and in the following we investigate whether this is coincidence or a more general property of the generalized multilevel Rasch model.

	Baseline		1st follow-up		2nd follow-up		Random effect	
	(T = 1)		(T = 2)		(T = 3)		Patient	Symptom
	Estimates of the regression parameters ζ_t of time (T)							
	Est.	s.e.	Est.	s.e.	Est.	s.e	SD	SD
Model 0 (empty)	−0.33	0.28	−2.23	0.29	−2.13	0.29	0.968	0.688
Model 1 (seperate time points)	−0.48	0.24	−2.22	0.24	−2.09	0.24	0.993	0.559
Model 2 (forward inclusion)	−0.57	0.30	−2.25	0.30	−2.14	0.30	1.000	0.712
Model 3 (simulated annealing)	1.10	0.36	−2.05	0.27	−1.87	0.27	0.998	0.624
Model 4 (restricted simulated annealing)	−1.05	0.28	−1.93	0.25	−1.90	0.20	0.997	0.414
Model adjusted for gender, age and living alone	−0.28	0.29	−2.17	0,29	−2,08	0,30	0,946	0,687
	Estimates of the regression parameters ζ_t^S of SHR-time interaction (SRH*T)							
	Est.	s.e.	Est.	s.e.	Est.	s.e	SD	SD
Model 0 (empty)	0.48	0.07	1.44	0.10	1.21	0.13	0.881	0.692
Model 1 (seperate time points)	0.47	0.07	1.45	0.10	1.20	0.13	0.906	0.564
Model 2 (forward inclusion)	0.48	0.07	1.46	0.10	1.23	0.14	0.911	0.740
Model 3 (simulated annealing)	0.49	0.07	1.46	0.10	1.24	0.14	0.911	0.649
Model 4 (restricted simulated annealing)	0.48	0.07	1.47	0.10	1.23	0.14	0.910	0.445
Model adjusted for gender, age and living alone	0.48	0.07	1.45	0.10	1.19	0.13	0.864	0.693

Table 14.2. *Estimates of the model parameters for time (T) and the SRH-time interaction (SRH*T) in the models resulting from the five model search methods, and additionally for a model where there is gender for adjustment, age and living alone (at baseline) in the usual manner of multivariable regression models*

14.4. Simulation study

To illustrate the dependence of the estimates of the model parameters in the presence of certain specific violations of the Rasch model – DIF and LD – we conduct a simulation study. Specifically, we simulate data with increasing magnitude of DIF and/or LD effects and estimate the model parameters ζ_t of the time variables and the parameters ζ_t^s of the relationship between symptom burden and SRH in a model where we do not allow for DIF and LD, that is, in the empty model

(Model 0), presented in equation [14.6]. We then investigate whether these estimates are biased, differ structurally from the values the data were simulated with, and whether inference becomes inefficient, whether the variance increases. In addition, we investigate whether the heterogeneity, the variance σ_{ε}^2 of the person random effect, changes when DIF and LD are erroneously omitted from the model.

For each simulation we simulate SRH data for $n = 1{,}000$ patients through random sampling from a binary distribution with probability $p = 0.5$, and subsequently binary item data for three time points from the model

$$\eta_{vit} = \zeta_t T_{vit} + \zeta_t^s \text{SRH}_{vit} T_{vit} + \varepsilon_v + \beta_i + \zeta_{12t}^{\text{LD}} W_{v12t} + \zeta_{3t}^{\text{DIF}} W_{v3t} \quad [14.13]$$

where the parameters ζ_t are chosen $\zeta_1 = -0.3$, $\zeta_2 = -2.2$ and $\zeta_3 = -2.1$ and the parameters ζ_t^s are chosen $\zeta_1^s = 0.5$, $\zeta_2^s = 1.4$ and $\zeta_3^s = 1.2$. The item parameters β_i of the six binary symptom items are chosen $\beta_1 = -0.5$, $\beta_2 = -0.5$, $\beta_3 = -0.5$, $\beta_4 = 0.5$, $\beta_5 = 0.5$ and $\beta_6 = 1$, implying a standard deviation of the symptom random effect of $\sigma_\beta = 0.69$. The standard deviation of the patient random effect is chosen $\sigma_\epsilon = 0.88$ and the 1,000 effects ε_v are drawn randomly from a Gaussian distribution with mean zero and with the indicated standard deviation. The choices for these parameters reflect approximately the estimates in the DCGP data as shown in Table 14.2, so that we can think of the simulations in terms of the relationship between symptom burden and SRH over the natural course of diabetes. In model [14.13] there are three parameters ζ_{12t}^{LD} (one for each time point) included for an LD between symptoms one and two, and three parameters ζ_{3t}^{DIF} for a DIF between symptom three and a binary (baseline) covariate Z_v that is simulated through random draws from a binary distribution with probability $p = 0.5$ Each of the four following simulation studies now comprises three scenarios where the magnitude c of the DIF and/or LD effect is increased from zero to two in 20 steps (of magnitude 0.1):

– Scenario I (only LD): $\zeta_{12t}^{\text{LD}} = c, \ \forall t$.

– Scenario II (only DIF): $\zeta_{3t}^{\text{DIF}} = c, \ \forall t$.

– Scenario III (LD and DIF): $\zeta_{12t}^{\text{LD}} = \zeta_{3t}^{\text{DIF}} = c, \ \forall t$.

Hence, in Scenario I there is only LD, in Scenario II only DIF and in Scenario III both DIF and LD; these effects are of equal magnitude for the three time points. Each simulation study is then based on $21 \times 3 = 63$ simulations.

– *Simulation study 1 (parameters ζ_t of the time variable)*: The first simulation study illustrates that we cannot ignore LD or DIF for the estimation of the parameters ζ_t pertaining to the time variable. Figure 14.3 shows that the parameter estimates are biased, arguably most when both DIF and LD are present. This is not unexpected, since we have seen this happen in Table 14.2 and we argued in section 14.2.3 that this is because these parameters mean something else when DIF and LD are introduced to the data. Possibly also the heterogeneity between the patients is seen to increase slightly.

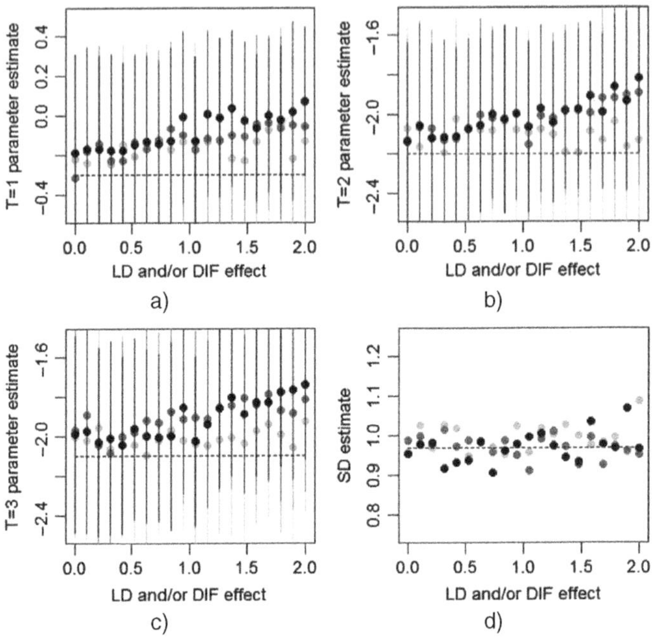

Figure 14.3. *Simulation study 1, estimates of ζ_t: Scenario I (only LD): light, Scenario II (only DIF): middle, Scenario III (LD and DIF): dark.*

– *Simulation study 2 (parameters ζ_t^s of the SRH variable)*: The second simulation study is essentially the same as the first simulation study except that now the parameters ζ_t^s pertaining to the relationship between symptom burden and SRH are estimated. The simulation results in Figure 14.4 show what already was suspected that these parameters are estimated unbiased even when DIF and LD effects are ignored. Also the efficiency of the estimation – the width of the confidence intervals – and the heterogeneity between the patients seem unaffected by the omission of DIF and LD terms in the model.

– *Simulation study 3 (parameters ζ_t^s of the SRH variable with covariate correlated to SRH)*: In the previous simulation study, the binary covariate Z_v was simulated independently from SRH – or any of the other variables in the model. Hence, the fact that, presumably, the covariate is balanced between the SRH categories may in itself cause the DIF effect to be balanced between SRH categories and thereby make possible biases cancel out when the difference between SRH categories is examined. In the third simulation study, a dependence between the binary covariate Z_v was induced by first generating Z_v as before and thereafter SRH_v through

$P(\mathrm{SRH}_v = 1) = \mathrm{logit}(2Z_v - 1)$; the marginal distribution of SRH stays the same. Figure 14.5 shows that indeed, when the covariate for which there is DIF is also associated with SRH, ignoring this DIF leads to biased parameters ζ_t^s; ignoring LD gives – as before – unbiased estimates. In general, we cannot ignore DIF.

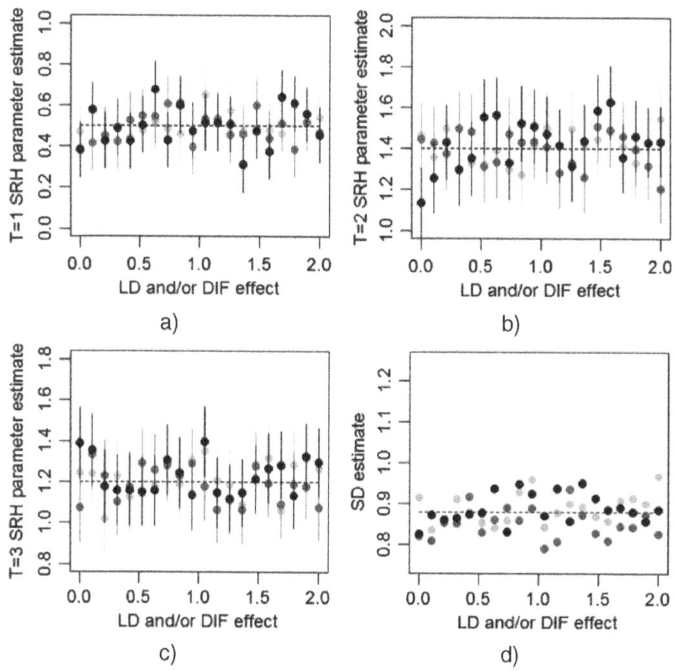

Figure 14.4. *Simulation study 2, estimates of ζ_t^s: Scenario I (only LD): light, Scenario II (only DIF): middle, Scenario III (LD and DIF): dark*

– *Simulation study 4 (parameters ζ_t^s of the SRH variable adjusting for a covariate correlated to SRH)*: Can we remove the bias in the estimates of the parameters ζ_t^s seen in the third simulation study without specifically modeling the DIF effect? In this last simulation study, we attempt to do this by simply adding the covariate Z to the linear term in equation [14.6] as if we were adjusting for a known confounder; the data are simulated as in the third simulation study. Figure 14.6 shows that this seems to remove the bias due to the DIF effect as shown in Figure 14.5. This is good news since the variables that are typically investigated for DIF are also the variables that are typically adjusted for in analyses on cohort data of the type we have in the DCGP study, for example gender and age.

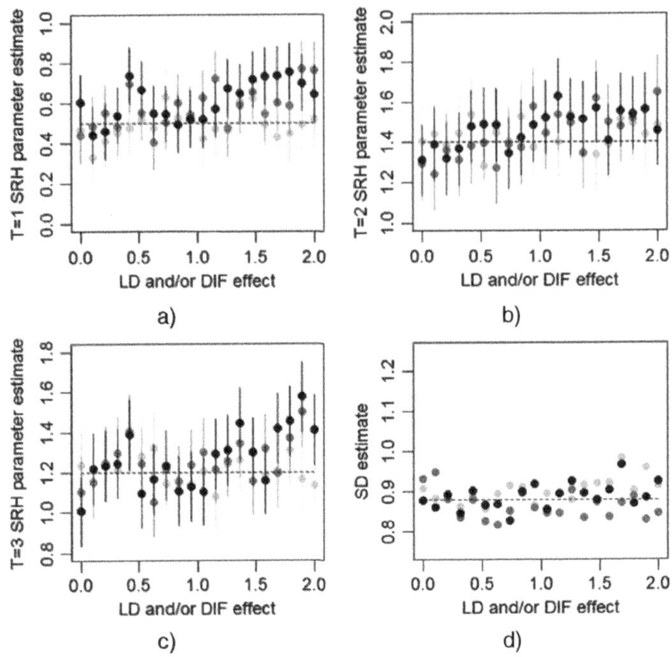

Figure 14.5. *Simulation study 3, estimates of ζ_t^s: Scenario I (only LD): light, Scenario II (only DIF): middle, Scenario III (LD and DIF): dark*

14.5. Discussion

The results from the various model search heuristics in Table 14.2, and the ensuing simulation study, seem to indicate that for adequate analyses of the parameters that are of primary importance for our research question, ζ_t^s, the presence of LD or DIF may be largely ignored. This then implies that we do not have to venture into a time-consuming process of identifying LD and DIF effects, with no guarantee that some "true" configuration of such effects is found. We only should adjust our analysis for enough covariates so that any bias because of DIF effects is gobbled up by these adjustments, but such adjustments are often demanded already by epidemiology so as to correct for possible confounding. Such analysis is performed alongside the analyses in the models based on model search heuristics in Table 14.2. Indeed, the results for the parameters that indicate the relationship between SRH and symptom burden are very similar to the results for the other models; the results for the time parameters are different from the other models. Hence, the conclusion from the above has to be that *ad hoc* scales may well be analyzed in a multilevel Rasch model of the type as in equation [14.6] without too much thought about violations of the assumptions of the Rasch model such as uniform LD and/or uniform DIF.

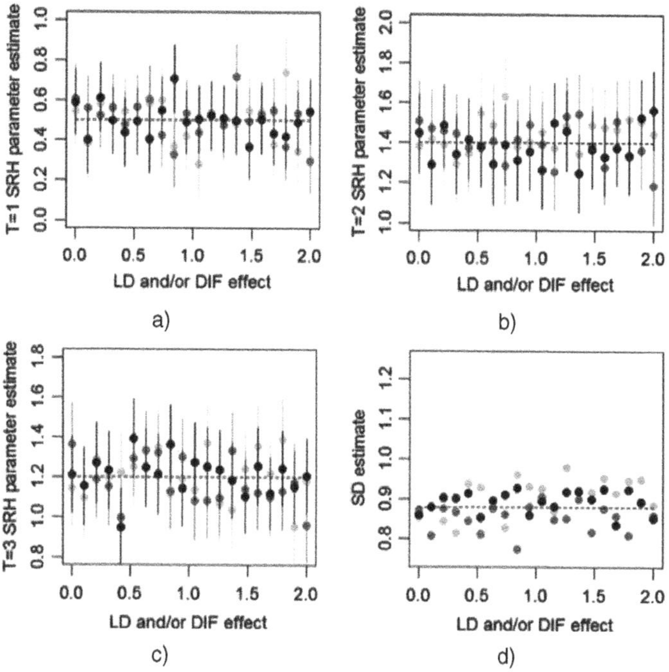

Figure 14.6. *Simulation study 4: Scenario I (only LD): light; Scenario II (only DIF): middle; and Scenario III (LD and DIF): dark*

Can we understand why the analysis is so insensitive to the presence of LD and DIF? In [14.9] and [14.12] we argue that for a given person v, item i, time point t and any given values for the dummy variables representing LD and DIF effects, the parameters ζ_t^s pertaining to the relationship between symptom burden and SRH are just the differences [14.14] of the probabilities (on logit scale) of a positive indication on a symptom between the two SRH indications:

$$\zeta_t^s = \eta_{vit}|_{\text{SRH}=1} - \eta_{vit}|_{\text{SRH}=0} \qquad [14.14]$$

Then, the parameters ζ_t^s are not only interpreted as the average differences as argued in section 2.3, but can also be adequately estimated as such. In the presence of DIF for a certain covariate Z, we estimate the probabilities by averaging the binary item indicators within the classes of SRH and Z, calculate the logit values of these, calculate the differences of these within each category of Z and construct the weighted average of these differences. But this is – roughly, because we ignore the random effects – how these parameters are estimated in a model that ignores DIF, but adjusts for the covariate in the fashion of a multivariate regression model, just as we propose. Why then do we not have to somehow adjust for some kind of item covariate in the presence of LD? And why do we not have to adjust for a covariate for which there is DIF when this variable is independent of SRH? As can be seen from [14.8] and [14.11], we envision DIF and LD effects that, in the presence of a positive indication for the covariate or the other item, respectively changes the logit η_{vit} of the probability for a positive answer on item i with a constant value; and DIF and LD effects of such type are used in the simulation studies. If this is indeed the case, taking the overall average of the binary item indicators will bias the estimate of the logit, but, since the DIF or LD effect does not depend on SRH, this bias is in the same direction and of the same magnitude for SRH $=1$ and SRH $=0$. Hence, the bias cancels out in the difference [14.14].

The optimistic account in this discussion so far demands some footnotes, some of them will have been seen coming by the attentive reader. First, the DIF and LD effects presented in section 2.3, the additions to the generalized multilevel Rasch model that repair these effects, and the argument that we often may ignore these effects, all assume a type of effect that shifts the logit values with a constant. The argument fails if the DIF and LD effects are not of this type, for example they assume a constant shift in the probabilities, or the shift depends on a third covariate (tentatively correlated to SRH). However, also the model elements presented in section 14.2.3 that aim to repair LD and DIF cannot immediately deal with such alternative formulations. Of course, we could introduce more dummy variables that deal with some other specific situations, but that would increase the search space for model search heuristics considerably, and thereby the convergence time and possibly the quality of the solution, and even then we could easily find situations not covered by the model. However, we feel confident that in many cases the assumed types of uniform DIF and LD are enough to adjust for the majority of instances of violations of the assumptions of the Rasch model. Second, items and covariates may be dependent between time points that may undermine the interpretations of the parameters ζ_t^s as indicating a development over time; for example, some of the differences may be because a positive indication of a certain item at a certain time point is correlated to a positive indication of the same item at another time point beyond what may be expected from the general development of the construct. This is not investigated in the present study. Third, and possibly most serious, is the possible presence of DIF with regard to SRH, the variable of interest. Certainly here we cannot ignore DIF as we proposed since we cannot adjust for SRH in an analysis where SRH is the variable of interest. However, we can for specific items construct the dummy variable [14.7] with SRH in the role of Z and in this way adjust for DIF. While this may affect the interpretation of the parameters ζ_t^s, the investigation of DIF with respect to SRH is certainly something that is advisable to do; if only to be able to conclude that there is no DIF connected to SRH and we do not have to worry about it.

We then conclude that it is often possible to use *ad hoc* scales based on binary items, provided the correct research questions are investigated, and some minimal precautions are observed, for example adjusting one's analysis for variables that may be involved in DIF effects. This is done in a multilevel Rasch model that now does not necessarily have to be generalized to incorporate violations to the Rasch model; only adjustments for confounding multivariable regression style. Beyond being a vehicle of inference in the present case, the multilevel Rasch model inherits many advantages from general mixed models. For example, Bayesian analysis is natural to implement for this class of models, and missing data due to dropout is dealt with in an appropriate way [VER 00].

14.6. Bibliography

[ADA 97] Adams R.J., Wilson M., Wu M., "Multilevel item response models: an approach to errors in variable regression", *Journal of Educational and Behavioral Statistics*, vol. 22, pp. 47–76, 1997.

[BON 01] Bond T.G., Fox C.M., *Applying the Rasch Model: Fundamental Measurement in the Human Sciences*, Lawrence Erlbaum Associates, Inc., Mahwah, NJ, 2001.

[BUR 98] Burnham K.P., Anderson D.R., *Model Selection and Inference: A Practical Information-Theoretic Approach*, Springer-Verlag, New York, NY, 1998.

[DEB 04] De Boeck P., Wilson M., *Explanatory Item Response Models: A Generalized Linear and Nonlinear Approach*, Springer, New York, NY, 2004.

[DOR 07] Doran H., Bates D., Bliese P., Dowling M., "Estimating the multilevel rash model: with the lme4 package", *Journal of Statistical Software*, vol. 20, pp. 1–18, 2007.

[FIS 95] Fischer G.H., Molenaar I.W., *Rasch Models: Foundations, Recent Developments and Applications*, Springer-Verlag, New York, NY, 1995.

[HOL 93] Holland P.W., Wainer H., *Differential Item Functioning*, Lawrence Erlbaum Associates, Hillsdale, NJ, 1993.

[KIR 83] Kirkpatrick S., Gelatt C.D., Vecchi M.P., "Optimization by Simulated Annealing", *Science*, vol. 220, pp. 671–680, 1983.

[KRE 03] Kreiner S., Introduction to Digram, Department of Biostatistics Research Report 03/10, University of Copenhagen, 2003.

[KRE 11] Kreiner S., Christensen K.B., "Item screening in graphical loglinear Rasch models", *Psychometrika*, vol. 76, pp. 228–256, 2011.

[NIE 11] Nielsen A.B.S., Gannik D., Siersma V., Olivarius N.F., "The relationship between HbA1c level, symptoms and self-rated health in type 2 diabetic patients", *Scandinavian Journal of Primary Health Care*, vol. 29, pp. 157–164, 2011.

[OLI 01] Olivarius N.F., Beck-Nielsen H., Andreasen A.H., Hørder M., Pedersen P.A., "Randomised controlled trial of structured personal care of type 2 diabetes mellitus", *British Medical Journal*, vol. 323, pp. 970–975, 2001.

[RAS 60] Rasch G., *Probabilistic Models for Some Intelligence and Attainment Tests*, Danish National Institute for Educational Research, Copenhagen, 1960.

[VER 00] Verbeke G., Molenberghs G., *Linear Mixed Models for Longitudinal Data*, Springer-Verlag, Berlin, 2000.

PART 5

Creating, Translating and Improving Rasch Scales

Introduction

In the previous parts of this book, we have described the Rasch model, the way of estimating its parameters, the way of validating the fit of a data set to the model, applications, and the way of creating and improving Rasch scales. Some of the topics covered are quite technical. This part describes more practical subjects, namely how to analyze responses to a set of items using the Rasch model and how to report the results of those analyses.

Chapter 15

Writing Health-Related Items for Rasch Models – Patient-Reported Outcome Scales for Health Sciences: From Medical Paternalism to Patient Autonomy

One must always respect the autonomy of the patient. The patient's views and priorities must always be paramount.

Parmenter, 1994 [PAR 94]

15.1. Introduction

Advances in medical technology and improvements in public health have eradicated, or reduced the significance of, many life-threatening infectious diseases in the developed world. Western health care systems are now increasingly concerned with the treatment of chronic, disabling conditions associated with an aging population. Furthermore, the past 30 years have seen a significant change in perceptions of illness within the medical sector. The move toward a biopsychosocial model of illness has led to an increased awareness of the importance of the views of the patient. Patients' perceptions of the impact of illness and treatment effectiveness are being given greater consideration, as it is recognized that they have an ultimate responsibility for major decisions taken in relation with their health. Within general medicine, the clinical interview remains the predominant means by which the clinician

Chapter written by John BRODERSEN, Lynda C. DOWARD, Hanne THORSEN and Stephen P. MCKENNA.

gathers information from the patient. However, the medical sector is increasingly demanding standardized tools to collect data from patients as an adjunct or aid to the clinical interview. The purpose of this chapter is to outline the value of patient-reported outcome (PRO) questionnaires to our understanding of the impact of disease and to describe the nature and development of such PROs. The chapter also considers the generation of questionnaire items for PRO's.

15.1.1. *The emergence of the biopsychosocial model of illness*

Despite the World Health Organization (WHO)'s 1947 declaration that health is "...a state of complete physical, mental and social well-being and not merely the absence of disease or infirmity" [WHO 47, WHO 48], illness paradigms have focused predominantly on the biomedical model of health until relatively recently. Under the biomedical model, the individual was regarded as a passive participant living or dying at the mercy of their biological hereditary material. However, by the 1970s, researchers presented increasingly convincing evidence that a person's state of health does not depend solely on his or her genetic makeup. Evidence was also emerging of the importance of environmental factors in explaining both illness and lifespan. These environmental factors related both to environmental factors affecting the development of the fetus in the womb and those affecting the development and lifestyle during childhood, youth and adulthood. In the late 1970s and early 1980s, George Engel proposed that health professionals should expand their view of illness from the monocausal, static and reductionist biomedical model of illness and adopt a dynamic biopsychosocial model [ENG 77, ENG 80]. Unlike the biomedical model, the biopsychosocial model considers individuals to be active participants in their health, who are both influenced by their environment and, in turn, influence their surroundings [IVE 02]. Clearly, the model is of less significance in the face of natural disasters, famine, war and similar catastrophes. However, for countries adopting a "Western" lifestyle, the interaction between the individuals and their surroundings is decisive for their state of health. Here, the individual's genetic predisposition, psychological state and social interactions are the decisive factors that jointly influence that individual's state of health. Research conducted over the past three decades has confirmed Engel's hypotheses that health is not solely biologically determined but results from the interplay of many factors.

The biopsychosocial model has increasingly influenced the way medical science views illness. This has resulted in numerous research projects seeking to illuminate and explain the causal connections between different variables, domains and concepts that affect our health. A prominent area of biopsychosocial research has been the investigation of links between the individuals' self-rated health and their future morbidity and mortality. Indeed, a global question on self-assessed illness has been shown to be a strong predictor of mortality [COA 97].

Similarly, epidemiological studies have confirmed strong correlations between sociodemographic parameters (educational level, income and employment status) and morbidity and mortality [IDL 97]. Lower levels of these sociodemographic parameters are clearly associated with greater morbidity and mortality [DIE 97, SMI 97, SMI 98, BOS 01, PIC 01].

15.1.2. *Changes in the consultation process in general medicine*

An evidence-based foundation for Engel's biopsychosocial model has been established over the past 30 years using research methods borrowed from across a spectrum of academic disciplines including the natural and social sciences and humanities. Arguments have been presented against the relegation of the subjective components of the clinical interview (specifically introspection on the part of the clinician and dialogue between clinician and patient) to a non-scientific status [ENG 90]. It is now generally recognized that the utilization of health services is more closely linked to the way people *feel* about their clinical condition than to the objective presence of symptoms or functional limitations [HUN 92a, CEL 94]. It has been pointed out that two patients sharing identical clinical criteria can have dramatically different responses to their condition [GUY 93]. Thus, whether or not individuals seek medical attention is less dependent on the "objective" presence of symptoms than on their response to these or to their general perception that something is faulty.

As a result, the past 30 years have seen a paradigm shift in the way doctors view their patients. It is no longer considered acceptable for medicine to operate a "beneficence model" of health care, with the assumption that health professionals are best placed to determine what promotes or protects the best interests of the patient [PAR 94]. Clearly, few clinicians today would support Morgan's assertion that "the subject's own opinion of his condition is not to be relied upon" [MOR 34]. Instead, the paternalistic physician role has been replaced by a more dialogue-oriented approach in which primacy is given to the patient's autonomy.

This trend is clearly seen in McWinney's patient-centered communication model [MCW 97], which has been developed further in a Danish setting by three general practitioners (GPs); Ole Risør, Jan-Helge Larsen and Klaus Witt [ØST 07]. Here, the consultation process is described as a communication between patient and doctor, and is divided into three phases. In the first phase, the GP's task is to listen actively and pose open questions designed to help patients tell their narrative in their own words. This allows the clinician to uncover a patient's view of his or her illness, associated fears and expectations of the consultation. The second phase is initiated by the doctor and represents a summary of what he has heard and obtaining further details about the case history through elucidatory diagnostic questions. This may lead to a clinical examination of the patient. The third phase begins with the doctor providing the patient with an explanation of his or her symptoms on the basis of the narrative, the findings from the clinical examination and the doctor's assessment. The doctor will include convergences and divergences between the patient's and the doctor's views of illness. The doctor's assessment will take note of the patient's fears and expectations and help put these into perspective. The consultation should end with a safety net, in which the doctor checks that the patient has understood the treatment plan, if there is one, and that the patient knows what to do if things do not go as expected. The three phases can be seen as the patient's phase, the doctor's phase and a joint phase. This model ensures that the focus is on the patient throughout and that the doctor continuously checks that both (s)he and the patient understand one another and agree on the decisions that are made.

It can be seen that there has been a radical change in medical culture from the doctor's paternalism toward the patient's autonomy. At the same time, there has been a change away from a monocausal, static, reductionist biomedical way of thinking about the occurrence, worsening, alleviation, treatment, prognosis and possibly healing of disease toward a more dynamic, interactive, holistic and complex biopsychosocial model. There has been a clear recognition that successful treatment depends on the education and the kind of life patients have, the resources available to them and the life stresses to which they are subjected. The treatment of a person who is ill cannot be separated from that person's life situation.

15.2. The use of patient-reported outcome questionnaires

As a result of this paradigm shift, it is necessary to identify new ways of determining what is important to the patients about their illness, its impact on their life and whether they believe that they have been benefitted from prescribed medical interventions. This information is increasingly captured using PRO questionnaires. PRO is an umbrella term that covers a whole range of potential measurement outcomes but is used specifically to refer to those collected directly from the patient, without interpretation by clinicians or others [DOW 04]. Thus, PROs are a means of gathering patient rather than clinical or other views on the content covered by the questionnaire.

PRO data are collected via standardized questionnaires designed to measure an explicit underlying characteristic. These measurement "characteristics" are called *constructs* and the questionnaires used to collect them are called *instruments, measures, scales or tools*. Although these terms are often used interchangeably, they all refer to a questionnaire designed to assess an underlying construct. A questionnaire that measures a single construct is called *unidimensional*. Items (questions) in a unidimensional questionnaire can be added to provide a single-scale score. However, it cannot be assumed that a questionnaire is unidimensional simply because the author intended it to be so. This must be demonstrated mathematically. A questionnaire that measures multiple different constructs is called *multidimensional*. A multidimensional questionnaire is used to provide a profile of scores; that is, each scale is scored and reported separately. It is not appropriate to produce an overall single summary score for a multidimensional questionnaire (akin to adding apples and pears together). Each scale (dimension) within a multidimensional questionnaire should have been shown by the authors to be unidimensional.

Within the medical sector, PROs may be used to cast light on and measure the views and experiences of patients and the general population with respect to biopsychosocial aspects of their contact with the health care system (e.g. in relation to preventive initiatives, diagnosis and treatment of diseases). Thus, PROs may be used to glean an insight into the state of health of individuals and/or patients. PRO questionnaires can be of importance in research studies ranging from, for example, the identification of patients' medical morbidity (including physical and psychiatric problems) or the quantification of patients' quality of life (QoL), health-related quality of life (HRQL) or functional status. PROs do not necessarily assess constructs that are of importance to the patient – they may collect information that is required by the doctor or health services.

15.2.1. *Defining PRO constructs*

In selecting a PRO instrument for use in a study, it is essential to be clear about the nature of the constructs addressed. This will ensure that the most appropriate tool is selected to measure the outcome of interest. It should be noted that the title of the instrument can sometimes be misleading as there has been a tendency in the past for instrument developers to refer to any questionnaire as a measure of QoL, irrespective of the constructs actually assessed. The most common PRO constructs used in clinical studies are measures of:

- impairment (symptoms);
- activity limitations (functioning);
- participation restrictions;
- health status/HRQL;
- quality of life;
- treatment satisfaction.

These are described in more detail below.

15.2.1.1. *Measures of impairment, activity limitations and participation restrictions*

The constructs of impairments (symptoms), activity (limitations) and participation (restrictions) are clearly defined in the International Classification of Functioning, Disability and Health [WHO 01, ICF] and are widely accepted.

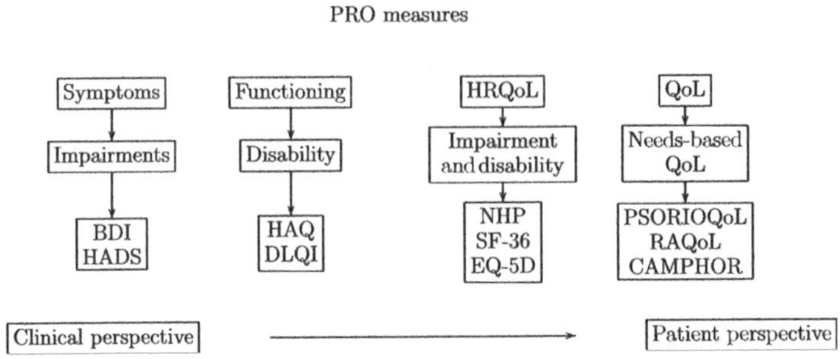

Figure 15.1. *PRO measures different constructs in clinical studies: clinical versus patient perspective*

Impairment is defined as any loss or abnormality of psychological, physiological or anatomical structure or function and largely equates to symptoms and signs. This outcome relates to disturbances at the level of the organ, and examples include anxiety, depression, pain and sleep disorder. Impairment is seen as representing some deviation from the norm in the individual's biomedical status. Measures that assess impairments tend to address the presence, severity or frequency of symptoms rather than the patient's reactions or responses to these elements. It should be noted that even where the patient is aware of impairment, it may not be of any particular concern to them.

Activity limitations are defined as any restriction or lack of ability to perform activities in the manner or within the range that is considered normal. Examples include problems with dressing, walking or personal care. Again, disability is seen as being a deviation from the norm and there is no need for an individual to consider this deviation a limitation. Activity limitations equate to what is often called *disability* or *functional status* – constructs that play a major part in the assessment of HRQL (see below). Thus, instruments that assess the impact of disease or its treatment at this level typically assess the construct of activity. The assessment of activity is essential where the objective of a study is to assess activities of daily living (ADL).

Participation is defined as a person's involvement in life situations and participation restrictions are problems that prevent an individual from involvement in life situations. The construct of participation is closely related to that of activity but differs from it insofar as it emphasizes the extent to which a person is able to take part in areas of life, regardless of the extent to which his or her ability to perform activities is limited. Again, the construct does not inform on the patient's response to such problems.

The constructs of activity and participation are of importance in determining and planning interventions and rehabilitation services or the need for provision of social services such as housing and social security. Similarly, it is an essential outcome to assess in studies of interventions intended to improve patients' participation in life.

15.2.1.2. *Health status/health-related quality of life*

Health status and HRQL, as defined by different authors, equate primarily to impairment and activity. HRQL instruments assess a combination of aspects of impairment and/or activity and (less often) participation. HRQL has been defined as the capacity to perform the usual daily activities for a person's age and major social role [PAT 71]. Thus, deviation from normality results in a reduced HRQL [PAT 93]. There is a general agreement that HRQL is multidimensional. Although there is no consensus on the constructs that should be assessed, it is common for researchers to include domains such as physical functioning, psychological well-being, social interactions and activities of daily living.

The main value of HRQL measurement lies in the assessment of health status, levels of impairment and activity limitation. Such information is valuable for clinical assessment of outcome. However, the focus on fulfillment of "normal" roles creates problems in that groups, such as the unemployed and disabled are automatically devalued. The emphasis on physical functioning found in HRQL instruments determines that disabled people cannot have a good "QoL"; this is a notion that is not borne out by experience.

15.2.1.2.1. Quality of life

Clear distinctions have been made between HRQL and QoL. The needs-based QoL model designed by Hunt and McKenna in 1992 goes beyond impairment and designed by asking about the patient's ability to fulfil their needs. It is important to note that HRQL is only one of the influences on QoL. Several authors have discussed the nature of the QoL construct but the needs-based model is the most widely applied in instrument development. The theory underlying this approach is that individuals are driven or motivated by their needs and the fulfillment of these needs provides satisfaction. Thus, functions are only important insofar as they allow needs to be fulfilled. From this, the needs-based model of QoL states that life derives its quality from the ability and capacity of the individual to satisfy certain human needs. QoL is good when most of the needs are fulfilled and poor when a few needs are satisfied.

Rather than relying on the literature or experts to determine those needs that are important to patients, the content of instruments measuring needs-based QoL is derived from qualitative interviews conducted with relevant patients. In this way, the needs that are relevant to the patients will be identified. This maximizes the instruments' content validity and ability to detect the change. The needs-based model has been used in the development of over 30 disease-specific QoL instruments (see e.g. [MCK 92, WHA 97, MCK 03, DOW 03, KEE 08]. The main value of needs-based QoL measures is that they provide information on the impact of disease and its treatment that is known to be of importance to the patient, rather than that which is of interest to professionals.

15.2.1.2.2. Treatment satisfaction

The construct of treatment satisfaction has become increasingly popular as a study outcome. Satisfaction with treatment affects a variety of health outcomes, including compliance, treatment success and continued use of health services. However, there is currently no consensus on how best to measure treatment satisfaction and no adequate definition of what "satisfaction" means.

The term "Satisfaction" is taken from the Latin word for "enough" – something that satisfies sufficiently, fulfills expectations, requirements or needs, and leaves no reason for complaint. Satisfaction with a treatment or service does not imply superior quality; rather it implies that an adequate or sufficient standard has been achieved. However, true satisfaction can only be assessed accurately by taking into account an individual's prior expectations, requirements or needs. A treatment that leaves one individual satisfied may leave another (with higher or different expectations) dissatisfied.

Several researchers have commented on the importance of clarifying the difference between satisfaction measures since the conclusions drawn about satisfaction are dependent on the characteristics of the measures used. Most authors agree that treatment satisfaction incorporates patient's satisfaction into the direct experience of a particular treatment (rather than attitudes to treatment) and include items about efficacy and side effects. However, others argue that distinctions should be made between "satisfaction with medication" and "satisfaction with treatment". These suggest that satisfaction with treatment encompasses the whole treatment experience (i.e. including issues of doctor–patient interaction, mode of administration or other therapies such as rehabilitation), whereas satisfaction with medication focuses on the issues surrounding a specific medication.

15.2.1.3. *Generic and specific questionnaires*

PROs may be either generic or specific. The generic PROs are designed to capture and quantify one or more general health-related constructs and to be, as their name suggests, suitable for use in any disease population or with populations made up of patients with different conditions. In contrast, specific questionnaires are designed for use with a well-defined population such as individuals with the same problem and disease. Most medical questionnaire studies use generic questionnaires.

15.2.1.3.1. Generic questionnaires

Generic instruments are designed to be used in any disease population and they cover a broad aspect of the construct measured. Some of the more widely known health status or HRQoL instruments are generic. Examples include the Sickness Impact Profile (SIP) [BER 76], the Nottingham Health Profile [EUR 93, NHP], the Short Form 36 [WAR 92, SF-36], Psychological General Well-Being Index [HUN 92b, PGWBI] and the EuroQoL [RAB 01, EQ-5D]. Such instruments usually assess several domains and provide a profile of scores. Advocates of generic questionnaires cite several key advantages for these scales. As they are widely used, they are regarded as having recognized and well-established validity. The widely used measures are reported to address important health-related aspects of patient's lives. Finally, they are promoted as a means of comparing the impact of interventions and diseases or to compare data to population normative values. However, such claims are now widely disputed. The use of generic questionnaires for cross-disease comparisons is scientifically flawed because questionnaire items work in different ways with different patient groups. Furthermore, a number of studies show that the validity of such scales is not consistent when we "move" a generic questionnaire from one population to another [HOB 02, BAR 06, HAG 08, COM 08, TWI 12]. Furthermore, generic instruments are not designed to capture the areas of concern to particular patient populations. In addition, they are likely to enquire about issues that are irrelevant for certain patient groups. Consequently, they are seen as less relevant by patient groups. For example, questions that address physical functioning or physical pain will only be relevant if these are a feature of the disease under study. Asking patients to answer questions that are irrelevant is likely to alienate respondents and increase the potential for missing data. This becomes, in particular, problematic in relation to the patients who are most ill [HAG 09].

A further consideration is the age of the content of the commonly used generic instruments. The most widely used instruments (the SIP, SF-36 and NHP) were developed over the past 30 years. Indeed, the SF-36 incorporates content derived from questionnaires that are over 50 years old [DOW 97]. However, the way in which patients conceptualize their problems and the terms through which they express themselves can change in a generation. Moreover, certain issues may become less important with time. For example, the lack of mobility may be compensated by advances in technology. Furthermore, these generic instruments have not benefited from modern improvements in test construction methodology and scaling techniques. Consequently, their reliability and responsiveness fall far short of that required for sensitive instruments suitable for use in clinical studies and trials.

The many pitfalls associated with the use of generic questionnaires have led to an increased use of specific measures.

15.2.1.3.2. Specific questionnaires

Condition and disease-specific PRO instruments are developed to measure those aspects of outcome that are of importance for a particular population. The primary advantage of specific instruments is that they provide more detailed information than generic instruments and are likely to be more sensitive to disease- or treatment-specific effects [WIE 03]. Specific questionnaires are better able to capture the relevant areas that the particular group of respondents experience in connection with illness or other significant events. This makes it possible to measure at a more refined level whether there is, for example, difference between alternative interventions. Addressing the specific concerns of a particular patient group also maximizes respondent acceptability and minimizes the potential for missing data. New approaches to instrument development incorporating item response theory allow the co-calibration of disease-specific diseases that are based on the same measurement model (such as the needs-based model and the biopsychosocial model). This overcomes the apparent disadvantage of specific questionnaires, that is they cannot be used to compare the impacts of different diseases.

Evidence clearly shows that specific questionnaires are the most valuable tools for gathering patient's views in the medical sector. This change from generic to more sensitive and specific outcome measures has led to an increase in the number of publications on the development and validation of disease-specific or condition-specific questionnaires in the past 10–15 years.

15.2.2. *Quality requirements for PRO questionnaires*

There are a number of requirements that any instrument intended to collect information from patients should meet if the data collected are to be meaningful and allow for valid inferences [DOW 03]. Quality standards relate to both the development and testing of instruments. This has recently been confirmed by the Food and Drug Administration (FDA) and European Medicines Agency (EMEA) in their development of scientific guidelines for PRO standards [EUR 05, FOO 06].

15.2.2.1. *Instrument development standards*

15.2.2.1.1. Theoretical basis

Any PRO instrument must be based on a stated model or theory of the construct being measured. It should be noted that this requirement is sometimes neglected in the development of PRO measures. This raises two, related, problems. First, unless instrument developers provide an explicit definition of the construct assessed, it is not possible to determine whether their definition is reasonable. Second, without such information, it is not possible to establish that an instrument has face, content, and construct validity.

15.2.2.1.2. Derivation of content

The content of any instrument should be derived from the most appropriate source, both in terms of the coverage of the measure and the actual wording of items used to elicit patient responses. For example, measures of symptoms (impairments) may be derived from patients but clinical input is also important. However, clinical expertise is not required for deriving the content of QoL measures; it should be derived directly from the relevant patients. This applies both to the areas included in the instrument and (as far as possible) to the actual wording of the items. The content of an instrument should also be appropriate to the culture and lifestyle of the countries in which it will be used. Instruments developed in a single country reflect the language and culture of that particular society, which may cause problems when adapting the measure into other languages. Deriving the content from relevant sources in different countries maximizes the cultural relevance of the measure (see Chapter 16).

15.2.2.1.3. Practicality

Instruments must be practical to administer in the clinical setting and easy to complete. For self-administered instruments, complex response systems must be avoided. Interviewer-based assessments should include clear instructions for the interviewer to maximize the standardization of administration. Wherever possible, patient-completed measures should be selected over interviewer-administered tools in order to avoid interviewer bias.

15.2.2.1.4. Acceptability to respondents

The content of any patient-completed instrument must be perceived as relevant by the respondents. One of the major disadvantages of many generic health status instruments is that they include items that do not apply to many specific health problems. By deriving the content of the instrument from relevant sources, problems of non-applicability are avoided and face and content validity are maximized.

15.2.2.2. *Psychometric and scaling standards*

Evidence should be available to demonstrate that scales are reliable, and they represent what they are intended to measure and are capable of detecting clinically meaningful change [HOB 01, HOB 03]. Such properties cannot be assumed but must be empirically established.

15.2.2.2.1. Unidimensionality

Any scale from which a summary (total) score is produced must be unidimensional and invariant if it is to provide valid change scores. This applies to both single-scale instruments and to individual scales within multidimensional instruments. Item response theory (predominantly the Rasch models) is now considered to be the most effective means of establishing invariant unidimensionality.

15.2.2.2.2. Reliability

The term "reliability" refers to the extent to which a measure yields the same number or score each time it is administered, all other things being equal (i.e. no true change has occurred in the attribute being measured). Any instrument designed to measure a construct that cannot be measured directly, such as HRQL and QoL, will contain a true score component, a systematic error component and a random error component. Basically, this is analogous to a signal-to-noise ratio where more reliable scores have less noise or random error. A good instrument should have good reliability (i.e low random measurement error) in order to have a good ability to detect differences between treatment groups. The most appropriate method of determining reliability is to assess the correlation between repeated measurements, as stability over time (or reproducibility) is the crucial variable. This is, in general, called test–retest reliability. Where reliability is low (i.e where the correlation coefficient is below 0.85), an instrument will unlikely show changes in the value of the measured construct associated with an improvement in the patient's condition. It should be noted that a quality standard of 0.70 is occasionally quoted by instrument developers as sufficient for demonstrating reliability. However, health economists should be aware that an instrument with a reliability correlation coefficient of 0.85 will contain 27.75% random measurement error whereas an instrument with a reliability correlation coefficient of 0.70 will contain 51% random measurement error [DRA 98].

15.2.2.2.3. Internal consistency

Cronbach's coefficient α [CRO 51] is often used as an indicator of reliability because of its interpretation as a lower bound of the test–retest correlation. Values of α should be ≥ 0.70, and preferably ≥ 0.90 [CRO 04], but can also be used as a measure of consistency because it is a function of the average inter-item correlations. Internal consistency reliability represents the homogeneity of items making up of the PRO scale or measure. However, it would be necessary to demonstrate first that the scale is unidimensional and that items are locally independent before relying on this statistic. Another issue is that Cronbach's coefficient α depends on the number of items in the scale. Although it is a useful indicator, internal consistency alone is not sufficient for judging the reliability of a scale designed to measure the change over time (see other chapters).

15.2.2.2.4. Validity

Instruments should be relevant, understandable and acceptable to potential respondents (face validity) and should provide adequate coverage of the construct assessed (content validity). Scores yielded by a PRO scale should also be meaningful and interpretable representations of the construct they are assumed to measure (construct validity). Three prerequisites of it are that the instrument is based on a coherent theory or model, the scale is unidimensional and it has a good reproducibility. Where these criteria are met, it is possible to infer that the instrument provides a valid assessment of the construct defined in the model. However, it is still necessary to assess construct validity formally. This can be supported externally by, for example, demonstrating that scores correlate with other variables in a hypothesized and expected pattern (concurrent validity) and that scores differentiate between subgroups of patients that are expected to differ ("known groups" validity). Internal validity refers to evidence supporting that the items within a scale depend on a common unidimensional latent variable and that the items represent a wide range of that variable.

Another important aspect of validity is differential item functioning (DIF). It is well known that items do not always function equally in different groups, for example across genders, languages and cultures [GRO 95, PET 03, TEN 04, SCO 06, SCO 07, BRO 07a, BRO 07b, BRO 10] or even across time [SPE 11]. For example, in most industrialized countries, it is more culturally acceptable for women to express their feelings than men. Hence, a woman who cries after receiving a diagnosis of cancer is not necessarily more sad or anxious than a man diagnosed with the same disease who does not cry. Consequently, in studies where PROs are used and different groups are compared, it is important to check for DIF in relation to covariates. When questionnaires are translated into different languages or even when the same language version of a questionnaire is used in different countries (e.g. an English questionnaire used in the UK, United States, Canada and Australia), it is also important to be aware of the possibility of DIF between cultures and local languages across national borders [BRO 07b].

15.2.2.2.5. Responsiveness

Any instrument intended for use in clinical trials must be responsive, that is, it must be able to detect changes in the measured construct associated with a change in the condition of the patient. Technically, responsiveness is a component of criterion validity. However, it is generally called a separate property as it is critical for PROs used to assess the change following the treatment. Non-responsive PRO measures are of little use in evaluating treatment effects. The responsiveness of PROs can be evaluated using multiple means, such as the application of a treatment of known efficacy (a treatment known to have an impact on the latent variable), relating changes in the PRO to changes in clinical status and relating changes in the PRO to patient- or clinician-rated changes in clinical status. However, a crucial problem here is that there is always no gold standard and therefore it can be hard to interpret whether a small or large difference in a summary score of a scale results from actual clinical change or it is due to the unreliability of the scale. Measures with poor reproducibility have poor responsiveness. This is true for many of the older generic health status measures, such as the Nottingham Health Profile and the SF-36 that have inadequate reproducibility.

In order for an instrument to be responsive, it requires an adequate range of coverage of the construct. Scales should also be well targeted to the intended population. It is important that scores on the scales are not skewed and the extent of floor and ceiling effects (the proportion of people obtaining minimum and maximum scores, respectively) should not be excessive. Skewed data sets with large floor or ceiling effects underestimate actual changes over time and differences between patients. This decreases the ability of an instrument to reflect changes in the patients' condition and differences in outcome between treatment arms in clinical trials accurately.

15.3. Writing new health-related items for new PRO scales

The development of new items for new PRO scales requires two fundamental processes:

1) Consideration of measurement issues:

   i) identification of target population;

   ii) identification of key measurement construct(s).

2) Questionnaire development:

   i) identification of suitable theoretical measurement model;

   ii) generation of questionnaire content;

   iii) assessment of psychometric and scaling properties.

15.3.1. *Consideration of measurement issues*

The first stage in developing a questionnaire is identifying the target population – the patient group of interest and the constructs to be measured. These can range from symptoms and functioning to QoL or satisfaction.

15.3.2. *Questionnaire development*

The stages required for the development of a new PRO questionnaire are summarized below and shown in Figure 15.2. The new instrument should meet the quality standard criteria described above.

– *Identification of theoretical model*: all PRO instruments should be based on a stated model or a theory of the construct being measured. Without this, it is not possible to prove that an instrument is valid. For example, measures of symptoms or functioning may be based on the WHO International Classification of Impairments, Disabilities and Handicaps (ICIDH) classification for impairments and disability, respectively (ICF) [WHO 01]. A measure of QoL is likely to be based on the needs-based model of QoL [HUN 92a].

– *Generation of questionnaire content*: the content of the questionnaire should be derived from the most appropriate source, both in terms of the coverage of the measure and the actual wording of items used to elicit responses. For example, measures of symptoms (impairments) may be derived from patients but clinical input is also important. However, clinical input would not be required for measures of QoL, which should be derived directly from the relevant patients. This applies both to the areas included in the instrument and (as far as possible) to the wording of the items.

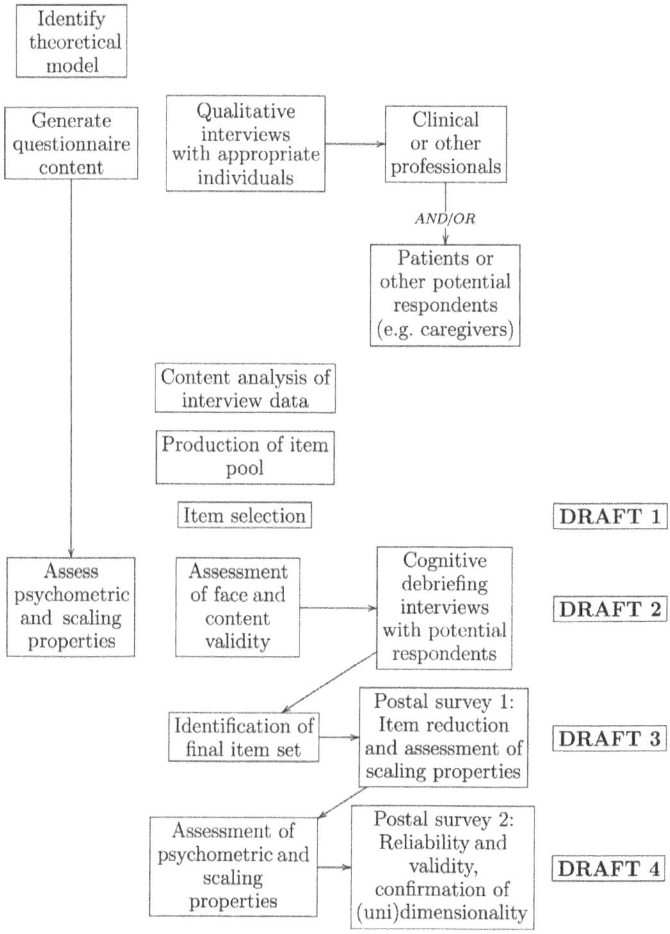

Figure 15.2. *Stages in the development of PRO outcome measures*

The content of an instrument should also be appropriate to the culture and lifestyle of the countries in which it will be used. Instruments developed in a single country reflect the language and culture of that particular society, which may cause problems when adapting the measure into other languages.

Content for patient-based PROs should be derived from qualitative interviews conducted with individuals face-to-face or in focus groups. The participants should be representative of those who will ultimately complete the questionnaire. Such interviews should be designed to allow interviewees to raise those issues that they consider important to, for example, their QoL. The most useful means of achieving this is conducting unstructured interviews, exploring the constructs that are intended to be covered by the measure. Rather than starting with a list of potential areas that should be assessed, the interviewer prompts and guides the interviewee to go beyond a simple listing of symptoms and loss of functionality. In this way, it is possible to look at how these direct impacts of the disease actually impact the needs of patients. For example, interviews conducted as part of the development of a QoL measure for psoriasis may reveal that the patient considers his or her skin disease to be unsightly. The interviewer would then investigate further to determine whether this affects needs related to fashion, self-image, socialization or other areas of experience. The aim is always to allow the interviewee to dictate the direction of the interview and to express the issues in his or her own words.

Interviews should be audio recorded and transcripts produced. Each transcript should be analyzed independently by at least two experienced researchers. Their task is to identify statements related to the construct to be measured, for example, symptoms experienced and needs that are affected by the disease in question. These statements are then grouped according to the topic. For the needs-based QoL instrument for psoriasis [MCK 01], this group may constitute issues related to control over the disease, identity, time structure, self-esteem, self-consciousness, independence, impact on relationships and social life, reaction of others and fears about the future.

For a measure of symptoms or functioning, the areas of impact can be used to construct questions for the measure, although it is often possible to use the actual words of interviewees for these types of outcome also. For a measure of QoL, the wording of items selected for the instrument should be taken, as far as possible, directly from the interview transcripts. This process helps to ensure that the items have relevant intensity or severity.

The first draft of the questionnaire will be produced at the end of this stage.

– *Assessment of psychometric and scaling properties*: cognitive debriefing interviews should be conducted with a sample of relevant respondents to establish face and content validity for the new questionnaire. Interviews will be semi-structured and will be designed to assess the respondents' views on relevance, comprehensiveness, applicability and comprehensibility. Items found to be problematic may be removed at this stage or the item wording may be altered, resulting in the second draft version of the questionnaire. It should be noted that questionnaire wording will not be altered during the remaining development stages. Consequently, where time is limited, instruments that have been field-tested may be included in clinical trial dossiers and the remaining stages conducted in parallel to a clinical trial.

– *Identification of final item set and assessment of scaling and psychometric properties*: ideally, where time and funds allow, two separate postal surveys should be conducted. The first survey should be a single administration survey designed to assess scaling properties (unidimensionality) and to reduce the number of items. For the second survey, the instrument should be administered on two occasions, two weeks apart, allowing the assessment of reproducibility (reliability), construct validity and confirmation of unidimensionality of scale/subscales. For both surveys, the application of item response theory to the data collected is crucial to ensure unidimensionality and the quality of the final scale.

15.4. Selecting PROs for a clinical setting

The process involved in selecting an appropriate instrument for a clinical setting involves first identifying the PRO constructs to be measured. To achieve this, it is necessary to formulate a precise and clear research questionaire. For example, if the intention is to measure the QoL of patients with leukemia while they are receiving chemotherapy, it is necessary for the researcher to be clear about the nature of quality of life. Irrespective of the choice of measurement construct selected, the researcher must be able to justify and describe the choice of definition used [MCK 04]. The second stage is to conduct a review of the literature to identify whether a suitable instrument already exists [STR 08]. The review should take account of the instrument quality criteria described above. The choice of the instrument should first be guided by its ability to measure the construct required in a reliable and valid manner. The next stage is to see whether the required language versions are available and then, whether the appropriate adaptation procedure has been used. Finally, it should be determined whether or not the new language version has psychometric properties comparable to the original version. Where no suitable translation is available, it is necessary to arrange for this work to be completed.

Where no suitable instruments are identified, it will be necessary to develop a new PRO instrument. This section sets out the optimum process for adapting an instrument for use in a new culture and the stages required to develop a new instrument.

15.5. Conclusions

The adoption of the biopsychosocial model of illness has led to the need to learn directly from patients both how their environment and lifestyle affect their health and how they perceive the symptoms and limitations that they experience. This, in turn, has resulted in the widespread use of PRO measures. Available measures vary considerably in quality and it is not often true that the best PROs are the most widely used. This chapter has attempted to summarize the different types of PROs, their required scaling and psychometric properties and their development. Underlying the quality of PROs is the need for a clear theoretical underpinning and the application of modern statistical techniques in their development – among which is the application of item response theory – especially the Rasch models.

15.6. Bibliography

[BAR 06] BARON R., ELASHAAL A., GERMON T., HOBART J., "Measuring outcomes in cervical spine surgery: think twice before using the SF-36", *Spine*, vol. 31, pp. 2575–2584, 2006.

[BER 76] BERGNER M., BOBBIT R.A., KRESSEL S., POLLARD W.E., GILSON B.S., MORRIS J.R., "The sickness impact profile: conceptual formulation and methodology for the development of a health status measure", *International Journal of Health Services*, vol. 6, pp. 393–415, 1976.

[BOS 01] BOSMA H., VAN DE MHEEN H.D., BORSBOOM G.J., MACKENBACH J.P., "Neighborhood socioeconomic status and all-cause mortality", *American Journal of Epidemiology*, vol. 153, pp. 363–371, 2001.

[BRO 07a] BRODERSEN J., THORSEN H., KREINER S., "Validation of a condition-specific measure for women having an abnormal screening mammography", *Value in Health*, vol. 10, pp. 294–304, 2007.

[BRO 07b] BRODERSEN J., MEADS D., KREINER S., THORSEN H., DOWARD L., MCKENNA S.P., "Methodological aspects of differential item functioning in the Rasch model", *Journal of Medical Economics*, vol. 10, pp. 309–24, 2007.

[BRO 10] BRODERSEN J., THORSEN H., KREINER S., "Consequences of screening in lung cancer: development and dimensionality of a questionnaire", *Value in Health*, vol. 13, pp. 601–612, 2010.

[CEL 94] CELLA D.F., "Quality of life: concepts and definition", *Journal of Pain and Symptom Management*, vol. 9, pp. 186–192, 1994.

[COA 97] COATES A., PORZSOLT F., OSOBA D., "Quality of life in oncology practice: prognostic value of EORTC QLQ-C30 scores in patients with advanced malignancy", *European Journal of Cancer*, vol. 33, pp. 1025–1030, 1997.

[COM 08] COMINS J., BRODERSEN J., KROGSGAARD M., BEYER N., "Rasch analysis of the knee injury and osteoarthritis outcome score (KOOS): a statistical re-evaluation", *Scandinavian Journal of Medicine and Science in Sports*, vol. 18, pp. 336–345, 2008.

[CRO 04] CRONBACH L.J., SHAVELSON R.J., "My current thoughts on coefficient alpha and successor procedures", *Educational and Psychological Measurement*, vol. 64, pp. 391–418, 2004.

[DIE 97] DIEZ-ROUX A.V., NIETO F.J., MUNTANER C., TYROLER H.A., COMSTOCK G.W., SHAHAR E., COOPER L.S., WATSON R.L., SZKLO M., "Neighborhood environments and coronary heart disease: a multilevel analysis", *American Journal of Epidemiology*, vol. 146, pp. 48–63, 1997.

[DOW 97] DOWARD L.C., MCKENNA S.P., "Evolution of quality of life assessment", in: RAJAGOPALAN R., SHERETZ E.F., ANDERSON R.T. (eds), *Care Management of Skin Diseases: Life Quality and Economic Impact*, Marcel Dekker, New York, pp. 9–33, 1997.

[DOW 03] DOWARD L.C., SPOORENBERG A., COOK S.A., WHALLEY D., HELLIWELL P.S., KAY L., MCKENNA S.P., TENNANT A., VAN DER HEIJDE D., CHAMBERLAIN M.A., "The development of the ASQoL: a quality of life instrument specific to *ankylosing spondylitis*", *Annals of the Rheumatic Diseases*, vol. 62, pp. 20–26, 2003.

[DOW 04] DOWARD L.C., MCKENNA S.P., "Defining Patient-Reported Outcomes", *Value in Health*, vol. 7, Issue s1, pp. S4–S8, 2004.

[DRA 98] DRAPER N.R., SMITH H., *Applied Regression Analysis*, 3rd ed., Wiley-InterScience, New York, NY, 1998.

[ENG 77] ENGEL G.L., "The need for a new medical model: a challenge for biomedicine", *Science*, vol. 196, pp. 129–136, 1977.

[ENG 80] ENGEL G.L., "The clinical application of the biopsychosocial model", *American Journal of Psychiatry*, vol. 137, pp. 535–544, 1980.

[ENG 90] ENGEL G.L., "On looking inward and being scientific. A tribute to Arthur H Schmale, MD", *Psychotherapy and Psychosomatics*, vol. 54, pp. 63–69, 1990.

[EUR 93] EUROPEAN GROUP FOR QUALITY OF LIFE ASSESSMENT AND HEALTH MEASUREMENT, *European Guide to the Nottingham Health Profile*, Brookwood Medical Publications, Brookwood, Surrey, 1993.

[EUR 05] EUROPEAN MEDICINES AGENCY, *Reflection paper on the regulatory guidance for the use of the health-related quality of life measures in the evaluation of medicinal products*, EMEA, London, 2005.

[FOO 06] FOOD AND DRUG ADMINISTRATION, "Patient-reported outcome measures: use in medicinal product development to support labelling claims", *Federal Register*, vol. 71, pp. 5862–5863, 2006.

[GRO 95] GROENVOLD M., BJORNER J.B., KLEE M.C., KREINER S., "Test for item bias in a quality of life questionnaire", *Journal of Clinical Epidemiology*, vol. 48, pp. 805–816, 1995.

[GUY 93] GUYATT G.H., FEENY D.H., PATRICK D.L., "Measuring health-related quality of life", *Annals of Internal Medicine*, vol. 118, pp. 622–629, 1993.

[HAG 08] HAGELL P., TORNQVIST A.L., HOBART J., "Testing the SF-36 in Parkinson's disease. Implications for reporting rating scale data", *Journal of Neurology*, vol. 255, pp. 246–254, 2008.

[HAG 09] HAGELL P., RELMER J., NYBERG P., "Whose quality of life? Ethical implications in patient-reported health outcome measurement", *Value in Health*, vol. 12, pp. 613–617, 2009.

[HOB 01] HOBART J.C., LAMPING D.L., FREEMAN J.A., LANGDON D.W., MCLELLAN D.L., GREENWOOD R.J., THOMPSON A.J., "Evidence-based measurement: which disability scale for neurologic rehabilitation?", *Neurology*, vol. 57, pp. 639–644, 2001.

[HOB 02] HOBART J.C., WILLIAMS L.S., MORAN K., THOMPSON A.J., "Quality of life measurement after stroke: uses and abuses of the SF-36", *Stroke*, vol. 33, pp. 1348–1356, 2002.

[HOB 03] HOBART J.C., "Rating scales for neurologists", *Journal of Neurology, Neurosurgery and Psychiatry*, vol. 74, no. Suppl IV, pp. 22–26, 2003.

[HUN 92a] HUNT S.M., MCKENNA S.P., "The QLDS: a scale for the measurement of quality of life in depression", *Health Policy*, vol. 22, pp. 307–319, 1992.

[HUN 92b] HUNT S.M., MCKENNA S.P., "A British adaptation of the general well-being index: a new tool for clinical research", *British Journal of Medical Economics*, vol. 2, pp. 49–60, 1992.

[IDL 97] IDLER E.L., BENYAMINI Y,. "Self-rated health and mortality: a review of twenty-seven community studies", *Journal of Health and Social Behaviour*, vol. 38, pp. 21–37, 1997.

[IVE 02] IVERSEN L., KRISTENSEN T.S., HOLSTEIN B., DUE P., *Medicinsk sociologi*, 1st ed., Munksgaard, Copenhagen, 2002.

[KEE 08] KEENAN A-M., MCKENNA S.P., DOWARD L.C., CONAGHAN P.G., EMERY P., TENNANT A., "OAQoL: the development and validation of a quality of life instrument for osteoarthritis", *Arthritis Care and Research*, vol. 15, pp. 841–848, 2008.

[MCK 92] MCKENNA S.P., HUNT S.M., "A new measure of quality of life in depression: testing the reliability and construct validity of the QLDS", *Health Policy*, vol. 22, pp. 321–330, 1992.

[MCK 01] MCKENNA S.P., COOK S.A., WHALLEY D., DOWARD L.C., VAN ASSCHE D., "Testing the psychometric properties of the PSORIQoL: a psoriasis-specific quality of life instrument", *Quality of Life Research*, vol. 10, pp. 262, 2001.

[MCK 03] MCKENNA S.P., COOK S.A., WHALLEY D., DOWARD L. C., RICHARDS H.L., GRIFFITHS C.E.M., VAN ASSCHE D., "Development of the PSORIQoL, a psoriasis-specific measure of quality of life designed for use in clinical practice and trials", *British Journal of Dermatology*, vol. 149, pp. 323–331, 2003.

[MCK 04] MCKENNA S.P., DOWARD L.C., "The needs-based approach to quality of life assessment", *Value in Health*, vol. 7, pp. S1–S3, 2004.

[MCW 97] MCWINNEY I.R., *A Textbook of Family Medicine*, 2nd ed., Oxford University Press, New York, NY, 1997.

[MOR 34] MORGAN A.E., "An attempt to measure happiness", *International Journal of Medical Ethics*, vol. 44, pp. 271–274, 1934.

[PAR 94] PARMENTER T.R., "Quality of life as a concept and measurable entity", *Social Indicators Research*, vol. 33, pp. 9–46, 1994.

[PAT 71] PATRICK D.L., BUSH J.W., CHEN M.M., "Methods for measuring levels of well-being for a health status index", *Health Services Research*, vol. 8, pp. 228–245, 1973.

[PAT 93] PATRICK D.L., ERIKSON P., *Health Status and Health Policy*, Oxford University Press, Oxford, 1993.

[PET 03] PETERSEN M.A., GROENVOLD M., BJORNER J.B., AARONSON N., CONROY T., CULL A., FAYERS P., HJERMSTAD M., SPRANGERS M., SULLIVAN M., "Use of differential item functioning analysis to assess the equivalence of translations of a questionnaire", *Quality of Life Research*, vol. 12, pp. 373–385, 2003.

[PIC 01] PICKETT K.E., PEARL M., "Multilevel analyses of neighbourhood socioeconomic context and health outcomes: a critical review", *Journal of Epidemiology and Community Health*, vol. 55, pp. 111–122, 2001.

[RAB 01] RABIN R., DE CHARRO F., "EQ-5D: a measure of health status from the EuroQol Group", *Annals of Medicine*, vol. 33, pp. 337–343, 2001.

[SCO 06] SCOTT N.W., FAYERS P.M., BOTTOMLEY A., AARONSON N.K., DE GRAEFF A., GROENVOLD M., KOLLER M., PETERSEN M.A., SPRANGERS, M.A., "Comparing translations of the EORTC QLQ-C30 using differential item functioning analyses", *Quality of Life Research*, vol. 15, pp. 1103–1115, 2006.

[SCO 07] SCOTT N.W., FAYERS P.M., AARONSON N.K., BOTTOMLEY A., DE GRAEFF A., GROENVOLD M., KOLLER M., PETERSEN M.A., SPRANGERS, M.A., "The use of differential item functioning analyses to identify cultural differences in responses to the EORTC QLQ-C30", *Quality of Life Research*, vol. 16, pp. 115–129, 2007.

[SMI 97] SMITH G.D., HART C., BLANE D., GILLIS C., HAWTHORNE V., "Lifetime socioeconomic position and mortality: prospective observational study", *British Medical Journal*, vol. 314, pp. 547–552, 1997.

[SMI 98] SMITH G.D., HART C., BLANE D., HOLE D., "Adverse socioeconomic conditions in childhood and cause specific adult mortality: prospective observational study", *British Medical Journal*, vol. 316, pp. 1631–1635, 1998.

[SPE 11] SPECHT K., LEONHARDT J.S., REVALD P., MANDOE H., ANDRESEN E.B., BRODERSEN J., KREINER S., KJAERSGAARD-ANDERSEN P., "No evidence of a clinically important effect of adding local infusion analgesia administrated through a catheter in pain treatment after total hip arthroplasty", *Acta Orthopaedica*, vol. 82, pp. 315–320, 2011.

[STR 08] STREINER D.L., NORMAN G.R., *Health Measurement Scales: A Practical Guide to Their Development and Use*, 4th ed., Oxford Medical Publications, 2008.

[TEN 04] TENNANT A., PENTA M., TESIO L., GRIMBY G., THONNARD J.L., SLADE A., LAWTON G., SIMONE A., CARTER J., LUNDGREN-NILSSON A., TRIPOLSKI M., RING H., BIERING-SØRENSEN F., MARINCEK C., BURGER H., PHILLIPS S., "Assessing and adjusting for cross-cultural validity of impairment and activity limitation scales through differential item functioning within the framework of the Rasch model: the PRO-ESOR project", *Medical Care*, vol. 42, no. Suppl 1, pp. I37–I48, 2004.

[TWI 12] TWISS J., MEADS D.M., PRESTON E.P., CRAWFORD S.R., MCKENNA S.P., "Can we rely on the dermatology life quality index (DLQI) as a measure of the impact of psoriasis or atopic dermatitis?", *Journal of Investigative Dermatology*, vol. 132, pp. 76–84, 2012.

[WAR 92] WARE J.E., SHERBOURNE C.D., "The MOS 36-item short-form health survey (SF-36)", *Medical Care*, vol. 30, pp. 474–483, 1992.

[WHA 97] WHALLEY D., MCKENNA S.P., DE JONG Z., VAN DER HEIJDE D., "Quality of life in rheumatoid arthritis", *British Journal of Rheumatology*, vol. 36, pp. 884–888, 1997.

[WIE 03] WIEBE S., GUYATT G., WEAVER B., MATIJEVIC S., SIDWELL C., "Comparative responsiveness of generic and specific quality-of-life instruments", *Journal of Clinical Epidemiology*, vol. 56, pp. 52–60, 2003.

[WHO 47] WORLD HEALTH ORGANIZATION, *Constitution of the World Health Organization*, WHO, Geneva, 1947.

[WHO 48] WORLD HEALTH ORGANIZATION, *Preamble to the Constitution of the World Health Organization as adopted by the International Health Conference*, New York, 19–22 June, 1946; signed on 22 July 1946 by the representatives of 61 States (*Official Records of the World Health Organization*, no. 2, pp. 100) and entered into force on 7 April 1948.

[WHO 01] WORLD HEALTH ORGANIZATION, "International Classification of Functioning, Disability and Health", WHO, Geneva, 2001.

[ØST 07] ØSTERGAARD I., ANDERSEN J.S., CHRISTENSEN B., DAMSBO N., LAURITZEN T., WITT K., *Almen medicin*, 2nd ed., Munksgaard Denmark, Copenhagen, 2007.

Chapter 16

Adapting Patient-Reported Outcome Measures for Use in New Languages and Cultures

...Translation is like a woman. If it is beautiful, it is not faithful. If it is faithful, it is most certainly not beautiful.

Yevgeny Yevtushenko (born 1933)

16.1. Introduction

Translating a questionnaire appears to be a simple task. The language and concepts used should not be very "technical" – particularly if it is designed to be completed by the average patient. From the perspective of the translator, it will be a quick job as the word count will be low and, consequently, will not be well paid [SWA 04]. In fact, translating a questionnaire is a highly "technical" task that goes well beyond finding the right words.

16.1.1. *Background*

In an ideal world, new patient-reported outcome measures (PROMs) would be developed from the start in a wide range of languages. Such parallel development overcomes the problems related to cultural differences, as items (questions) that work poorly in one culture can be deleted from the initial item pool [DOW 98, MCK 99].

Chapter written by Stephen P. MCKENNA, Jeanette WILBURN, Hanne THORSEN and John BRODERSEN.

However, such parallel development is rare due to its cost and the possibility that the PROM will not be widely adopted.

Consequently, it becomes necessary to produce new language versions of available PROMs. It is now increasingly common for clinical trials to be conducted in multicountry (or multicultural) settings. This, together with the recognition of the need to determine health outcomes from the patients' perspective, means that consideration has to be given to how best to produce the required adaptations.

A further consideration is the present move of clinical trial programmes from Western Europe and North America to Eastern Europe, South and Central America and Asia. This requires adaptations of PROMs for use in quite different cultures from those in which they were developed. Little is known about the success of such adaptations although it is generally conveniently assumed that they will work perfectly well.

Depending on the number of language versions required, the production of new language versions of PROMs will be costly in terms of both money and time. Given the cost of running multinational clinical studies and trials and the need to compare findings from different countries, it is important that adaptations of PROMs produced are of a very high standard.

Health authorities have started to specify how PROMs should be adapted [EME 05, BUR 08], but the recommendations are far from clear and are generally interpreted by practitioners in a way that suits the approach that they prefer to use. In particular, although the recommendations state that the adaptations should be equivalent to the original questionnaire and that they should be valid and reliable, few adequate validation studies are ever completed. Despite this, a handful of patient interviews are reported as being evidence of the validity of adaptations (e.g. see [HER 09, LEG 10]). The use of the term "linguistic validation" (generally shortened in the literature to "validation") has become common ([ACQ 03, ABB 12]). This term is used to imply that the adaptation has been validated. Even if the results of a "linguistic validation" are positive, it does not imply that the new language version either works or that it has equivalent psychometric properties to the original measure.

16.1.2. *Aim of the adaptation process*

The aim of the adaptation process is to achieve new language versions of PROMs that are conceptually equivalent to, and that meet the same psychometric and acceptability standards as, the original. Adaptation of an instrument into a new language involves four main stages:

– Consideration of suitability for adaptation into target languages.

– Translation into target language.

– Assessment of acceptability to the new culture.

– Establishing psychometric and scaling properties of the new language version.

16.2. Suitability for adaptation

Most PROMs were developed in the United States or in the United Kingdom for individuals whose primary language is English. A measure produced in one language, for use with one cultural group within a national population, will reflect the values, experiences and preoccupations of that societal group. Before adapting a PROM, consideration should be given to the acceptability of the content to the target population. Its content must be appropriate to the culture and lifestyle of the target country. Successful adaptation of a measure into a different language or for use with a different cultural group can only be achieved if the content of the measure reflects experiences that are common across the source and target cultures.

16.3. Translation process

The adaptation of an instrument for use in another language highlights a number of linguistic, conceptual and technical issues.

16.3.1. *Linguistic issues*

It is inappropriate to produce a new language version of a PROM by simply translating the content (literal translation). Cultural factors are often central to the spoken language. In addition, language contains numerous subtle nuances that are not always clear to non-native speakers. Thus, although a literal translation may produce an item that *appears* identical to the original, it may have missed some subtlety of *meaning* in the source item. As a result, the *concept* addressed by the source and translated items may be very different. Hopefully, items such as "I have trouble passing water" are no longer translated as "I am unable to step over a stream".

Any given language may contain words for which there is no commonly accepted meaning among speakers of another language. For example, in English, words such as "occasionally" or "often" – commonly used in PROMs, are not understood in the same way in other European languages. Other words such as "sex" can convey very different meanings depending on the context in which they are used. In English, "sex" may be used to describe gender or it can be ascribed to sexual behavior and any of the feelings, desires or urges associated with it. During the development of the Recurrent Genital Herpes Quality of Life (RGHQoL) questionnaire [DOW 98] difficulties were encountered in translating items containing the word "sex". In French, Italian and Spanish, "sex" would have been translated literally as "gender" whereas in the context of the RGHQoL, the intended meaning was "sexual activity".

16.3.2. *Conceptual issues*

Measures that are comparable across languages require *conceptually* equivalent items. Conceptual equivalence ensures that the *meaning* of the original item is preserved by the translation of the concept or idea covered by that item. It may be possible to translate an item using the same expression as in the original language, thus producing an item that is *conceptually* and *linguistically* equivalent. Conversely, it may be possible to produce an item with conceptual equivalence that uses quite different wording. For example, during the development of the QoL in Growth Hormone Deficiency Assessment (QoL-AGHDA) questionnaire [MCK 99] – which was developed simultaneously in seven European languages – the English item "I am easily irritated by other people" was conceptually translated as "People give hits on my nerves" in Italian. Thus, although the Italian version used very different wording to the UK original, it conveyed the same conceptual meaning.

16.3.3. *Technical issues*

Technical equivalence is composed of two parts: grammatical considerations and sociocultural acceptability of the questionnaire's content.

Care needs to be taken to ensure that the grammar and syntax of the original items are maintained in translation. It is good practice to avoid using double negatives when developing questionnaires. Although such statements often give the greatest immediacy for some questionnaire respondents, they can give rise to response ambiguity. Similarly, care should be taken to avoid double negatives when translating items. It is preferable for a translation to result in an item that sounds a little clumsy than to produce one that causes confusion for the respondent and the investigator.

The importance of cultural relevance when adapting questionnaires has already been discussed. Consideration should be given to the acceptability of the content to the target population. For example, during the early stages of the production of the QoL-AGHDA, the English item "I find it hard to get on with people" created difficulties in Italian. Some respondents did not consider it to be socially acceptable to answer "yes" to this item. The item was replaced in all language versions with "I avoid mixing with people I don't know well".

16.4. Translation methodology

In order to ensure high-quality adaptations, it is crucial for the test developer to be closely involved in the adaptation process. However carefully done, the original intention of an item may be lost as a result of the adaptation process. It is unwise to handover the adaptation task to an organization that has had no involvement in the development process, if this can be avoided. Despite this, it is common practice for the test developer to be overtly or covertly excluded from the process.

All adaptations must be based on the original source language version of the measure. For example, when an instrument developed in the United Kingdom has been adapted for use in France, the United Kingdom version should be used as the source measure for producing a French Canadian adaptation. This is because minor changes in meaning adopted for the French adaptation may not be appropriate for the French Canadian adaptation.

There are two main methods used in the adaptation of PROMs; forward–backward translation and dual-panel translation.

16.4.1. *Forward–backward translation*

When test developers first needed their measures to be adapted, they wanted a means of determining the quality with which the work had been done. They adopted a method that appeared to achieve this but was misleadingly simple. Such a method would never have been suggested by true experts in translation. In fact, translators might well consider forward–backward translation to be demeaning as it questions their ability.

Adaptations using forward–backward translation rely on the production of translated versions of the questionnaire into the new language and the subsequent "back translation" of these (by different individuals) into the source language. The two versions are then compared and if they appear similar, the source and target versions of the measure are considered equivalent. Translations are conducted by bilingual people who are usually professional translators. Although this method is commonly used it has a number of potential problems. If the translation is good, the back translation may look nothing like the source questionnaire. Consequently, little information of any value will be obtained from the back translation, whereas it may result in a lot of misleading impressions. Although this is intuitive to any competent translator, the pitfalls have been described by Swaine-Verdier and colleagues [SWA 04].

16.4.1.1. *Situation 1: The forward translation is good*

If questionnaire items are conceptually translated, the resulting version may appear very different in content and structure. Hence, a good back translation may differ considerably from the original. Comparing the two source language versions may not inform highly on the quality of the translation, unless the comparison is made by someone who has a good enough command of the target language to see that the match is in fact there. Because those testing the quality of the translation (the developers of the PROM) need to do so precisely because they do *not* have expertise in the target language, the exercise is of questionable value.

16.4.1.2. *Situation 2: The forward translation is good, but the back translation is poor*

There is no reason to suppose that back translators are better at their job than forward translators, yet this is assumed when the back translation is used to test the forward version. In this case, the back translation may suggest that the forward version is poor even when it is good. Such a situation is unproductive of useful information.

16.4.1.3. *Situation 3: The forward translation is poor*

The translation may be too literal or stay too close to the original in sentence structure or in choice of words. The back translator, doing his or her best to produce something readable in the source language, may find the exact wording of the original item. This would not happen by chance, as poor translations are easy to identify. This means that the back translation, intended to assess the quality of the translation, will mistakenly indicate that it is good.

16.5. Dual-panel translation

This method aims to produce quality *in* the translation, rather than checking it *a posteriori*. Producing quality requires checking and rechecking throughout the process (as well as after it, to see whether the instrument functions as required with "real" people). The method assumes that the verification and acceptability of translations should rest with people who are typical of the patients who will later be asked to complete the questionnaire. Two translation panels are conducted sequentially in the target country: a "bilingual" panel and a "lay" panel. Where instruments are required for the same language but for use in a different country (e.g. use of a US-English instrument by UK-English speakers) it is still generally necessary to conduct a formal translation procedure. However, only the second (lay) panel is required.

Another important difference of the dual-panel and forward–backward methodologies is that the former is conducted in the country where the measure is required. Forward–backward translations can be produced anywhere in the world – often in a offices of a translation agency. Consequently, the language used can be out of date not having developed with the culture of the people who actually live in the country.

16.5.1. *Bilingual panel*

The first translation is produced by a panel of people who are fluent in both the target and source language. The panel should represent the target audience of the questionnaire in terms of age and gender. Professional translators and clinically trained individuals are generally excluded from the panel. It is essential for one of the test developers to attend and participate in this panel meeting. This is because it is important that the participants are made aware of the context in which the items were generated. This will aid in selecting from alternative translations.

Emphasis in the bilingual panel is placed on the production of conceptually equivalent translations. Linguistic equivalence is of secondary importance. It is also vital that the new items are expressed in common (everyday) language that will appeal to future respondents. The panel works together as a group to agree on the most appropriate translation. This process is more efficient than the production of separate translations/back translations by individuals working in isolation. The panel members have the opportunity to discuss alternatives and the final decision on translations is taken by the group as a whole rather than a single translator. Alternative wordings can be produced for consideration by the lay panel.

16.5.2. *Lay panel*

This step is an integral part of a quality translation procedure. The translations produced by the bilingual panel are then considered by a group of local people of average educational attainment who are not proficient in the source language (the "lay" panel). Again, sufficient participants should be included to ensure that the group is varied enough, while allowing adequate discussion. Ideally, participants should meet the following criteria:

– There should be a balance between the genders and age groups unless the target population for the instrument is biased by gender or age.

– It is preferable for the participants to be of average educational attainment with some of a lower educational status included to test the questionnaire adequately for comprehensibility.

– They should represent varied occupational and social backgrounds.

– Individuals with the disease covered by the questionnaire are omitted. This is because they tend to be too concerned about themselves (or their disease) when they asses the suitability of the questionnaire content (which cannot be changed) and too little about the appropriateness of the wording. Furthermore, the next stage of the adaptation process involves testing with patients.

Participants discuss the items as a group, rewording them where it is considered necessary. This process allows a check on whether the appropriate concepts have been captured and whether individual items are comprehensible and acceptable in content and wording. Other outcomes are also possible:

– Wordings that the first panel were searching for but were unable to find are frequently identified.

– Other wordings that are considered questionable can be shown to be acceptable and well understood.

– Unforeseen connotations may be identified. Translators may not be aware that members of the lay panel can unexpectedly and wrongly associate words with certain ideas. Such associations are a reality due to cultural differences in conceptual meaning and should be taken into account.

It is possible for the panel to suggest testing out alternative wordings with actual patients. The group leader (who has been involved in all stages of the translation procedure) ensures that the original meaning of the items is maintained. The second panel has priority over the first. The new version of the instrument is next tested for face and content validity by conducting cognitive debriefing interviews with relevant patients.

It is important that a detailed report is prepared on the two panels. The test developer is not present at the second panel, which is conducted in the target language. Where changes to wording are recommended, this must be explained in detail and approved by the authors.

The adaptation process, using the dual panel method for translation, is summarized below.

16.6. Assessment of psychometric and scaling properties

Psychometric and scaling properties of the new language version should be assessed in the target culture. It cannot be assumed that the new language version shares the same psychometric properties as the original; this must be tested. The process should involve at a minimum the assessment of face and content validity (via cognitive debriefing interviews), reliability (reproducibility), construct validity and unidimensionality.

16.6.1. *Cognitive debriefing interviews*

The purpose of the interviews is to assess the relevance, acceptability, comprehensiveness and understandability of questionnaire items and instructions by patients in the target country. Face-to-face interviews are conducted with up to 15 relevant patients by suitably trained and qualified interviewers. The patients should be literate and, if possible, they should represent a range of severity of the condition in question, gender and age.

16.6.1.1. *Interview setting*

Interviews can be completed in the respondent's home, in the interviewer's office or in a clinic. They should be conducted in a quiet private room where the door can be shut and where the interview will not be disturbed by other people. The interviewer should ensure that the patient has everything necessary to complete the measure; a pen or pencil, reading glasses (if needed) and something to place the questionnaire on (preferably a desk). Members of the respondent's family or their friends should not be present during interviews.

16.6.1.2. *Materials*

The interview schedule includes standardized questions on understandability, acceptability and comprehensiveness plus any additional questions arising from the lay translation panel. This includes demographic information on the patient in order for the surveyed population to be described.

The interviewee is asked to complete the questionnaire in the presence of the interviewer but as if he or she were on his or her own. They are discouraged from asking questions before they have finished completing the measure – because it is a self-completed measure. The interviewer observes and notes any obvious problems the patient has completing the questionnaire. Questions are then asked about any problems observed and the interviewee's opinion of the measure. In particular they should be asked:

– whether the questions were relevant, easy to understand and acceptable;

– whether they found any of the questions ambiguous or inappropriate;

– whether they thought that any important aspect of their experience has been omitted; and

– any specific questions arising from the lay panel such as how specific items are understood or preferences for alternative wordings.

16.6.1.3. *Reporting on the interviews*

Reports are needed to feed back the results to the test developers and should summarize all information recorded during the interviews. The interviewer is also asked to comment on the importance of these findings. It is particularly important to note any suggested changes in the wording of items made as a result of (or during the course of) the interviews. The reasons for these changes should be made clear and the new wording's relation to the English original should be discussed.

16.6.2. *Determining the psychometric properties of the new language version of the measure*

Any translation produced must be tested by means of a validation survey to establish that it is both reliable and that it has construct validity. However, this step is rarely conducted.

The validation study can usually be conducted by mail to keep the costs as low as possible. However, in some countries the postal system may not be reliable or the idea of receiving questionnaires through the mail may be alien. The larger the sample included in the validation study the more accurate are the estimates of reproducibility and construct validity produced. Testing reproducibility involves administering a scale on two occasions, assuming that no change in health status has occurred in between. It would be expected that the responses to questions will be the same on each occasion. The new language version is administered to appropriate individuals on two occasions, approximately two weeks apart. This standard period is used, as it minimizes the risk of respondents remembering their first set of answers while making it unlikely that major changes in health status have occurred.

The mode of administration should be standard at both time points as should be the location of completion. Packs posted to the participants at each time point will include a demographic questionnaire, an appropriate comparator instrument and, for postal surveys, a self-addressed postage-paid envelope in addition to the new questionnaire adaptation.

Scores of the two administrations of the new measure are correlated. Adequate reproducibility is indicated by a correlation of 0.85 or above [WEI 84]. A correlation of 0.7 (often claimed to be adequate by test developers) indicates that half the variance measured by the scale is error variance.

Construct validity is shown by fit to the Rasch model (see below) and adequate reproducibility. Additional indications of construct validity are derived from convergent and divergent validity and known group validity. As their names suggest, convergent and divergent validity are tested by relating scores on the new adaptation to those on comparator measures assessing related or distinct outcomes. Known group validity investigates whether scores for specific subgroups of patients on the new adaptation differ as expected. For example, patients with a mild disease might be expected to have a lower score than those with severe disease.

As mentioned above, it cannot be assumed that the new language version shares the same psychometric properties as the original; this must be tested. When establishing dimensionality, it is important to ensure that the new language version of the scale measures the same construct as the original. The easiest way to test this is to merge data collected with the original and adapted questionnaire as though the two data sets were collected with the same questionnaire. A variable indicating language is included in the data-matrix. A test of unidimensionality is then conducted to see whether the items in the combined data set fit a Rasch model. If fit is revealed, then differential item functioning (DIF) related to the language is tested. Often DIF analyses indicates that some individual items function differently in the two languages. This often results from uniform DIF. If uniform DIF due to language is found, it is possible to estimate the difference in function of the different language versions of the scale, using Rasch models. Adjustments can then be made to cope with this difference [BRO 07].

It is now also possible to test whether adapted measures are equivalent to the original source version by application of item response theory [TEN 04]. The probability of being able to affirm a PROM item for patients at the same level of ability (or, e.g. with the same level of QoL) should remain the same across language versions. Thus, comparability of language versions is dependent on both the conceptual equivalence of items and also on the construct value equivalence of those items. An item may cover the same concept in both source and target language but it may well be valued differently in each culture. Assessment of such "DIF" yields crucial information about the equivalence of language versions and provides valuable information on the validity of pooling data across countries; an issue that is of particular importance for multicenter clinical trials [SMI 92]. But why should it be expected that well-translated questionnaires will be equivalent across languages?

16.6.3. *Practice guidelines*

Practice guidelines have been produced for adapting PROMs (e.g. see [BUL 98, WIL 05]). Unfortunately, rather than presenting "principles of good practice" they provide a synthesis of the opinions of a number of organizations on how to translate PROMs [MCK 05]. Indeed, in several instances more than one opinion is expressed. No scientific evidence is provided to support these opinions, and the suggested methodology (forward–backward translation) falls short of including an assessment of the quality of the adaptations produced or of their equivalence to the original.

Rather than reviewing all published translation recommendations (as claimed), the authors have neglected the considerable body of literature that uses the dual panel method (e.g. see [HUN 91, EUR 93, SWA 04]). This approach has been used in the adaptation of more than 30 disease-specific PROMs in to up to 60 languages [MCK 04].

A classic example of the problem with relying on back translation was provided by Fukuhara and colleagues, whose attempt to translate the SF-36 into Japanese failed and they had to resort to using the equivalent of a lay translation panel to overcome the problems [FUK 98]. The researchers concluded that adherence to the International Quality of Life Assessment project guidelines [BUL 98] did not ensure an adequate translation, reflecting the linguistic and cultural differences between Japan and the United States.

A language is a specific way of putting life into words; and words change with their context. They generate representations that may be universal or culturally specific. Therefore, it is more appropriate to consider the process as one of adaptation rather than translation [SWA 04]. Extending this idea, it is likely that in the relatively near future it will be recognized that translating source measures into new languages is both inefficient and scientifically unhelpful.

Where carefully constructed unidimensional scales are produced on the basis of a coherent measurement model, it is possible to develop language versions that consist of items that are specific to, and work well in, each country. These need not be the same items – although it is likely that there will be items in common across languages. The aim would be to have a set of items that had the same value in each language (derived from the application of item response theory). Only then would construct equivalence be guaranteed.

Although such work is currently being piloted, it is likely to take some time before such a radical (but necessary) development is acceptable to health authorities. In the meantime, how is it possible to determine the most appropriate method of translating PROMs? An opportunity arose to conduct a blind study to compare two different Swedish versions of the Rheumatoid Arthritis Quality of Life (RAQoL) questionnaire [DEJ 97, WHA 97]. An unauthorized Swedish translation of the RAQoL [EBE 02] was conducted simultaneously with the production of an authorized adaptation [MCK 03]. Neither research team was aware of the activities of the other.

Eberhardt and colleagues applied forward and backward translation and the official adaptation used the two-panel methodology to produce the translations. Assessments of the final item translations were made by Swedish bilinguists and patients with rheumatoid arthritis (RA) who were not aware of the different translation methods used. Although the standard psychometric properties of the two methodologies were similar, the study found that items translated using the two-panel method were statistically significantly preferred to those produced using forward–backward translation and produced a higher response rate. This is the initial evidence that the two-panel method has better face validity than the use of back translation. Acceptability of questionnaires to patients is crucial if they are to be accurately completed.

It is clearly important to produce evidence before asserting that the forward–backward translation methodology, an untested method, however widely implemented, represents "principles of good practice".

16.7. Bibliography

[ABB 12] ABBRUZZESE G., ANTONINI A., BARONE P., STOCCHI F., TAMBURINI T., BERNARDI L., AMBONI M., VACCA L., POSOCCO V., COLOMBO D., "Linguistic, psychometric validation and diagnostic ability assessment of an Italian version of a 19-item wearing-off questionnaire for wearing off-detection in Parkinson's disease", *Neurological Science*, 4 February 2012.

[ACQ 03] ACQUADRO C., BERZON R., DUBOIS D., LEIDY N.K., MARQUIS P., REVICKI D., ROTHMAN M., PRO HARMONIZATION GROUP., "Incorporating the patient's perspective into drug development and communication: an ad hoc task force report on the patient-reported outcomes (PRO) harmonization group meeting at the food and drug administration, February 16, 2001", *Value in Health*, vol. 5, pp. 522–531, 2003.

[BRO 07] BRODERSEN J., MEADS D.M., KREINER S., THORSEN H., DOWARD L., MCKENNA S.P., "Methodological aspects of differential item functioning in the Rasch model", *Journal of Medical Economics*, vol. 10, pp. 309–324, 2007.

[BUL 98] BULLINGER M., ALONSO J., APOLONE G., LEPLÈGE A., SULLIVAN M., WOOD-DAUPHINEE S., GANDEK B., WAGNER A., AARONSON N., BECH P., FUKUHARA S., KAASA S., WARE J.E. Jr., "Translating health status questionnaires and evaluating their quality: the IQOLA project approach. International quality of life assessment", *Journal of Clinical Epidemiology*, vol. 51, pp. 913–23, 1998.

[BUR 08] BURKE L.B., KENNEDY D.L., MISKALA P.H., PAPADOPOULOS E.J., TRENTACOSTI A.M., "The use of patient-reported outcome measures in the evaluation of medical products for regulatory approval", *Clinical Pharmacology Therapeutics*, vol. 84, pp. 281–283, 2008.

[DEJ 97] DE JONG Z., VAN DER HEIJDE D., MCKENNA S.P., WHALLEY D., "The reliability and construct validity of the RAQoL: a rheumatoid arthritis-specific quality of life instrument", *British Journal of Rheumatology*, vol. 36, pp. 878–883, 1997.

[DOW 98] DOWARD L.C., MCKENNA S.P., KOHLMANN T., NIERO M., PATRICK D., SPENCER B., THORSEN H., "The international development of the RGHQoL: a quality of life measure for recurrent genital herpes", *Quality of Life Research*, vol. 7, pp. 143–153, 1998.

[EBE 02] EBERHARDT K., DUCKBERG S., LARSSON B.M., JOHNSON P.M., NIVED K., "Measuring health related quality of life in patients with rheumatoid arthritis—reliability, validity, and responsiveness of a Swedish version of RAQoL", *Scandinavian Journal of Rheumatology*, vol. 31, pp. 6–12, 2002.

[EME 05] EMEA, Committee for medicinal products for human use (CMHP), Reflection paper on the regulatory guidance for the use of health-related quality of life (HRQL) measures in the evaluation of medicinal products, Doc. Ref. EMEA/CHMP/EWP/139391/2004, London, 27 July, 2005.

[EUR 93] EUROPEAN GROUP FOR QUALITY OF LIFE ASSESSMENT AND HEALTH MEASUREMENT, *European Guide to the Nottingham Health Profile*, Brookwood Medical Publications, Brookwood, Surrey, 1993.

[FUK 98] FUKUHARA S., BITO S., GREEN J., HSIAO A., KUROKAWA K., "Translation, adaption, and validation of the SF-36 health survey for use in Japan", *Journal of Clinical Epidemiology*, vol. 51, pp. 1037–1044, 1998.

[HER 09] HERTRAMPF K., WENZ H.J., KOLLER M., SPRINGER I., JARGOT A., WILTFANG J., "Assessing dentists' knowledge about oral cancer: translation and linguistic validation of a standardized questionnaire from American English into German", *Oral Oncology*, vol. 45, pp. 877–882, 2009.

[HUN 91] HUNT S.M., ALONSO J., BUCQUET D., NIERO M., WIKLUND I., MCKENNA S.P., "Cross-cultural adaptation of health measures", *Health Policy*, vol. 19, pp. 33–44, 1991.

[LEG 10] LE GAL M. MAINGUY Y., LE LAY K., NADJAR A., ALLAIN D., GALISSIÉ M., "Linguistic validation of six patient-reported outcomes instruments into 12 languages for patients with fibromyalgia", *Joint Bone Spine*, vol. 77, pp. 165–170, 2010.

[MCK 99] MCKENNA S.P., DOWARD L.C., ALONSO J., KOHLMANN T., NIERO M., PRIETO L., WÍREN L., "The QoL-AGHDA: an instrument for the assessment of quality of life in adults with growth hormone deficiency", *Quality of Life Research*, vol. 8, pp. 373–383, 1999.

[MCK 03] MCKENNA S.P., HEDIN P.J., "Adapting the rheumatoid arthritis quality of life instrument (RAQoL) for use in Sweden", *Scandinavian Journal of Rheumatology*, vol. 32, pp. 1–3, 2003.

[MCK 04] MCKENNA S.P., DOWARD L.C., MEADS D.M., PATRICK D., TENNANT A., "Summary of needs-based quality of life instruments", *Value Health*, vol. 7, no. suppl. 1, pp. S39–S40, 2004.

[MCK 05] MCKENNA S.P., DOWARD L.C., "The translation and cultural adaptation of patient-reported outcome measures", *Value in Health*, vol. 8, pp. 89–91, 2005.

[SMI 92] SMITH R.M., *Applications of Rasch Measurement*, JAM Press, Sacramento, 1992.

[SWA 04] SWAINE-VERDIER A., DOWARD L.C., HAGELL P., THORSEN H., MCKENNA S.P., "Adapting quality of life instruments", *Value in Health*, vol. 7, no. suppl. 1, pp. S27–S30, 2004.

[TEN 04] TENNANT A., MCKENNA S.P., HAGELL P., "Application of Rasch analysis in the development and application of quality of life instruments", *Value in Health*, vol. 7, no. suppl. 1, pp. S22–S26, 2004.

[WEI 84] WEINER E.A., STEWART B.J., *Assessing Individuals*, Little Brown, Boston, 1984.

[WHA 97] WHALLEY D., MCKENNA S.P., DE JONG Z., VAN DER HEIJDE D., "Quality of life in rheumatoid arthritis", *British Journal of Rheumatology*, vol. 36, pp. 884–888, 1997.

[WIL 05] WILD D., GROVE A., MARTIN M., EREMENCO S., MCELROY S., VERJEE-LORENZ A., ERIKSON P., ISPOR TASK FORCE FOR TRANSLATION AND CULTURAL ADAPTATION, "Principles of good practice for the translation and cultural adaptation process for patient reported outcomes (PRO) measures: report of the ISPOR task force for translation and cultural adaptation", *Value in Health*, vol. 8, pp. 94–104, 2005.

Chapter 17

Improving Items That Do Not Fit the Rasch Model

17.1. Introduction

Development of measurement scales (hereafter test development) is a time- and resource-consuming process with many stages. The number, order and exact nature of these stages depend on the approach chosen, see for example DeVellis' guidelines for scale development with eight stages [DEV 03] or Nielsen, Kreiner and Styles' adapted approach with four main stages and 10 substages [NIE 07a]. Irrespective of the approach used, the larger part of time and resources are used in the first stages of the process to get to the point where a first data sample is available for the initial psychometric analysis and evaluation. The expenditure of that many resources on developing an initial test version stands in sharp contrast to the most commonly used strategy for determining the final test version, namely the so-called salami method where poor performing items are simply sliced away and discarded. This method will occasionally mean that the resulting scale consists of very few items so that entirely new items need to be developed, evaluated and so on, by the same time- and resource-consuming process as the initial items. Accordingly, a strategy is needed that will help test developers to preserve as much of the initial item pool by identifying items in need of only minor modifications and items in need of being exchanged, as well as providing some input toward how to modify or exchange items.

This chapter introduces a systematic approach to improving poor performing items based on Nielsen and Kreiner's strategy for scale improvement [NIE 05c].

Chapter written by Tine NIELSEN and Svend KREINER.

This strategy combines the results from graphical log-linear Rasch modeling [KRE 02, KRE 04] with the results of a subject matter analysis of items within the particular theoretical framework to facilitate systematic decisions about which items should be modified and which items should be exchanged with new items in order to improve the scale psychometrically, that is toward functioning as a pure Rasch model (RM) [RAS 60]. Before we introduce the strategy for scale improvement, this chapter briefly covers the assumptions and requirements of the graphical log-linear Rasch model (GLLRM) and the effects of local response dependence (LD) and differential item functioning (DIF) in such a model on the reliability and validity of the scale in question (section 17.2). The strategy for scale improvement is described in detail and some results of applications of the strategy are presented in section 17.3. In section 17.4, the strategy is applied to the Physical Functioning (PF) scale of the SF-36 [WAR 93] and suggestions as to how this scale might be improved are given.

17.2. The RM and the graphical log-linear RM

The purpose of item analysis by the RMs is to evaluate the psychometric quality of measurement scales. At the general level, item analysis by RMs can result in two outcomes:

– *Item responses fit the RM*. When this happens, the measurement is close to ideal, because the measurement is both criterion and construct valid [ROS 89], free of DIF [HOL 88, HOL 93], specifically objective [RAS 66, RAS 77], statistically sufficient [AND 77, FIS 95] and as reliable as it can be with the given number of items [BAR 96]. Stated in more general terms, fit to the pure RM means that a number of desirable psychometric quality claims about the measurement scale in question can be made, of which the first is unique to RMs: (1) The total score is statistically sufficient in the conditional distribution of item responses given the latent trait (statistical sufficiency), which means that the score holds as much information as the items put together or that no information has been lost by adding the items to the total score. (2) Items and included exogenous variables are conditionally independent given the latent variable (no DIF), which means that the scale functions in the same way for subgroups so that these groups can be compared fairly in subsequent inference analysis. (3) Within a specific frame of reference, measurement is not confounded by arbitrary choices related to selection of items and sampling of persons (specific objectivity), which means that the level of what is measured reflects the actual level of a person and is not dependent on the items used to measure this, whereas the location of items reflect the actual location of an item and does not depend on the sample of persons. All that remains in this case is to decide whether the reliability of the scale in question is acceptable.

– *Item responses do not fit the RM*. When this is the case, there is a list of problems cataloguing the departures from the RM, that can be used to improve the psychometric quality of the scale in question [KRE 04, KRE 11, NIE 05c]. This is a common situation when evaluating health-related scales. However, whether items have to be revised, discarded or exchanged with new items depends on the nature of misfit [NIE 05c]. Therefore, careful investigation is required, because it does not automatically follow that items have to be revised or discarded if they do not fit the RM. Measurement by items that do not fit the RM will be less than optimal, but careful examination of the departures from the RM is required to decide whether this difference is severe enough to warrant such action.

The GLLRMs provide a useful framework for investigating the exact nature of the departures from the pure RM. Within this framework of analysis, where a loglinear RM is embedded in the larger framework of graphical models, it is possible to model uniform DIF and uniform LD, while retaining statistical sufficiency of the total score [KRE 02, KRE 04]. Here, "uniform" means that the interaction between items (or between items and exogenous variables) *does not* depend on the latent variable. Partial γ coefficient can provide a measure of the degree of local dependence between items (see Chapter 8).

The presence of uniform LD, in particular, is not a problem for validity and objectivity, but it may lead to reduced reliability compared to locally independent items. To calculate the reliability of the scale the methods proposed by Hamon and Mesbah [HAM 02] can be used. The presence of uniform DIF is more problematic because it requires that information about the exogenous variables generating DIF is always available together with the item responses in order to adjust for the confounding of the measurement. If this requirement is fullfilled, it is, as illustrated by [KRE 07], easy to estimate the degree to which measurement is confounded by the exogenous covariate and to adjust scores if the effect is sizeable. However, for the practitioner administering and scoring a test they will always need to have available tables in order to transform the score so that the DIF is adjusted for specific testing situations. We therefore recommend that efforts are made to eliminate DIF in scales whenever possible.

The overall strategy for the investigation of the nature of the departure from the RM attempts to model departures from the model in terms of uniform LD and DIF. If not successful, care must be taken to take note of the difficulties and other departures from the RM encountered in the analysis, so that this information may be used in future in improving the quality of the scale. If successful, items are accepted as essentially valid and objective, and the information about departures can be used for improving the quality of the scale, but the presence of DIF and LD affects the validity and reliability of the scale.

To calculate the reliability of the scale the methods proposed by Hamon and Mesbah [HAM 02] can be used.

17.3. The scale improvement strategy

The scale improvement strategy presented in this section was developed in connection with Nielsen's doctoral work concerned with the development of the Danish Self-Assessment Learning Styles Inventory [NIE 05a] and the learning styles of Danish university students [NIE 05b]. A detailed account as well as application of the strategy to 13 learning style scales are given in [NIE 05c].

GLLRMs [KRE 02, KRE 04] enable the researcher to model departures from the RM in terms of uniform DIF and uniform LD. If a GLLRM is not possible for the complete set of items, the option then is to eliminate items in order to fit a GLLRM with fewer items. Once a GLLRM is found, this can serve as one of two bases on which the decision of rewriting (in the sense modify) or replacing items to improve the scale, while retaining both simplicity and reliability, can be made. The other basis for these decisions is a subject matter analysis where the items are analyzed within the particular theoretical framework of the study/scale in order to determine problems with or between items on the theoretical level. The scale improvement strategy attempts to systematize the relationship between the results of the statistical analysis by GLLRMs, the subject matter analysis and the decision to rewrite or replace items into an applicable strategy for scale improvement. There are two concerns that override the strategy. The first is that evidence from subject matter analysis suggesting theoretical errors during item construction should always lead to elimination of items. The second is that a very complicated structure with extensive DIF and LD always indicates serious problems with the fundamental notion of a construct-valid score. The strategy therefore basically address the situation where the departures from the RM are limited and where the face validity of items is plausible even after careful rethinking of the theoretical foundations in the light of the results of the initial analysis.

As illustrated on the left in Figure 17.1 and in the rows of Table 17.1, the *GLLRM analysis* can result in a pure RM where there are no apparent problems with the items of the scale. The analysis can also pinpoint a number of problems resulting in inability to fit a GLLRM or a list of different departures from the RM. Analyses where GLLRM is not possible are also relevant for the modification strategy. The reason for the failure of the GLLRM may be that DIF and/or LD is non-uniform, that discrimination differs across items or that one or more items are seriously defective. The worst possible case – lack of construct validity – could, of course, also be a possibility. In such cases the analysis provides hints to why a GLLRM fails, but the reason for the failure can only be determined by examination of items in the subject matter analysis. Finally, the results of the GLLRM analysis point out what items should receive special attention in the subject matter analysis. It should, however, be stressed that all items should be subjected to subject matter analysis if the GLLRM analyses show any problem with a scale.

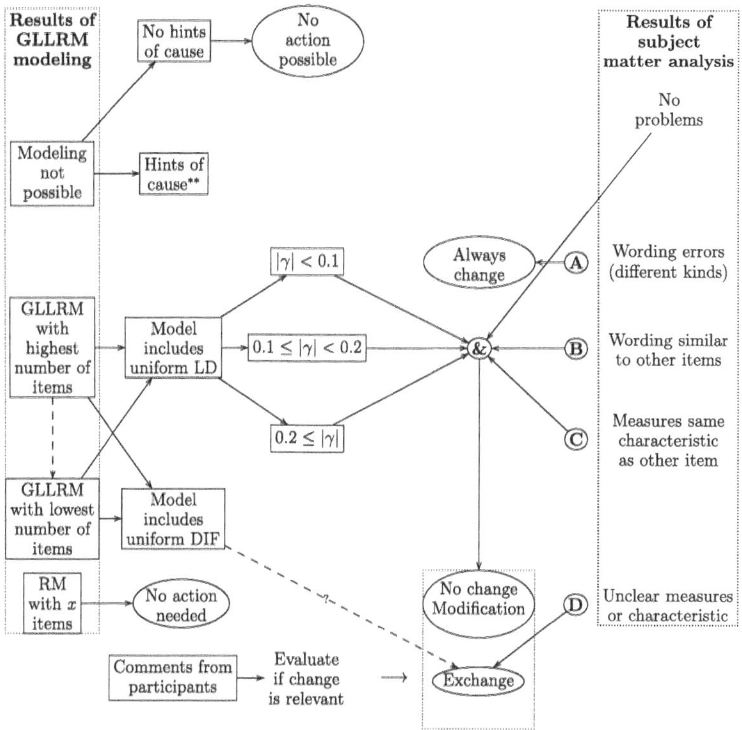

Figure 17.1. *The modification strategy. "&" signifies that different analysis results are combined into the decision of modification action. **The hints can in principle refer to, guessing, discrimination, distribution, local dependence and DIF issues*

As illustrated on the right in Figure 17.1 and in the columns of Table 17.1, the *subject matter analysis* can show that there are no problems with the items of the scale, in which case no changes to the scale are needed, or it can pinpoint a range of scale problems classified in four groups.

When applying the modification strategy, the starting point is the results of GLLRM analysis (the rows in Table 17.1). These results identify the items that need special attention during the subject matter analysis. The next step is the subject matter analysis (the columns in Table 17.1). During the last step, a modification is chosen on the basis of the results of the analyses (the cells in Table 17.1). Before going into detail with the specific relationships between results and choice of action, it should be noted that modification is only warranted for items pinpointed by both analyses, for example a GLLRM with high degree of uniform LD between items F and G together with subject matter analysis showing that these items measure the same characteristic (type C problem).

GLLRM analysis results	Subject matter analyses results				
	No problem	Type B wording similar	Type C measure same characteristic	Type D unclear measure	Type A wording error
RM (No problem with items)	No change	No change	No change	Exchange single item	Single item modification
GLLRM with *low* uniform LD[a]	No change	No change	No change	Exchange single item*****	Single item modification
GLLRM with *moderate* uniform LD[b]	No change	Mutual modification of items	Exchange single item	Exchange single item *****	Single item modification
GLLRM with *high* uniform LD[c]	No change	Mutual modification of items	Exchange single item	Exchange single item*****	Single item modification
GLLRM with uniform DIF[d]	No change	Exchange single item **	Exchange single item **	Exchange single item	Single item modification
Modeling not possible	No change	Exchange single item (consider additional problematic items for modification)	Exchange single item (consider additional problematic items for modification)	Exchange single item	Single item modification

Notes.
[a]Negligable problems = low uniform LD when $\gamma < |0.1|$.
[b]Moderate problems = moderate uniform LD when $0.1 \leq |\gamma| < 0.2$.
[c]Severe problems = high uniform LD when $|\gamma| > 0.2$.
[d]When resulting GLLRM includes uniform DIF, each case should be judged individually for two reasons: (1) the model might only be accepted when a certain DIF component is included but the size of the DIF (i.e. the gamma value) is negligible, (2) even with strong DIF, it is not certain that sense can be made of it conceptually. In both cases (1) and (2) DIF may be an error and can be considered irrelevant.
** Logically incompatible combinations of GLLRM with uniform DIF and type B or C problems.
***** Logically incompatible combinations of type D and GLLRM with any degree of uniform LD.

Table 17.1. *Choice of modification action, based on analyses results*

17.3.1. *Choice of modification action*

In Table 17.1, the choice of action depends on combinations of results of the GLLRM analyses and the subject matter analyses in a general pattern, where increasing severity of the problems detected in the two types of analysis warrant increasing degrees of changes made to items. Because of the difference in nature of the two types of analyses, some combinations are logically incompatible (marked ** and *****), and the choice of modification action in these cases must depend on the results of single regime of analysis.

Incompatible results are also possible, where the nature of one problem warrants a certain type of modification regardless of the result of the other analysis. In this case, choice of modification depends on the results of a single analysis.

The cases where the choice of modification action depends solely on the *results of the subject matter analysis* are as follows:

– When the subject matter analysis reveals the presence of less severe *(type A) problems* with items, this should always lead to modification of the relevant item(s) regardless of the results of the GLLRM analysis, because these problems effect the reliability of the scale and can contribute to generating spurious problems with other items. These problems should preferably be eliminated before new data collection takes place. If type A problems occur in combination with the more severe problems (type B and C) we recommend that the type A problem is corrected and the other problems are ignored, if an extra phase of data collection, required if type B and C problems persist, is a possibility.

– When the subject matter analysis does *not reveal problems* with items, no change is recommended regardless of the problems pointed out by the GLLRM analysis. This recommendation is made because the problems revealed by statistical analysis could be caused by type I errors., when they are not reflected in the subject matter analysis. Even if these problems are not due to error it would be impossible to change items, without the information from the subject matter analysis.

– When the subject matter analysis reveals the most severe *(type D) problems* with an item, we recommend that the item be exchanged with an item measuring another (in the sense more precise) characteristic of the construct regardless of the results of the GLLRM analysis, due to the effect the inclusion of unclear measures has on the scale's validity. The recommendation includes type D problems discovered in combination with data fitting a pure RM, because the theoretical foundation of the model is then imprecise. The recommendation also extends to the logically incompatible combinations of type D and GLLRM with any degree of uniform LD (marked ***** in Table 17.1), because in these cases we expect the LD to be caused by statistical type I error and therefore not contributing information to the decision of modification action.

The cases where the choice of modification action depends solely on the results of the *GLLRM analysis* are as follows:

– When the GLLRM includes *low uniform LD* (i.e. $\gamma < |0.1|$), no modification action is needed. This recommendation is based on the consideration that this type of problem may be due to type I error. The results of the subject matter analysis in the development study support this consideration in that we found that a low degree of LD was related with finding no problems or problems of type C involving only one of the items contributing to the LD – none of which warrant modification of the pair of items involved in the LD.

– When the GLLRM includes *uniform DIF*, we recommend that the item be exchanged with an item measuring another characteristic to avoid the inconveniences of dealing with biased items during calculation of scores. This recommendation also extend to the logically incompatible combinations of GLLRM with uniform DIF and type B or C problems (marked ** in Table 17.1), because the subject matter problems cannot contribute any information on the nature of the changes needed to eliminate DIF. Of course, other options outside the framework of this modification strategy are available: to perform additional GLLRM analysis and thereby choosing another model, as the basis of the modification strategy; to perform more advanced qualitative investigations into the nature of the DIF problem; or to retain the item without modifying it, using subsequent score equating to determine the correct scale score for the different groups defined by the exogenous variable involved in the DIF.

The cases where the choice of modification depends on combinations of the results of both the GLLRM and subject matter analyses are the cases where the subject matter analysis reveals problems of type B or C and the GLLRM analysis either reveals no problems or moderate or high uniform LD. Different modification actions are recommended as follows:

– No change is recommended when the GLLRM analysis reveals that data fits a *pure RM* combined with subject matter analysis revealing a *type B or type C problem* with items included in the GLLRM. The recommendation is based on the finding in the development study [NIE 05c] that no problems revealed in the statistical analysis is reflected in the subject matter analysis as no problems in the majority of cases in this study – in a few cases the subject matter analysis revealed type A problems and in one case a type D problem – leading us to the conclusion that type B and type C problems can be so slight that they will not turn up as problems (of LD) in the statistical analysis.

– Mutual modification of involved items is recommended when the subject matter analysis reveals a *type B problem* (similar wording as other items) with the items pointed out as contributing to *moderate* (i.e. $0.1 =< |\gamma| < 0.2$) *or high* (i.e. $|\gamma| >= 0.2$) *uniform LD* by the GLLRM analysis. It is then of course up to the researcher to decide the exact modifications to be made to the items, based on a thorough analysis of the wording of the items mutually and in relation to the remaining items in the scale.

– Exchange of a single item is recommended when the subject matter analysis reveals a *type C problem* (measures same characteristic as other items) with the items pointed out as contributing to *moderate* (i.e. $0.1 =< |\gamma| < 0.2$) *or high* (i.e. $|\gamma| >= 0.2$) *uniform LD* by the GLLRM analysis. Again, it is up to the researcher to decide which of the two items is to be exchanged, based on a thorough analysis of their relationships to the other items in the scale and their precision of measurement.

– Mutual modification or exchange of a single item is recommended, when the GLLRM analysis shows *moderate* (i.e. $0.1 =< |\gamma| < 0.2$) *or high* (i.e. $|\gamma| >= 0.2$) *uniform LD* combined with the subject matter results of *type B* (similar wording) or *type C* (measure same characteristic) problems. This is based on the finding that high LD in the majority of cases in the development study [NIE 05c] was reflected in the subject matter analysis as either type B or type C problems or a combination of both – and vice versa – the analyses results thereby verifying each other. We then extend the recommendation to include moderate LD, because we consider moderate LD to be problematic if the problem is indeed reflected in the subject matter analysis.

– Exchanging a single item with an item measuring a different characteristic of the style with possible modification of other involved items is recommended when the subject matter analysis reveals a *type B* problem (similar wording in items) or a *type C* problem (measures same characteristic as other items), if the item(s) are pointed out as possibly causing *modeling problems* by the GLLRM analysis, because specific departures from RMs generate spurious evidence of other types of problems.

It should be noted that if both type B and type C problems relating to an item are found in the cases above, we recommend that modification action is always chosen on the basis of the type C problem (and the specific problem pointed out by the GLLRM analysis), because a type C problem is considered the more severe of the two.

17.3.2. *Result of applying the scale improvement strategy*

In the study where the scale improvement strategy was developed, the strategy was applied to 13 Danish learning style scales, which had been translated from American English, adapted to Danish culture and evaluated by an expert panel, in order to improve their psychometric quality [NIE 05c]. The results showed considerable improvement in 10 scales. In seven scales, a higher number of items were included in the "best" revised scale model, whereas in three scales, the model had improved from being a GLLRM to being a pure RM with the same number of items. One scale had not changed (psychometrically) in any noteworthy way. The last two scales had declined slightly in quality from the initial to the revised version: one scale had an additional LD component in the GLLRM, and the other scale had unfortunately been revised in a manner that had added a DIF component (by gender) to the GLLRM for the scale.

The scale improvement strategy has also been applied as part of the process to develop the democratic learning style scale [NIE 07a], and in the development of six scales measuring different dimensions in a student semester evaluation, with good results [NIE 07b].

17.4. Application of the strategy to the Physical Functioning Scale of the SF-36

The PF scale of the SF-36 [WAR 93] comprises 10 items with three response categories; "no, not limited at all", "yes, limited a little" and "yes, limited a lot". The items are shown in Table 17.2.

Item	Item wording
PF1	Vigorous activities, such as running, lifting heavy objects and participating in strenuous sports
FF2	Moderate activities, such as moving a table, pushing a vacuum cleaner, bowling and playing golf
PF3	Lifting or carrying groceries
PF4	Climbing several flights of stairs
PF5	Climbing one flight of stairs
PF6	Bending, kneeling or stooping
PF7	Walking more than a mile
PF8	Walking several blocks
PF9	Walking one block
PF10	Bathing or dressing yourself

Table 17.2. *The 10 items of the PF sub-scale of the SF-36. Items are presented under the common heading "The following items are about activities you might do during a typical day. Does your health now limit you in these activities? If so, how much?" (response categories: "no, not limited at all", "yes, limited a little" and "yes, limited a lot")*

17.4.1. *Results of the GLLRM*

Kreiner and Christensen's analysis of the PF scale showed items PF2 to PF10 to fit a GLLRM with LD between four item pairs and five items functioning differentially relative to three exogenous variables: gender, age and self-reported health (SRH). Modeling was not possible when including item PF1 [KRE 07]. The magnitudes of the LD and DIF in the nine-item PF-scale fitting a GLLRM are shown in Table 17.3.

Note that two of the DIF departures in the final GLLRM were insignificant, and one was marginally significant. Also, note that the great number and the complexity of the departures from the RM in the PF-scale, and the fact that it was not possible to reach an RM in the analyses, makes the scale a perfect candidate for modification, as a traditional item elimination strategy would leave us with no scale.

Item showing DIF	Exogenous variable	γ	p
PF2	BMI	0.27	0.000
PF3	SRH	0.21	0.013
PF3	Sex	−0.38	0.000
PF8	Age	−0.04	0.747
PF10	SRH	−0.15	0.254
Item pairs showing LD		γ	p
PF2 and PF3		0.75	0.000
PF4 and PF5		0.76	0.000
PF7 and PF8		0.53	0.000
PF8 and PF9		0.95	0.000

Table 17.3. *Local response dependence and differential item functioning in nine-item PF-scale*

17.4.2. *Results of the subject matter analysis*

The GLLRM identified nine items requiring special attention during the subject matter analysis, because the only item not involved in either LD or DIF was PF6. However, as pointed out earlier, all items should be investigated in this phase, as evident from the results of the subject matter analysis.

PF1 (*vigorous activities*, such as running, lifting heavy objects and participating in strenuous sports) was found to be an *unclear measure* (type D problem). This in the sense that the listed example activities are very different from each other with regard to the stamina required to perform these activities, the involved body parts and being rare versus more common activities.

PF2 (*moderate activities*, such as moving a table, pushing a vacuum cleaner, bowling and playing golf) was found to be an *unclear measure* (type D problem). As with PF1, the listed example activities are very different from each other with regard to the stamina required to perform these activities and being everyday versus rare activities.

PF2 (*moderate activities*, such as moving a table, pushing a vacuum cleaner, bowling and playing golf) and PF3 (lifting or carrying groceries) were found to be *measuring the same characteristic*, physical activities (type C problem).

PF4 (climbing *several* flights of stairs) and PF5 (climbing *one* flight of stairs) were found to be *measuring the same characteristic*, stair climbing, (type C problem) and to be very *similar in wording* (type B problem).

PF6 (bending, kneeling or stooping) was found to be an *unclear measure* (type D problem), in the sense that the item is asking for a common answer to three quite different physical actions involving different body parts.

PF7 (walking *more than a mile*), PF8 (walking *several blocks*) and PF9 (walking *one block*) were found to be *measuring the same characteristic*, walking, (type C problem) and to be very *similar in wording* (type B problem).

PF10 (bathing or dressing yourself) was found to be an *unclear measure* (type D problem). This in the sense that even though these two activities often follow each other, they require quite different levels of physical functioning; bathing involves slippery floors, the ability to reach every part of your body, etc., whereas dressing yourself is a more safe activity that can be performed mostly seated and does not require as much physical mobility as bathing. Also, these two activities are for many people undertaken at quite different time intervals; bathing maybe as rarely as once a week, whereas dressing for many is at least a daily activity.

17.4.3. *Suggestions according to the strategy*

The combined results of the GLLRM and subject matter analyses and how these point to different modifications of items are given in Table 17.4, which shows that several items are involved in more than one type of departure from the RM and also suffer from more than one problem according to the subject matter analysis. To determine the specific changes needed for a single item, we have to simultaneously consider all the findings of problems concerning this item as well as other items that are involved in these problems. The rest of this chapter attempts to do so.

PF1 (vigorous activities, such as running, lifting heavy objects and participating in strenuous sports): The combination of the facts that modeling fails when this model is included and that the measurement properties of the item are unclear (type D problem) suggests that the item should be replaced by a new item. On the basis of the information gained in the subject matter analysis, our specific suggestion is that the new item is constructed of vigorous activities that are more similar or without examples at all.

PF2 (moderate activities, such as moving a table, pushing a vacuum cleaner, bowling and playing golf): This item is involved in both several departures from the pure RM and several content-wise problems. First, the combination of strong DIF relative to body mass Index (BMI) together with the item being an unclear measure (type D problem) motivates that the item be exchanged with a clearer one. Second, the strong LD between this item and item PF3 (lifting or carrying groceries) together with the finding that these two items measure the same characteristic (type C problem) also suggests that one of the two items should be exchanged. Because the first combination of problems is the more severe one, usually we would replace PF2 with a more precisely measuring item. However, as the two items also measure the same characteristic, we also need to make changes in order to differentiate these items better. This could, of course, be done by replacing PF2 with an item measuring another characteristic of physical functioning, but as item PF3 was also found to be suffering from DIF, both relative to SRH (though only marginally significant) and relative to gender in combination with no content-wise problems found in the subject matter analysis, we have to think more about the meaning of these DIF departures as well, before specific decisions on how to modify the questions are made.

GLLRM analysis results	Subject matter analyses results				
	No problem	Type B wording similar	Type C measure same characteristic	Type D unclear measure	Type A wording error
RM (No problem with items)			**PF6** Exchange single item		
GLLRM with *low* uniform LD					
GLLRM with *moderate* uniform LD					
GLLRM with *high* uniform LD		PF4 + PF5 PF7 + PF8 PF8 + PF9 Mutual modification of items	**PF2 + PF3** **PF4 + PF5** **PF7 + PF8** **PF8 + PF9** Exchange single item		
GLLRM with uniform DIF	**PF3, (PF8)** No change			**PF2, (PF10)** Exchange single item	
Modeling not possible				**PF1** Exchange single item	

NOTE. *Bold* item names signify that the suggested modification action is chosen. Item names in normal text signify that the suggested modification action is *not* chosen. Parentheses () signify that the departure from the RM is insignificant.

Table 17.4. *Specific suggestions for modification actions on the SF-36 items, based on analyses results*

The DIF of PF3 relative to SRH means that respondents reporting the highest levels of SRH are more inclined to say that they have no difficulties lifting or carrying groceries than respondents at the same general level of physical functioning but at lower levels of SRH. Because this DIF departure is only marginally significant and because we did not find any content-wise problems we suggest that item PF3 is not modified on the basis of these findings.

The DIF of PF3 relative to sex implies that male respondents are less inclined to say that they are limited compared to women at the same level of physical functioning.

Even though we found no problems during the subject matter analysis of this item, we consider the DIF to be genuine due to the fact that there are probably gender-related differences with regard to how usual it is to be carrying groceries and because males – everything else being equal – are expected to be stronger than women. To avoid these problems, we suggest that PF3 is exchanged with an item asking about a more gender–neutral physical activity in a way that should be closely related to the solution chosen for item PF2.

The DIF of PF2 relative to BMI implies that respondents with high levels of BMI are more inclined to say that they are more limited than respondents at the same level of physical functioning, but at lower levels of BMI. Therefore, and because PF2 measures across very different activities (hence the unclear measure), we suggest that the item is replaced with an item listing example activities that are all everyday activities that all respondents need to perform as part of their everyday lives. In this way, all respondents regardless of BMI should be equally inclined toward the different answer possibilities at different levels of physical functioning, so that the DIF might be eliminated. If this solution is chosen, care should be taken to ensure that the new item PF2 does not measure the same characteristic as the new item PF3. An alternative – and probably a better – suggestion could be to split this item up into a number of items, each asking about one single everyday activity. If this solution is chosen, then item PF3 could be included in this array of "different daily activities" items.

PF4 (climbing several flights of stairs): A strong degree of LD was found between this item and item PF5 (climbing one flight of stairs) in combination with the finding of both similar wording of these items (type B problem) and measurement of the same characteristic by both items (type C problem) (Table 17.2). According to the strategy, the more severe type C problem should be the one attended to. As such, it should be determined which of the two items (PF4 + PF5) should be exchanged. Because the items measure exactly the same characteristic of physical functioning, namely stair climbing, we suggest that the two items are combined into one single item measuring this characteristic.

PF6 (bending, kneeling or stooping): This item was not found to suffer from any problems in relation to the log-linear Rasch analyses, but in the subject matter analysis it was found to be an unclear measure (type D problem). According to the strategy, we suggest that the item is exchanged with a new and more precisely item measuring one physical function rather than several different ones.

PF8 (walking several blocks): This item is involved in several departures from the pure RM, and the subject matter analysis point to the item being involved in several content-wise problems as well. The question therefore is that the modification of the item should be based on which problems. First, there is the combination of weakly significant evidence of DIF relative to age and no problems found in the subject matter analysis for the item alone. Second, there is the strong LD between this item and item PF7 (walking more than a mile) as well as item PF9 (walking one block) in combination with the finding of both similar wording of these three items (type B problem) and measurement of the same characteristic by these three items (type C problem). According to the strategy, the more severe type C problem should be the one attended to. Accordingly, it should be determined which of the two pairs of items (PF7 + PF8, PF8 + PF9) should be exchanged. Because the three items indeed measure exactly the same characteristic of physical functioning, namely walking distance, we suggest that the three items are combined into one single item measuring this characteristic. PF10 (bathing or dressing yourself): The DIF of this item relative to SRH was found in combination with the item being an unclear measure (type D problem). According to the strategy, this suggests that the item should be exchanged with a more precisely formulated item (Table 17.2). Our suggestion is to replace PF10 with an item measuring the ability to bathe yourself, an item measuring the ability to dress yourself or both. However, as the DIF departure is less than conclusive because some of the DIF statistics are insignificant, the patient researcher could leave this change for a possible second round in the scale modification process – our choice would be to make the appropriate changes in a first round though.

17.5. Closing remark

The PF items violate a number of the fundamental assumptions of Rasch and IRT models. The GLLRM model found by Kreiner and Christensen [KRE 07] suggests that measurement despite this is essentially valid and objective. Items belonging to a pure RM are however, preferable and it would be interesting to see if the suggested changes will lead to improved psychometric quality of the physical functioning scale. We hope that someone will take on the challenge of changing the SF-36 and reporting on the results.

17.6. Bibliography

[AND 77] ANDERSEN E.B., "Sufficient statistics and latent trait models", *Psychometrika*, vol. 42, pp. 69–81, 1977.

[AND 04] ANDRICH D., STYLES I., Report on the psychometric properties of the Early Development Inventory (EDI), Unpublished report for Institute for Child Health Research, Perth, Western Australia, 2004.

[BAR 96] BARTHOLOMEW D.J., *The Statistical Approach to Social Measurement*, Academic Press, London, 1996.

[DEV 03] DEVELLIS R.F., "Scale development. Theory and applications", *Applied Social Research Methods Series*, vol. 26, 2nd ed., Sage Publications, London, 2003.

[FIS 95] FISCHER G., "The derivation of polytomous Rasch models", in FISCHER G., MOLENAAR I. (eds), *Rasch Models: Foundations, Recent Developments and Applications*, Springer Verlag, New York, pp. 293–306, 1995.

[HAM 02] HAMON A., MESBAH M., "Questionnaire reliability under the Rasch model", in MESBAH M., COLE B.F., LEE M.T. (eds), *Statistical Methods for Quality of Life Studies. Design, Measurement and Analysis*, Kluwer Academic Publishers, London, pp. 155–168, 2002.

[HOL 88] HOLLAND P.W., THAYER D.T., "Differential item performance and the Mantel-Haenszel procedure", in WAINER H., BRAUN H.I. (eds), *Test Validity, Lawrence Erlbaum Associates*, Hillsdale, NJ, pp. 129–245, 1988.

[HOL 93] HOLLAND P.W., WAINER H., *Differential Item Functioning*, Lawrence Erlbaum Associates, Hillsdale, NJ, 1993.

[KRE 02] KREINER S., CHRISTENSEN K.B., "Graphical Rasch models", in MESBAH M., COLE B.F., LEE M.T. (eds), *Statistical Methods for Quality of Life Studies*, Kluwer Academic Publishers, Dordrecht, pp. 187–203, 2002.

[KRE 04] KREINER S., CHRISTENSEN K.B., "Analysis of local dependence and multidimensionality in graphical loglinear Rasch models", *Communication in Statistics. A Theory and Methods*, vol. 33, pp. 1239–1276, 2004.

[KRE 07] KREINER S., CHRISTENSEN K.B., "Validity and objectivity in health reelated summated scales: analysis by graphical loglinear Rasch models", in VON DAVIER M., CARSTENSEN C. (eds), *Multivariate and Mixture Distribution Rasch Models – Extensions and Applications*, Springer Verlag, New York, pp. 329–346, 2007.

[KRE 11] KREINER S., CHRISTENSEN K.B., "Item screening in graphical loglinear Rasch models", *Psychometrika*, vol. 76, pp. 228–256, 2011.

[NIE 05a] NIELSEN T., Spørgeskema og tolkningsmanual til selvvurdering af læringsstile, Unpublished, 2005.

[NIE 05b] NIELSEN T., Learning styles of Danish university students, Doctoral Thesis, Department of Educational Psychology, Danish University of Education, Copenhagen, 2005.

[NIE 05c] NIELSEN T., KREINER S., "Modifying or replacing items: a suggestion for a strategy", in NIELSEN T. (ed.), *Learning Styles of Danish University Students*, Doctoral Thesis, Department of Educational Psychology, Danish University of Education, Copenhagen, 2005, Paper 1.

[NIE 07a] NIELSEN T., KREINER S., STYLES I., "Mental self-government: development of the additional democratic learning style scale using Rasch measurement models", *Journal of Applied Measurement*, vol. 8, pp. 124–148, 2007.

[NIE 07b] NIELSEN T., RAVN J., Test af nyt evalueringsskema på Cand. Merc., Report for the Cand. Merc. study board at Copenhagen Business School, Unpublished, 2007.

[NIE 11] NIELSEN A.B.S., GANNIK D., SIERSMA V., OLIVARIUS N.D.F., "The relationship between HbA1c level, symptoms and self-rated health in type 2 diabetic patients", *Scandinavian Journal of Primary Health Care*, vol. 29, pp. 157–164, 2011.

[RAS 60] RASCH G., *Probabilistic Models for Some Intelligence and Attainment Tests*, The Danish Institute for Educational Research, Copenhagen, 1960.

[RAS 66] RASCH G., "An informal report on the present state of a theory of objectivity in comparisons", *Proceedings of the NUIFFIC International Summer Session in Science at the Het Onde Hof*, The Hague, pp. 14–28, 1966.

[RAS 77] RASCH G., "On Specific objectivity: an attempt at formalizing the request for generality and validity of scientific statements", *Danish Year Book of Philosophy*, vol. 14, pp. 58–94, 1977, Reprinted in D.J. Bartholomew, Measurement, vol. II, Sage Publications, London, pp. 3–42, 2006.

[ROS 89] ROSENBAUM P.R., "Criterion-related construct validity", *Psychometrika*, vol. 54, pp. 625–633, 1989.

[WAR 93] WARE J.E. JR., SNOW K.K., KOSINSKI M., GANDEK B., *SF-36 Health Survey. Manual and Interpretation Guide*, The Health Institute, New England Medical Center, Boston, MA, 1993.

PART 6

Analyzing and Reporting Rasch Models

Chapter 18

Software for Rasch Analysis

18.1. Introduction

The measurement and analysis of latent variables is of great importance in clinical research. The use of patient reported outcomes in clinical research and epidemiology has increased during the past decades. Such increase was partly due to the phenomenal development of hardware and software in computing. Computer programs nowadays can analyze large data sets of more complexity.

In the recent past, general statistical packages did not allow users to perform item analysis or to estimate parameters of most common models in this specific field. The practitioners were obliged to use various specific software to analyze measurement properties of a questionnaire. Moreover, each of these were often very limited, and often practitioners were obliged to use several software packages to perform a valid analysis, because no single package contained all necessary analyses.

Well-known statistical packages, such as Statistical Analysis System (SAS), SPSS, S-plus R and Stata, have recently (since the end of the 1990s) developed procedures that allow estimating the parameters of linear or generalized linear fixed or mixed models. This very late appearance is certainly due to the increasing complexity of algorithms used in such fields.

In this chapter, we first present software packages for Rasch analysis and describe briefly what each package can do. The reader can find more information about each software package on the Internet. Next, we present and discuss a SAS macro and an R package that programmers in SAS or R language can use. Finally, we present simple

---

Chapter written by Mounir MESBAH.

SAS programs that can be used to estimate Rasch or partial credit model parameters, or to generate Rasch or partial credit items.

18.2. Stand alone softwares packages

This section briefly presents stand-alone Rasch software. The list is far from complete, and a more complete list, including direct links to each software Website, can be found at `www.rasch.org/software.html`. All of the discussed packages provide estimates of item and person parameters, and fit statistics. They differ with respect to the inference frame. DIGRAM is free software, while the others are proprietary.

18.2.1. *WINSTEPS*

WINSTEPS is a widely used Rasch software program for the windows platform. It uses the joint maximum likelihood (JML) method of estimation of parameters. Originally developed at the University of Chicago, its latest update is from 2009 by Linacre [LIN 09]. In addition to the standard Rasch variable maps, person and item measures, and fit statistics, WINSTEPS also provides many advanced analytical features, such as distractor analysis, principal component analysis of Rasch residuals for assessing unidimensionality and analysis of differential item functioning. It reports tables, files, plots and graphs. A free student version is also available.

18.2.2. *RUMM*

RUMM was developed at the RUMM Laboratory in Perth, Australia. A time-limited version is usually provided as part of a popular online course offered periodically by several universities. RUMM provides an all-graphical interface that uses familiar point and click set-up features, as found in commercial statistical packages such as SPSS and JMP. It can output a wide range of multicolor charts and graphs, and fit a variety of Rasch models, including dichotomous, rating scale and partial credit models. It is also highly interactive, providing easy reanalysis following diagnosis of previous analyses. The latest version is RUMM2030 [AND 10]. The estimation is based on pairwise conditional maximum likelihood.

18.2.3. *CONQUEST*

CONQUEST was developed by Wu *et al.* [WU 07] at the Australian Council for Educational Research as an improved update of Quest, an older software program. Besides the standard dichotomous, rating scale, partial credit and many-facet Rasch models, CONQUEST also estimates a multidimensional Rasch model using MML methods. It outputs a wide range of informative graphs, charts and variable maps. It is a powerful and flexible program that combines Rasch with latent regression model.

18.2.4. *DIGRAM*

DIGRAM is part of a larger statistical package, SCD, supporting Statistical analysis of Categorical Data. The program dates back to 1980s and is dedicated to analysis of high-dimensional contingency tables by block recursive chain graphical models. It has since then been expanded to cover other types of models and problems as well, while still focusing on problems that could be solved complete or partly by simple tests for conditional independence. The current version of DIGRAM supports item analysis by graphical and log-linear Rasch models for dichotomous and polytomous items using the conditional frame of inference. Importantly, DIGRAM provides exactly the same tests of fit for the GLLRM as for the pure Rasch model. DIGRAM also provides a number of routines that can be used to construct a GLLRM using an item screening procedure [KRE 11]. DIGRAM is free software, but is not as well-known as the three previously discussed software packages.

18.3. Implementations in standard software

Recently, software procedures, such as NLMIXED in SAS, the NLME library in Splus, and GLLAMM in STATA, have made nonlinear random effects models like the Rasch model in the marginal frame of inference, which is a standard tool. On the other hand the theoretical relationship between the Rasch model and the multiplicative Poisson model has been well-known for many years. This means that conditional maximum likelihood estimation can be done using generalized linear models [TJU 82, KEL 84] and can thus be implemented in standard statistical software.

The parameters of the Rasch model can thus be estimated in standard software like SAS [CHR 06]. This section describes software using these possibilities.

18.3.1. *SAS macro for MML estimation*

The SAS macro %ANAQOL was written by Hardouin and Mesbah [HAR 07]. It easily and automatically provides (1) indices like Cronbach coefficient α, (2) various useful graphical representations, including different kinds of item traces and Backward Reliability Curves, and (3) estimation of the parameters of five IRT models among the most famous (Rasch, Birnbaum, OPLM, partial credit model (PCM) and rating scale model (RSM)). Goodness of fit tests are implemented for dichotomous items, and the fit of the models can be evaluated by graphical comparison of the expected and observed item characteristics curves, as well as infit and outfit test statistics. Results are composed of outputs of SAS procedures, specific tables and graphical representations.

18.3.2. *SAS macros based on CML estimation*

Christensen and Bjorner [CHR 03] describe a number of SAS macros that can be used for latent variable models based on the Rasch model. They present macros for item parameters estimation using conditional maximum likelihood (CML), for testing the assumption of unidimensionality and for fitting regression models where either outcome variables or covariates are latent variables measured using (loglinear) Rasch models.

Most notably, their macro %RASCH can do CML estimation for dichotomous *and* polytomous items. Plots of observed and expected item category frequencies stratified by the total score are also available. The macro %LLRASCH fits some simple log-linear Rasch models and the Martin-Löf test described in Chapter 9 is implemented in their macro %PML. Christensen and Bjorner also present macros for latent regression.

18.3.3. *eRm: an R Package*

The eRm package (http://epub.wu.ac.at/332/) fits the following models: the Rasch model, the RSM and the PCM, as well as linear reparameterizations through covariate structures, such as the linear logistic test model (LLTM), the linear rating scale model (LRSM) and the linear partial credit model (LPCM). It uses an unitary, efficient CML approach to estimate the item parameters and their standard errors. Graphical and numerical tools for assessing goodness of fit are provided.

18.4. Fitting the Rasch model in SAS

Finally, we present a few simple programs illustrating how to (1) simulate a data set of 10 dichotomous Rasch items and (2) estimate, using different methods, their item parameters.

18.4.1. *Simulation of Rasch dichotomous items*

Responses to a set of Rasch dichotomous items can be simulated using the following program:

```
/* simulate theta */
%let N=1000;
data latent;
    do ind=1 to &N;
        theta=rannor(0);
        output;
    end;
run;
/* simulate item responses */
data Rasch;
    set latent;
    b1=quantile('NORMAL',.05);
    b2=quantile('NORMAL',.15);
    :
    b10=quantile('NORMAL',.95);
    L1=b1+theta; E1=exp(L1)/(1+exp(L1)); X1=ranbin(0,1,E1);
    L2=b2+theta; E2=exp(L2)/(1+exp(L2)); X2=ranbin(0,1,E2);
    :
    L10=b10+theta;E10=exp(L10)/(1+exp(L10)); X10=ranbin(0,1,E10);
    total=X1+X2+X3+X4+X5+X6+X7+X8+X9+X10;
run;
```

The purpose of the first data step is to fix the sample size N and simulate the latent variable with a normal distribution with zero mean and unit variance. The role of the second data step is to generate a sample of N responses of 10 binary Rasch items, with specified values for item parameters. We have chosen item parameters located in increasing positions on the normal scale, but other values can be choosen. We can, then, directly put the chosen value of the item parameter.

18.4.2. *MML estimation using PROC NLMIXED*

MML estimation using PROC NLMIXED is done as follows:

```
/* transpose */
data rasch1; set rasch; keep ind X1-X10; run;
proc sort data=rasch1; by ind; run;
proc transpose data=rasch1 out=outtable name=Question Prefix=resp;
by ind; run;
/* recode */
data TableRasch; set outtable;
    if Question="X1"  then X1 =1; else X1 =0;
    if Question="X2"  then X2 =1; else X2 =0;
    if Question="X3"  then X3 =1; else X3 =0;
    if Question="X4"  then X4 =1; else X4 =0;
    if Question="X5"  then X5 =1; else X5 =0;
    if Question="X6"  then X6 =1; else X6 =0;
```

```
    if Question="X7"  then X7 =1; else X7 =0;
    if Question="X8"  then X8 =1; else X8 =0;
    if Question="X9"  then X9 =1; else X9 =0;
    if Question="X10" then X10=1; else X10=0;
run;
/* estimate */
proc nlmixed data=TableRasch;
    parms beta1=0 beta2=0 beta3=0 beta4=0 beta5=0
                beta6=0 beta7=0 beta8=0 beta9=0 beta10=0 sigma=1;
    eta=theta-(beta1*X1+beta2*X2+beta3*X3+beta4*X4+beta5*X5
                    +beta6*X6+beta7*X7+beta8*X8+beta9*X9+beta10*X10;
    expeta=exp(eta); P=expeta/(1+expeta);
    model resp1 ~ binomial(1,p);
    random theta ~ normal(0,sigma*sigma) subject=ind;
run;
```

The sorted Rasch file is an SAS file with 11 columns, items `X1` to `X10` and `ind` the number (index) of each person. We create a new table, called OUTTABLE, with 10,000 rows and three column variables, where `Question` is a character variable containing the name of the corresponding item. Next, indicators variables are created. These are used by NLMIXED that does not support the CLASS statement. For an example of how to do this for polytomous items see [CHR 06].

18.4.3. *MML estimation of using PROC GLIMMIX*

MML estimation of the item parameters of the Rasch model can be done using PROC GLIMMIX:

```
proc glimmix data=TableRasch method=quad;
    class question ind;
    model resp1=question/noint dist=binomial link=logit solution cl;
    random intercept/subject=ind;
    output out=fic pred=p resid=r;
run;
```

18.4.4. *JML estimation using PROC LOGISTIC*

JML estimation of the item parameters of the Rasch model can be done using PROC LOGISTIC

```
proc logistic data=TableRasch;
    class question ind/PARAM=GLM;
    model resp1=ind question/noint TECH=NEWTON ABSFCONV=0.0001 cl;
run;
```

18.4.5. *CML estimation using PROC GENMOD*

CML estimation of the item parameters of the Rasch model can be done using PROC GENMOD

```
proc freq data=rasch;
    table X1*X2*X3*X4*X5*X6*X7*X8*X9*X10/sparse out=table noprint;
run;
data new; set table;
    sumscore=X1+X2+X3+X4+X5+X6+X7+X8+X9+X10;
    if COUNT=0 then COUNT=0.00000000001;
run;
ods output genmod.estimates=est;
/* estimate */
proc genmod data=new;
    where 0<sumscore<10;
    class sumscore;
    model count=sumscore X1 X2 X3 X4 X5 X6 X7 X8 X9 X10 / dist=p noint;
    estimate 'beta1'  X1  9 X2 -1 X3 -1 X4 -1 X5 -1 X6 -1 X7 -1 X8 -1 X9 -1 X10 -1;
    estimate 'beta2'  X1 -1 X2  9 X3 -1 X4 -1 X5 -1 X6 -1 X7 -1 X8 -1 X9 -1 X10 -1;
    estimate 'beta3'  X1 -1 X2 -1 X3  9 X4 -1 X5 -1 X6 -1 X7 -1 X8 -1 X9 -1 X10 -1;
    estimate 'beta4'  X1 -1 X2 -1 X3 -1 X4  9 X5 -1 X6 -1 X7 -1 X8 -1 X9 -1 X10 -1;
    estimate 'beta5'  X1 -1 X2 -1 X3 -1 X4 -1 X5  9 X6 -1 X7 -1 X8 -1 X9 -1 X10 -1;
    estimate 'beta6'  X1 -1 X2 -1 X3 -1 X4 -1 X5 -1 X6  9 X7 -1 X8 -1 X9 -1 X10 -1;
    estimate 'beta7'  X1 -1 X2 -1 X3 -1 X4 -1 X5 -1 X6 -1 X7  9 X8 -1 X9 -1 X10 -1;
    estimate 'beta8'  X1 -1 X2 -1 X3 -1 X4 -1 X5 -1 X6 -1 X7 -1 X8  9 X9 -1 X10 -1;
    estimate 'beta9'  X1 -1 X2 -1 X3 -1 X4 -1 X5 -1 X6 -1 X7 -1 X8 -1 X9  9 X10 -1;
    estimate 'beta10' X1 -1 X2 -1 X3 -1 X4 -1 X5 -1 X6 -1 X7 -1 X8 -1 X9 -1 X10  9;
run;
/* output */
data est;
    set est;
    estimate=LBetaEstimate/10; lower=LBetaLowerCL/10; upper=LBetaUpperCL/10;
    keep estimate lower upper;
run;
proc print data=est round noobs; run;
```

18.4.6. *JML estimation using PROC LOGISTIC*

JML estimation of the item parameters of the Rasch model can be done using PROC LOGISTIC

```
ods output logistic.clparmwald=est5;
proc logistic data=TableRasch;
    class question ind/PARAM=GLM;
    model resp1(EVENT='1')=ind question / noint TECH=NEWTON ABSFCONV=0.0001;
    output out=fic1 pred=p;
run;
ods rtf file='c:\file.rtf'; proc print data=est; run; ods rtf close;
```

18.4.7. *Results*

Results are shown in the table below. Values of true item parameters are in the second columns. All procedures (NLMIXED, GLIMMIX, GENMOD and LOGISTIC) provide confidence interval estimates including corresponding true value.

	True value	MML NLMIXED Est.	lower	upper	CML GENMOD Est.	lower	upper	MML GLIMMIX Est.	lower	upper	JML LOGISTIC Est.	lower	upper
β_1	−1.65	1.60	1.42	1.78	−1.64	−1.79	−1.48	−1.60	−1.78	−1.42	−0,93	−2,34	0,47
β_2	−1.04	0.99	0.83	1.15	−1.02	−1.16	−0.88	−0.99	−1.15	−0.83	−0.58	−1.99	0.82
β_3	−0.67	0.75	0.59	0.90	−0.78	−0.92	−0.64	−0.75	−0.90	−0.59	−0.45	−1.85	0.96
β_4	−0.39	0.32	0.17	0.47	−0.35	−0.49	−0.22	−0.32	−0.47	−0.17	−0.21	−1.61	1.20
β_5	−0.13	0.03	−0.12	0.18	−0.07	−0.20	0.06	−0.03	−0.18	0.12	−0.05	−1.45	1.36
β_6	0.13	−0.23	−0.38	−0.08	0.20	0.06	0.33	0.23	0.08	0.38	0.10	−1.30	1.50
β_7	0.39	−0.39	−0.54	−0.23	0.35	0.22	0.49	0.39	0.23	0.54	0.19	−1.22	1.59
β_8	0.67	−0.65	−0.80	−0.49	0.62	0.48	0.75	0.65	0.49	0.80	0.34	−1.07	1.74
β_9	1.04	−1.06	−1.22	−0.90	1.03	0.88	1.17	1.06	0.90	1.22	0.57	−0.84	1.97
β_{10}	1.65	−1.70	−1.89	−1.52	1.67	1.51	1.83	1.70	1.52	1.89	0.93	−0.47	2.34
σ	1	1.0042	0.9251	1.0832									

Table 18.1. *Comparison of item parameter estimates obtained using four different methods*

The table illustrates the advantages of MML and CML estimates compared to JML estimates because the confidence interval of the JML estimates is ten times larger than the confidence of the other estimates. Furthermore, the implementation in PROC LOGISTIC as shown here, is quite time consuming.

18.5. Bibliography

[AND 10] ANDRICH D., SHERIDAN B., LUO G., RUMM2030, Computer software and manual, RUMM Laboratory, Perth, Australia, 2010.

[CHR 03] CHRISTENSEN K.B., BJORNER J.B., SAS macros for Rasch based latent variable modelling, Research Report 13, Department of Biostatistics, University of Copenhagen, 2003.

[CHR 06] CHRISTENSEN K.B., "Fitting polytomous Rasch models in SAS", *Journal of Applied Measurement*, vol. 7, pp. 407–417, 2006.

[HAR 07] HARDOUIN J.B., MESBAH M., "The SAS macro-program %ANAQOL to estimate the parameters of item responses theory models", *Communication in Statistics—Theory and Methods*, vol. 36, pp. 437–453, 2007.

[KEL 84] KELDERMAN H., "Loglinear Rasch model tests", *Psychometrika*, vol. 49, pp. 223–245, 1984.

[KRE 03] KREINER S., Introduction to DIGRAM, Research report 03/10, Department of Biostatistics, University of copenhagen, Copenhagen, 2003.

[KRE 11] KREINER S., CHRISTENSEN K.B., "Item screening in graphical loglinear Rasch models", *Psychometrika*, vol. 76, pp. 228–256, 2011.

[LIN 09] LINACRE J.M., Winsteps (version 3.68), Computer Software and manual, Winsteps.com, Beaverton, OR, 2009.

[TJU 82] TJUR T., "A connection between Rasch's item analysis model and a multiplicative Poisson model", *Scandinavian Journal of Statistics*, vol. 9, pp. 23–30, 1982.

[WU 07] WU M.L., ADAMS R.J., WILSON M.R., HALDANE S., ConQuest (Version 2.0), Computer Software and manual, ACER, Camberwell, Australia, 2007.

Chapter 19

Reporting a Rasch Analysis

19.1. Introduction

19.1.1. *Objectives*

The Rasch model [RAS 60] is based on a philosophy of measurement that differs considerably from the predominant paradigm in the social sciences, understood as a collective term for sciences outside the domain of the natural sciences. Therefore, reporting a Rasch analysis raises questions as to what to include in a write-up. This chapter suggests a structure of a Rasch analysis report and its elements that corresponds to the philosophy of Rasch measurement. Although it is primarily meant for writing a manuscript, the concept also helps interpret and evaluate Rasch reports. The proposed scheme is on no account an empirical compilation of what sort of findings published Rasch papers actually report. Such an account would merely ensure compliance with what has been done up to now. By contrast, the orientation of this chapter is forward-looking. Furthermore, it is in no way implied that papers deviating from the suggested scheme are necessarily deficient. Conversely, there is no guarantee that papers that do follow the proposal are based on an adequate Rasch analysis. Throughout this chapter it is assumed that the instrument development and the underlying Rasch analysis are appropriate. Wolfe and Smith [WOL 07a] provide a good overview of proper instrument development, while Wolfe and Smith [WOL 07b] refer to measure validation using Rasch models. Tennant and Conaghan [TEN 07] focus on the fields of applications of the Rasch model in health and provide guidelines as to what to look for in a Rasch report. Hagquist *et al.* [HAG 09] demonstrate the potential of Rasch analysis in nursing research [HAG 09].

Chapter written by Thomas SALZBERGER.

19.1.2. *Factors impacting a Rasch analysis report*

To begin with, no single scheme meets the requirements of every Rasch analysis under all circumstances. The extent and the focus of a report primarily depend on the purpose of the Rasch analysis, but also on the characteristics of the particular scientific discipline and the fact how common Rasch analysis plays a role. Finally, restrictions and conventions of the research publication outlet have to be taken into consideration.

A Rasch analysis may either refer to an evaluation of an existing scale using Rasch methodology or to a new scale development project. In the first case, the audience is presumably familiar with the measurement instrument and its theoretical underpinnings but possibly less acquainted with the fundamentals of Rasch analysis. In the latter case, the report typically has to be more comprehensive and present the substantive theory of the construct in more detail.

Another distinction, which is certainly related to the issue of reanalysis versus new scale development, refers to the objective of the study being either substance driven or method driven. Substance-driven research aims at the measurement of a particular latent variable. It is more typical for applied research and new scale development, yet it also applies to studies that advance existing instruments to achieve a higher quality of measurement. In these cases, the report should be as comprehensive as possible and cover the substantive theory of the construct and a wide range of empirical evidence of the validity of the suggested scale. Alternatively, the research may investigate a methodological issue, for instance the assessment of multidimensionality or differential item functioning (DIF). In such studies, the latent variables considered are typically only illustrative. Consequently, the focus lies on selected properties or requirements of the Rasch analysis. While being of utmost importance to applications of Rasch methodology, applied researchers are rarely concerned with this type of fundamental research into Rasch measurement methodology. Yet another important determinant of a Rasch analysis report lies in the degree to which Rasch measurement is common and properly understood in a given scientific discipline. In education, for example, Rasch measurement is still more prevalent than in the health sciences [TEN 07] or in business studies [SAL 09]. If the audience is less familiar with Rasch measurement concepts, technical terms need to be defined and explained in more detail. For instance, the concept of reliability assessed by means of Cronbach's coefficient α [CRO 51] hardly requires any justification or explication in an empirical paper using standard methods rooted in classical test theory [LOR 68]. By contrast, the meaning of reliability in the context of a Rasch analysis or the definition of the person separation index [AND 82] cannot be taken for granted. The explanation of the item location parameter or, in the case of polytomous items, the threshold parameters often represents a special challenge, since there is no direct equivalent in classical test theory. Technical terms such as item difficulty that alludes to achievement testing should be avoided as they easily cause misunderstandings. What is more, publications in the social sciences often have to provide convincing arguments as to why the Rasch model has been applied at all. The consequences of the need for elaborating on the fundamentals of the Rasch measurement can be problematic when restrictions on space apply. Then the technical and philosophical underpinnings are explained at the expense of the substantive findings. Besides a lack of familiarity of journal reviewers, authors of Rasch papers often face paradigmatic resistance [AND 02, AND 04]. The reasons are manifold. The most important difference though seems to be related to the objective of measurement, which is, making things worse, hardly ever made explicit. Traditionally, measurement aims at an optimal fit of a measurement model to a given data set, which may be called the statistical paradigm (see [MIC 86]). The data takes precedence over the measurement model, which is chosen in a way as to best account for the data. Consequently, more flexible models, for example, item response theory models that allow for different item discrimination, are preferred. By contrast, the choice of the Rasch model of measurement is motivated by its unique properties that are considered indispensable to scientific measurement, for example the principle of specific objectivity [RAS 61, RAS 77, IRT 87, IRT 95] and the invariance property [AND 88] it entails, or raw score sufficiency [AND 77]. Thus, the Rasch measurement paradigm is in stark contrast to the statistical paradigm of traditional measurement.

In practice, arguing for the use of the Rasch model in non-Rasch media can be delicate. The exceptional position of the model has to be communicated while traditional patterns of thought have to be accommodated. It is important that authors refrain from overstating or misrepresenting the features of the Rasch model. In fact, its advantageous properties are requirements that data sets have to meet, rather than characteristics the Rasch model would deliver irrespective of data. The latter notion invites critics to claim that the Rasch model can be dismissed should the invariance property not hold across different samples.

If item misfit leads to discarding large parts of the original data set, the item scoring is modified or if many items are split in order to account for DIF, the analysis becomes to some extent exploratory when amendments are essentially data driven. It is a great virtue of the Rasch model that these problems are highlighted rather than hidden. However, it is imperative to try to provide, or at least suggest, theoretical explanations as to why items misfit, why response scales do not operate as expected or why items exhibit DIF.

19.1.3. *The role of the substantive theory of the latent variable*

The ambitious goals of a Rasch measurement analysis can only be fully met, if the substantive theory of the latent variables is sophisticated enough to not only suggest suitable items but also propose at least a theory-driven order of the items. Ideally the theory should identify a mechanism that allows for the prediction of quantitative relationships between item locations [STE 09]. In education, the Lexile framework for reading ability [STE 06] represents an example of a successful identification of a measurement mechanism. Whether such a level of substantive theory will be attained in attitudinal measurement remains to be seen. But it is definitely an objective worth striving for. In any case, if every order of item locations is *a priori* equally plausible, revealing a particular order is hardly informative. Then evidence of successful measurement is to all intents and purposes limited to statistical fit. In Popper's parlance, this resembles a cautious prediction rather than a bold conjecture, which drives scientific knowledge [POP 96]. Therefore, the Rasch analysis report should include a detailed account of the substantive theory (inasmuch as theory shapes expectations) as well as the implication of the empirical evidence for the theory. In practice, this claim may occasionally conflict with limitations of space in academic journals. Given that the predominant paradigm of measurement favors statistical evidence, this may lead to an overemphasis on numerical documentation.

The importance of the theoretical underpinnings of a suggested latent variable demonstrates the rather limited value of a reanalysis of an existing scale developed within the traditional paradigm of classical test theory compared to a Rasch-based scale development project. Since traditional construct theories normally lack any considerations in terms of the order of item locations, the Rasch analysis tends to be statistical in essence. Still the Rasch analysis may reveal anomalies in the data that raise doubts about the proper functioning of the items.

19.1.4. *The frame of reference*

The measurement of a quantitative latent variable always refers to a frame of reference [RAS 77], within which specific objectivity holds. Thus, the frame of reference is defined by the conditions under which comparisons are invariant. The specification of the frame of reference is an empirical problem. In other words, it has to be demonstrated that invariance actually holds across different conditions and for various respondents. It goes without saying that a wide frame of reference is desirable. Therefore, empirical evidence of invariance based on greatly diverse conditions is more informative than invariance assessment substantiated on marginally different conditions. In any case, the data set has to reflect the intended frame of reference to allow for its empirical investigation. Thus, the Rasch analysis report should provide information on the empirically established frame of reference.

19.2. Suggested elements

In the following, a comprehensive scheme for a Rasch analysis report is suggested that takes theoretical and empirical requirements into considerations. In a real data set, deviations from perfection as prescribed by the measurement model occur almost inevitably. Model violations are typically intertwined and eventually become manifest in misfit. Therefore, various reasons for misfit have to be disentangled, which can be an intricate task. As a rule, changes to the data set, for example the deletion of an item, rescoring of the responses or splitting an item, should be kept to a minimum at each stage of the analysis. Further diagnosis of misfit should then be based on a new estimation of model parameters and fit statistics. Some amendments to the data set might actually turn out to be inappropriate and consequently have to be revoked at a later stage. The Rasch analysis report can hardly reflect this multistage process adequately, but typically focuses on the final conclusion. Specifically, the order of suggested elements does not imply that the issues have to be dealt with in that order during the data analysis or that a unique order exists at all. However, regarding the whole scale development process, theoretical considerations have to precede data analysis. If empirical findings inform the theory, the research becomes exploratory and should therefore be marked as such.

19.2.1. *Construct: definition and operationalization of the latent variable*

The substantive theory of the latent variable is an integral part of a psychometric analysis. No sophisticated statistical procedure compensates theoretical deficiencies or omissions. Thus, a description of the construct is an indispensable element of the measurement report. As mentioned before, first of all the theory of the construct should inform the researcher as to how suitable items look like. Furthermore, the theory should suggest an expected order of the items on the latent continuum. In the long run, an elaborated theory of a construct should allow for concrete quantitative predictions in terms of the relationships between items. This would ensure that the empirical claim of the measurement of a quantitative latent variable is matched by an equally quantitative theory of the latent variable. A construct map [WIL 05] is one way to visualize the anticipated order of the items in terms of their location on the latent dimension.

The plausibility of the substantive theory is traditionally associated with content validity, which is assessed qualitatively and often suffers from a confirmation bias [KAN 01]. A substantive theory suitable for Rasch analysis goes beyond a merely qualitative description of the suggested construct. In particular, it allows for a testable hypothesis of the structure of the construct. It is the construct map that renders the subsequent statistical assessment of construct validity confirmatory, that is the theoretical construct map allows for a link between content and construct validity ("confirmation of theoretical item hierarchy", [WOL 07b, p. 212]). Table 19.1 summarizes this suggested element of a Rasch analysis report.

19.2.2. *Response format and scoring*

The report should present the characteristics of the response scale, for example the number of response categories, the direction of the response scale, the labeling of the categories and the scoring key. It should be noted that the suitable number of response categories can depend on the population of the respondents. Experts may be able to distinguish between more response options than patients.

Element	Report
Latent variable	Definition and substantive theory of the latent variable
Operationalization	Description of the instrument (items) based on the definition of the construct, construct map
Response format and scoring	Characteristics of response scale (scoring key, number of categories, direction, position in the instrument, verbal labeling or description, etc.)

Table 19.1. *Suggested elements of a measurement report 1: theory of the construct: definition and operationalization*

19.2.3. *Sample and sampling design*

The most important sample characteristics comprise its composition as a consequence of the sampling design, which is a qualitative property, and its size as a quantitative feature of the sample. Because of the invariance property of the Rasch model, the composition of the sample is less critical than in classical test theory. Specifically, no distributional assumptions of the person parameters have to be met in order to estimate the item parameters. This property is often referred to as sample-independence. However, invariance requires empirical evidence. Therefore, the sampling design has to take the intended frame of reference into consideration. Whenever theoretical considerations suggest items functioning differently for different groups of respondents (DIF), the sample has to include a sufficient number of respondents representing these subpopulations. Since, in practice, DIF analyses are often exploratory, a more heterogeneous sample offers more and stronger opportunities to test for DIF. Preferrably DIF assessment should be based on theoretical considerations as far as possible.

Targeting is another important issue that qualifies sample-independence. A mismatch of respondent and item locations implies bias, large measurement error, and poor power of the tests of fit. This problem is particulary relevant for screening instruments, which aim at identifying abnormal individuals in a population of respondents who mostly do not display the anomalous condition. A scale validation study should therefore overrepresent those who can be expected to exhibit the condition under scrutiny as only these respondents are properly targeted. The Rasch analysis report should expound to what extent the sample composition corresponds to the objectives of the study.

Finally, the overall sample size is an essential piece of information. It affects the power of the tests of fit in general, though the latter depends on the targeting as well. Furthermore, the setting and the context of data collection should be outlined. Table 19.2 summarizes this suggested element of a Rasch analysis report.

Element	Report
Total population	Definition of total population as a part of the intended frame of reference sampling frame (from which the sample has actually been drawn)
Intended sample	Design, sampling method sample size

Table 19.2. *Suggested elements of a measurement report 2: sample design*

19.2.4. *Data*

The description of the actual data set complements information on the sample composition and the total sample size. Specifically, the number and the distribution of missing responses have to be exposed and whether the missing values are structural (e.g. due to the non-administration of some items to some respondents) or unexpected. Furthermore, the report should highlight dependencies in the data as a result of repeated measurements. Finally, as a service to the scientific community, the data set should be made available upon request whenever feasible. Table 19.3 summarizes this suggested element of a Rasch analysis report.

Element	Report
Actual sample	Actual sample size Targeting (discuss potential problems due to poor targeting) Missing values (frequency, type and consequences) Sample characteristics (demographic variables)
Data dependency	Structure of the data in terms of dependency (e.g. repeated measurement) Consequences
Context factors	Context factors conditions and circumstances under which data were collected, to be considered when interpreting outcome of analysis

Table 19.3. *Suggested elements of a measurement report 3: data*

19.2.5. *Measurement model and technical aspects*

Rasch measurement theory offers different variants of the Rasch model suited for particular response formats and data structures. The probably most fundamental distinction is the one between dichotomous and polytomous responses and whether the latter are ordered or representing a multiple choice format. The most widely used polytomous Rasch models either use a common threshold structure across all items, often referred to as the rating scale model [AND 78a, AND 78b], or an item-specific threshold structure, frequently called the partial credit model [AND 78b, MAS 82]. In any case, the used version of the model has to be stated, including key references to the literature. Finally, the method of parameter estimation should be mentioned in conjunction with the software employed. The extent to which fundamental properties of Rasch measurement should be explained depends on the target audience, the degree of acceptance of the model in the field of research and on the available space. Tables 19.4 and 19.5 summarize these suggested elements of a Rasch analysis report.

Element	Report
Fundamentals of Rasch measurement	Fundamental elements of the Rasch model (model parameters and their meaning) Unique advantages of the Rasch model/Rasch measurement theory At least stress invariance property/specific objectivity as a requirement of measurement
Measurement model	Variant of model used (depending on given data/response format), cite relevant references (e.g. [AND 78a, AND 78b, MAS 82] for polytomous Rasch model)

Table 19.4. *Suggested elements of a measurement report 4: theoretical background of measurement and measurement model*

Element	Report
Estimation method	Estimation method used (e.g. conditional maximum likelihood (CML), marginal maximum likelihood (MML) for item parameter estimation), maximum likelihood (ML) or weighted maximum likelihood (WML) for person location estimation) Often a consequence of software chosen, be aware of theoretical consequences Provide references (e.g. [MOL 95, AND 03, ZWI 95, WAR 89])
Software	Software used for data analysis, provide reference

Table 19.5. *Suggested elements of a measurement report 5: technical aspects of analysis*

19.2.6. *Fit analysis*

The core of the Rasch analysis report consists of the summary of the fit assessment. In general, the evaluation of a measurement instrument should not be made purely on the basis of statistical evidence. Numerical results need to be accompanied by qualitative interpretation and theoretical considerations. On the basis of the rationale of the Rasch approach, anomalies in the data should not simply be accounted for but revealed and exposed. Attempts at plausible explanations are certainly advantageous for future revisions of the scale, should the necessity arise.

The assessment of fit frequently is a complicated issue. Different tests of fit are sensitive to different types of violations, which, in turn, have to be tackled differently. Besides the comparison of observed and expected responses, the report has to refer to the functioning of the response scale, multidimensionality, local dependence and DIF. Specifically, the authors should inform the readers about the method of assessment, the findings, potential problems and threats, and how the latter has been accounted for. Table 19.6 summarizes this suggested element of a Rasch analysis report.

Element	Report
Local independence	Method used to investigate local independence, extent of actual local dependence in the data, plausible explanation of why local dependence occurs, remedies undertaken (e.g. item removal and sub tests)
Unidimensionality	Method used to check for unidimensionality, extent of departure from unidimensionality and remedies undertaken to resolve multidimensionality
Functioning of response scale	Indicate order of threshold estimates and any problems with empirical threshold order, ideally along with plausible interpretation of why disordering occurs, report collapsing and new scoring scheme
Invariance	Method used to check independence of item (person) parameters from respondents (items), see also DIF

Table 19.6. *Suggested elements of a measurement report 6: measurement requirements*

19.2.7. *Response scale suitability*

The polytomous Rasch model offers the possibility to investigate the functioning of the response scale categories [AND 97]. If reversed threshold estimates indicate that the response scale does not work as intended, subsequent tests of fit might actually be misleading and hard to interpret. A proper analysis of the order of category thresholds has to be done in any case. A transparent account of the results is helpful to the reader and contributes to an advancement of the scale in the future. If categories are collapsed, the way this is done should be disclosed.

19.2.8. *Item fit assessment*

One of the most important approaches to item fit assessment is the comparison of expected and actual responses. The report should provide information on the particular test statistic used and the results for each item. Whenever possible and appropriate, graphics should be presented in order to visualize the way the items work. Overall fit statistics provides a summary measure of fit.

The report should mention the methods used to investigate local dependency and multidimensionality as well as summarize the findings. The results of all tests of fit have to be put into perspective, in particular regarding power issues and implications of misfit or marginal fit. Any amendments to the data carried out as a consequence of misfit (e.g. item deletion, rescoring and item splitting due to DIF) should be reported keeping the theoretical consequences in mind. Table 19.7 summarizes this suggested element of a Rasch analysis report.

Element	Report
Test of total fit	Type of test statistic(s) used, (e.g. χ^2 (item–trait interaction), interpretation based on sample size, targeting and person separation. Discuss theoretical implications of item deletion
Test of individual item fit	Type of test statistics used, complement fit analysis by investigating graphics
Differential item functioning (DIF)	Method used to assess DIF, measures undertaken to account for DIF, implications for substantive theory of construct and the frame of reference

Table 19.7. *Suggested elements of a measurement report 7: item fit assessment*

19.2.9. *Person fit assessment*

In general, person fit is an issue attracting less attention than item fit. Since the number of respondents usually outweighs the number of items by far, misfit of items can be revealed much more easily than misfit of persons. Person misfit implies that the measurement instrument does not work for some respondents as it does for most others. Strictly speaking, this is also a violation of the invariance property, which particularly matters when individual measures are of interest. But even if aggregate statistics like group means are considered, person misfit should not be simply ignored. If there are systematic patterns of person misfit, group means may be seriously distorted and mean comparisons invalidated. Person fit assessment is also a tool to identify response styles. The way person fit is investigated and the findings obtained should be reported. If respondents are deleted because of misfit, the authors have to disclose to what extent this is done and provide a convincing justification. In general, discarding respondents is questionable, most notably if there are no theoretical considerations whatsoever. Table 19.8 summarizes this suggested element of a Rasch analysis report.

Element	Report
Test of individual person fit	Type of test statistic used, number or proportion of respondents outside acceptable limits Considerations of factors responsible for person misfit if persons are deleted, provide a rationale and a description of discarded respondents

Table 19.8. *Suggested elements of a measurement report 8: person fit assessment*

19.2.10. *Information*

As mentioned above, fit statistics should never be interpreted without reference to the test information. A lack of information compromises the power of the test of fit and is, therefore, a limitation of the generalizability of the findings. The amount of information available also impacts the level of precision. A good way to provide evidence about information is a targeting plot that conjointly displays the distribution of item locations or thresholds, respondents and information.

The person separation index provides information on how well the scale differentiates between the respondents. The authors should give a definition of the reported index or at least reference the index used. Person separation corresponds to reliability in classical test theory. Although its meaning is not as pivotal in Rasch analysis as it is in classical test theory, the index provides some insight into the power of the analysis of fit. Table 19.9 summarizes this suggested element of a Rasch analysis report.

Element	Report
Targeting	Present targeting plot and/or verbal description, refer to purpose of scale when interpreting targeting, discuss consequences for person separation and power of the tests of fit
Precision	Provide estimate of person separation and standard errors at critical levels of the latent variable (e.g. at cutoff values considered important from a clinical perspective), discuss possible reasons for a low person separation index
Power of test of fit	Comment on limitations of the power of the test of fit due to, for example, targeting or sample size

Table 19.9. *Suggested elements of a measurement report 9: information*

19.2.11. *Validated scale*

Whether the purified scale represents a valid and generalizable instrument to measure a suggested latent variable depends on the degree to which the analysis actually was confirmatory. If a large set of items has been reduced to a relatively small subset and/or the data have been altered extensively (e.g. by rescoring or item splitting), we run the risk of capitalizing on chance. This is particularly true if the substantive theory of the construct does not give substance to an expected order of item locations. Such an analysis requires cross-validation and discloses the need for a more elaborated theoretical framework of the latent variable.

The specification of the overall item locations (mean of the threshold estimates) is essential, a full table of threshold estimates is desirable. If the actual item order deviates from the expected order, the measurement report should reflect on the implications for the construct definition and the meaning of the measures. The report should, furthermore, point out strong and weak points of the measurement instrument and it should contain recommendations for scale usage and future applications.

If different scales exist that purport measuring the same latent variable, a comparison of the instruments is beneficial. Ideally, measures based on different instruments are equated and placed onto the same metric. Thus, co-calibrations of instruments add to building up a coherent framework of scientific measurement of a latent variable. Table 19.10 summarizes this suggested element of a Rasch analysis report.

Element	Report
Fit of data to the model	*See measurement requirements and fit assessment*
Matching substantive theory of latent variable and empirical evidence	Compare actual item hierarchy with expected hierarchy based on substantive theory of the construct
Comparison with other instruments	Compare instrument with other scales measuring the same latent variable, findings related to deriving a common metric by linking existing instruments (if applicable)

Table 19.10. *Suggested elements of a measurement report 10: validity*

19.2.12. *Application and usefulness*

In the context of a Rasch analysis, validity requires adequate fit of the data to the measurement model and a sufficient agreement of the substantive theory of the construct and the empirical evidence. Traditionally, the relationship of the latent variable and other constructs or phenomena is also integrated into the concept of validity under the label of external validity [KAN 01]. However, the assessment of external relationships provides at best indirect evidence of validity. The concept of external validity confounds successful measurement and the tenability of the structural theory suggesting the relationship investigated. If the structural theory is wrong, a poor relationship of the latent variable with another variable does not necessarily imply an inadequate measurement instrument. Conversely, a strong relationship could be due to other unrevealed processes rather than acceptable measurement of the suggested latent variable. Thus, external relationships should be better viewed as aspects of a scale's usefulness. It cannot replace the investigation of the link between the substantive theory of the latent variable and the empirical evidence in the data, but rather builds upon a previous demonstration of validity.

However, given that measurement instruments are often developed with a specific purpose or application in mind, the suitability of a measurement instrument, for example as a predictor of a future state, frequently is of interest to readers. Therefore, it may be advisable to include evidence of external relationships, albeit not framed as evidence of validity.

Table 19.11 summarizes this suggested element of a Rasch analysis report.

Element	Report
Description of final instrument	List set of items in the final scale (after deletion of misfitting items) and, in case of rescoring, the final scoring scheme
Item parameters	Table of final threshold estimates and overall item locations
Person parameters	State person summary statistics (mean, SD) and describe shape of distribution
Theoretical implications	Reflect the consequences of scale purification (in particular item deletion) for theory of the construct
Application and usefulness of the scale	Findings related to the application of the scale and its relationship to other constructs
Recommendations	Provide recommendations for scale usage, stress strong and weak points of the instrument, suggest amending of scoring procedures in future applications when appropriate (e.g. decrease number of categories in case of disordered thresholds, increase number of categories if thresholds are properly ordered but precision is too low), propose changes to items that do not function properly

Table 19.11. *Suggested elements of a measurement report 11: final instrument*

19.2.13. *Further issues*

Finally, any particularities and extraordinary factors that are relevant to the analysis, to the interpretation of measures or to the application of the measurement instrument are to be documented.

19.3. Bibliography

[AND 77] ANDERSEN E.B., "Sufficient statistics and latent trait models", *Psychometrika*, vol. 42, pp. 69–81, 1977.

[AND 78a] ANDRICH D., "A rating formulation for ordered response categories", *Psychometrika*, vol. 43, pp. 561–573, 1978.

[AND 78b] ANDRICH D., "Application of a psychometric rating model to ordered categories which are scored with successive integers", *Applied Psychological Measurement*, vol. 2, pp. 581–594, 1978.

[AND 82] ANDRICH D., "An index of person separation in latent trait theory, the traditional KR-20 index, and the Guttman scale response pattern", *Education Research and Perspectives*, vol. 9, pp. 95–104, 1982.

[AND 88] ANDRICH D., Rasch models for measurement, series: quantitative applications in the Social Sciences, Sage University Paper 68, Sage Publications, Newbury Park, 1988.

[AND 97] ANDRICH D., DE JONG J.H.A.L., SHERIDAN B.E., "Diagnostic opportunities with the Rasch model for ordered response categories", in *Rost, Langeheine Applications of Latent Trait and Latent Class Models in the Social Sciences*, Waxman, Münster, pp. 59–72, 1997.

[AND 02] ANDRICH D., "Understanding Rasch measurement: understanding resistance to the data-model relationship in Raschs Paradigm: a reflection for the next generation", *Journal of Applied Measurement*, vol. 3, pp. 325–359, 2002.

[AND 03] ANDRICH D., LUO G., "Conditional pairwise estimation in the Rasch model for ordered response categories using principal components", *Journal of Applied Measurement*, vol. 4, pp. 205–221, 2003.

[AND 04] ANDRICH D., "Controversy and the Rasch model: a characteristic of incompatible paradigms?", *Medical Care*, vol. 42, pp. 7–16, 2004.

[CRO 51] CRONBACH L.J., "Coefficient alpha and the internal structure of tests", *Psychometrika*, vol. 16, pp. 297–334, 1951.

[IRT 87] IRTEL H., "On Specific objectivity as a concept in measurement", in ROSKAM E.E., SUCK R. (eds), *Progress in Mathematical Psychology 1*, Elsevier, Amsterdam, pp. 35–45, 1987.

[IRT 95] IRTEL H., "An extension of the concept of specific objectivity", *Psychometrika*, vol. 60, pp. 115–118, 1995.

[HAG 09] HAGQUIST C., BRUCE M., GUSTAVSSON J.P., "Using the Rasch model in nursing research: an introduction and illustrative example", *International Journal of Nursing Studies*, vol. 46, pp. 380–393, 2009.

[KAN 01] KANE M.T., "Current concerns in validity theory", *Journal of Educational Measurement*, vol. 38, pp. 319–342, 2001.

[LOR 68] LORD F.M., NOVICK M.R., *Statistical Theories of Mental Test Scores*, Addison-Wesley, Reading, MA, 1968.

[MAS 82] MASTERS G.N., "A Rasch model for partial credit scoring", *Psychometrika*, vol. 47, pp. 149–174, 1982.

[MIC 86] MICHELL J., "Measurement scales and statistics: a clash of paradigms", *Psychological Bulletin*, vol. 100, pp. 398–407, 1986.

[MOL 95] MOLENAAR I.W., "Estimation of item parameters", in FISCHER G.H., MOLENAAR I.W. (eds), *Rasch Models, Foundations Recent Developments, and Applications*, Springer, New York, pp. 39–51, 1995.

[POP 96] POPPER K.R., *Conjectures and Refutations the Growth of Scientific Knowledge*, 5th ed. (Reprint), Routledge, London, 1996.

[RAS 60] RASCH G., *Probabilistic Models for Some Intelligence and Attainment Tests*, Danish National Institute for Educational Research, Copenhagen, 1960.

[RAS 61] RASCH G., "On general laws and the meaning of measurement in psychology", *Berkeley Symposium on Mathematical Statistics and Theory of Probability*, vol. IV, University of California Press, Berkeley, CA, pp. 321–333, 1960.

[RAS 77] RASCH G., "On specific objectivity: an attempt at formalizing the request for generality and validity of scientific statements", *Danish Yearbook of Philosophy*, vol. 14, pp. 58–93, 1977.

[SAL 09] SALZBERGER T., *Measurement in Marketing Research: an Alternative Framework*, Edward Elgar, Cheltenham/Northampton, MA, 2009.

[STE 06] STENNER A.J., BURDICK H., SANFORD E.E., BURDICK D.S., "How accurate are Lexile text measures?", *Journal of Applied Measurement*, vol. 7, pp. 307–322, 2006.

[STE 09] STENNER A.J., STONE M.H., BURDICK, D.S., "The concept of a measurement mechanism", *Rasch Measurement Transactions*, vol. 23, pp. 1204–1206, 2009.

[TEN 07] TENNANT A., CONAGHAN P.G., "The Rasch measurement model in Rheumatology: what is it and why use it? When should it be applied, and what should one look for in a Rasch paper?", *Arthritis & Rheumatism (Arthritis Care & Research)*, vol. 57, pp. 1358–1362, 2007.

[WAR 89] WARM T., "Weighted likelihood estimation of ability in item response theory", *Psychometrika*, vol. 54, pp. 427–450, 1989.

[WIL 05] WILSON M., *Constructing Measures: An Item Response Modeling Approach*, Lawrence Erlbaum Associates, Mahwah, NJ, 2005.

[WOL 07a] WOLFE E.W., SMITH E.V. JR., "Understanding Rasch measurement: instrument development tools and activities for measure validation using Rasch models: part I instrument development tools", *Journal of Applied Measurement*, vol. 8, pp. 97–123, 2007.

[WOL 07b] WOLFE E.W., SMITH JR E.V., "Understanding Rasch measurement: instrument development tools and activities for measure validation using Rasch models: part II validation activities", *Journal of Applied Measurement*, vol. 8, pp. 204–234, 2007.

[ZWI 95] ZWINDERMAN A.H., "Pairwise parameter estimation in Rasch models", *Applied Psychological Measurement*, vol. 19, pp. 369–375, 1995.

List of Authors

David ANDRICH
University of Western Australia
Australia

Silvia BACCI
Finanza e Statistica
Dipartimento di Economia
University of Perugia
Italy

Francesco BARTOLUCCI
Finanza e Statistica
Dipartimento di Economia
University of Perugia
Itlay

John BRODERSEN
Unit and Section of General Practice
Department of Public Health
University of Copenhagen
Denmark

Karl Bang CHRISTENSEN
Department of Biostatistics
University of Copenhagen
Denmark

Lynda DOWARD
Galen Research
Manchester
UK

Paolo EUSEBI
Department of Stastics
University of Perugia
Italy

Mike HORTON
Academic Department of
Rehabilitation Medicine
Leeds Institute of Molecular
Medicine
University of Leeds
UK

Svend KREINER
Department of Biostatistics
University of Copenhagen
Denmark

Ida MARAIS
Graduate School of Education
University of Western Australia
Australia

Stephen P MCKENNA
Galen Research
Manchester
UK

Mounir MESBAH
Laboratoire de Statistique
Théorique et Appliquée
(LSTA)
University Pierre and Marie Curie
Paris
France

Tine NIELSEN
Department of Psychology
University of Southern Denmark
Denmark

Jørgen Holm PETERSEN
Department of Biostatistics
University of Copenhagen
Denmark

Thomas SALZBERGER
Wirtschaftsuniversität Wien
Institute for Statistics
and Mathematics
Vienna
Austria

Volkert SIERSMA
Unit and Section of General Practice
Department of Public Health
University of Copenhagen
Denmark

Hanne THORSEN
Department of General Practice
University of Copenhagen
UK

Jeanette WILBUNN
Galen Research
Manchester
UK

Index

T

U

V

W